Self-Healing with Chinese Medicine

"Jam-packed with practical insights, *Self-Healing with Chinese Medicine* provides a clear road map to restoring and maintaining your health and balance. This gem of a book distills beautifully and clearly the fundamentals of Chinese medicine and the world of nature and how we can apply them in our everyday life on our path to self-healing. Full of dietary recommendations, lifestyle advice, and detailed exercises and manual therapy that you can do at home, this will be one of those comprehensive and practical books that you will always refer back to."

— REBECCA BOND, L.Ac., MBAcC, classical acupuncturist and member of the British Acupuncture Council

"In this extensive and practical book, Clive Witham shares with us a deep perspective of health and self-healing with the natural world at its core. I recommend it to everyone who wants to live according to nature's patterns."

— PERE GARCIA, L.Ac., N.P., naturopath and licensed acupuncturist

"Why do I have this health problem? What can I do myself to contribute to a solution? And what are the things I can do to prevent more problems? If you ask yourself these questions, then *Self-Healing with Chinese Medicine* is a must-read. It shows how our body and mind are interwoven with the nature that surrounds us and how you can empower yourself by following the eternal and fundamental principles of nature to lead a healthy and balanced life."

— ELMAR PESTEL, M.D., licensed internist and doctor of traditional Chinese medicine, manual therapy, and hypnosystemic therapy

"Clive Witham brings a profound knowledge of Chinese medicine to treating yourself for some of the most common conditions we see in modern-day society. This book contains a good amount of theory followed by lots of practical tips and is the perfect guide to self-help for all those who do not wish to consult the doctor with every minor ailment."

— XAVIER FRICKER, L.Ac., licensed acupuncturist and practitioner of Chinese medicine

"In-depth knowledge beautifully balanced with an engaging writing style, *Self-Healing with Chinese Medicine* is different from other books about traditional Chinese medicine. Complex ideas are explained in a way that's easy to grasp, and I feel like reading it from cover to cover and then going back into the chapters to dig in more. Ultimately, this is a book that you'll return to time and again, rereading and checking things, as you maintain your health."

— ANETTE SELBERG, certified phytotherapist and herbal and massage therapist

SELF-HEALING WITH CHINESE MEDICINE

A Home Guide to Treating Common Ailments

Clive Witham,

L.Ac., M.Sc.

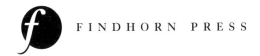

Findhorn Press
One Park Street
Rochester, Vermont 05767
www.findhornpress.com

Findhorn Press is a division of Inner Traditions International

Disclaimer
The information in this book is given in good faith and is neither intended to diagnose any physical or mental condition nor to serve as a substitute for informed medical advice or care. Please contact your health professional for medical advice and treatment. Neither author nor publisher can be held liable by any person for any loss or damage whatsoever which may arise from the use of this book or any of the information therein.

Cataloging-in-Publication Data for this title is available from the Library of Congress

ISBN 978-1-64411-705-7 (print)
ISBN 978-1-64411-706-4 (ebook)

Printed and bound in China by Reliance Printing Co., Ltd.

10 9 8 7 6 5 4 3 2 1

Edited by Nicky Leach
Illustrations by Clive Witham
Text design and layout by Damian Keenan
This book was typeset in Calluna sans, with Larken used as a display typeface.

To send correspondence to the author of this book, mail a first-class letter to the author
c/o Inner Traditions • Bear & Company, One Park Street, Rochester, VT 05767, USA, and we will forward to the author directly at **www.clivewitham.com**.

Contents

Introduction

I am not the same person who wrote the first edition of this book. How could I be? I started it 15 years ago in the early days of my North Africa adventure, and so much has passed since then. It is apt, therefore, that in this new edition, I take the skeleton of the old book and fill it afresh with ideas and approaches that better meet the needs of where we are now in this stage of the 21st century.

And be in no doubt we are not in a good place. The world has changed and is in danger of further change for the worse. It is time for a new approach, one that veers from the main narrative and brings us to where we should have been all along.

When I explain many of the concepts you will learn about in this book to the people I help in my clinics, it is a wonder to watch their faces. They just get it. Of course, we are built like trees. Of course, our bodies act like rivers. Of course, we live with breath motion. I can see that I am not talking to their intellect. They do not need to process complicated theories in their brains. I am speaking to their primal bodies. It is knowledge within them that has been suppressed within the strict boundaries of what we are supposed to learn about the world as we grow up.

This is the helplessness I referred to in the introduction to the first edition. With the standard view of our health—the one that fits in so well with the separation of our bodies into manageable parts so that they can be pharmaceutically monetized—our interaction in the process of healing is usually limited. We rarely have a deep understanding of what is happening inside our bodies and, truth be told, you will find that this includes many medical professionals, especially connected to areas of your body that are still relatively unknown, such as the brain.

I have never hidden my opinion. If I designed a system of healthcare, I would not entrust my wellbeing to an overworked practitioner who is running late, with a waiting room full of people and barely five minutes to scribble an unpronounceable drug on a stamped piece of paper and send me off to the pharmacy.

Surely, in an ideal world, any one of us can come up with a better plan than that. I do not want to spend a fortnight blindly taking an antibiotic "just in case" and then return to square one for another drug when it turns out to not, in fact, be the case. I want someone to investigate—to investigate properly, find the problem, and resolve it.

But we do not live in an ideal world, and for many of us this is where we find ourselves, our children, our partners, and the people we care most about in the world. We have to follow a system, not because it is right but because it is there and alternatives are not often freely available.

I needed this book a long time ago, as an eight-year-old kid with a bowl haircut and chubby cheeks living in the suburbs of London in the 1970s. One day I woke up with small blue bruises dotted all over my arms and legs. I remember counting them on just one arm and the number reached well over 40. With the other limbs covered in even more, it was quite clear to me and my parents that I was sick, and so I was sent to be an inpatient at Great Ormond Street Hospital in London, where the cream of Britain's pediatricians spent the best part of a week doing a series of inconclusive tests on what was going on inside my body.

In the absence of any better solution, it was decided that since I had had an aspirin a few days before the appearance of the bruises, it was very probably an allergic reaction. As with most families at the time, aspirin was the go-to pill when any member showed the slightest sign of sickness, and we had all grown up with the familiar foil packets and the fizzy sound as the flat white pills dissolved in water.

It was, therefore, a surprise that one of us was allergic, but when a man with lots of letters after his name, wearing a white coat and grasping a clipboard with scribbled numbers, tells you you are allergic to aspirin, well, you are allergic to aspirin. And with that I was promptly discharged and sent home.

So time moved on and the bruises gradually disappeared, and as flared trousers and polo-necks of the 70s changed to skin-tight jeans and leg-warmers of the 80s, they ceased to appear. I then grew up and continued to proclaim to any nurse with a sharp needle that I had an allergy to aspirin, but other than that the whole bruising incident was forgotten for many years.

That is, until the bruise-penny finally dropped in the brain of an older and wiser me. With the hindsight of someone in a very different place and time, I can now piece together what happened.

I was part of the school milk generation. And for anyone who is not familiar with this concept, you were force-fed milk on a daily basis for no apparent reason other than a date. My birthday hit during the summer holidays, and I had only just made it into that academic year, so along with the other "late" birthday people, I was obliged to ritually sip a bottle of milk a day through a stupidly small plastic straw. If I refused, then I could not go to playtime and waste 15 minutes trying to play soccer with a tennis ball with my friends.

The milk did not stop at school, though. My dairy consumption continued at home with a glass of bottled pasteurized milk (back then the milkman used to deliver them to the door) and a pile of ginger snaps, and this, added to the milk-soaked cereal from breakfast, and milky hot chocolate later on, meant that with just milk alone, I was drinking like a newborn calf.

Add to this my daily buttery sandwiches and my liking for potato chips, bananas, peanuts, tall glasses of orange juice, chocolate, and all things sweet, and it was no wonder I had developed into a barrel with cartoon chubby cheeks ("He's so cute! I could just squeeze him!").

What I know now, but what my mother (who like any mother had only the best intentions) did not know then, was that the food I was eating was proving too much for me to digest. It was getting stuck and slowly being processed through my steadily expanding body. This was quite literal, in the form of chronic constipation, but also meant that the other functions the digestive system would normally do with ease started to do the opposite.

One of these functions was connected with the containment of blood in my blood vessels. When the systems that control my digestion (the stomach and pancreas systems) became impaired, this had a domino effect on the liver system and the holding force to stop the blood from spilling out from veins—capillaries and the tiny vessels almost too small to see—was just not strong enough.

This is what was happening to me. I had bruises all over my arms and legs because of impaired digestion, which meant that it could not send enough strength around my body to control my blood from leaking out of the vessel walls. It was like a river systematically bursting its banks every few metres because they just collapsed.

Like any river system, if the flow of water is not strong enough, it cannot adequately support the farthest parts with enough flow, hence the symptoms specifically affected the four limbs. This was why the bruises appeared only on my arms and legs not my body (you will understand this better when I tell you about the root regions of your body).

If we had had this information back in the hot summer of 1977, the solution would have been simple: Stop the milk—and stop the orange juice, the bananas, the potato chips, the peanuts, and all the other food that was grinding my digestion to a halt.

If we had had this book back then, my mother could have borrowed a Chinese soup spoon from the local takeaway, spread Vicks Vaporub on my back, and scraped just below my shoulder blades to help digestion. She could have pressed and massaged key areas to help to strengthen my stomach and pancreas systems. I could have done some stretches to help harmonize the balance of the river systems in my body and been forced to stop playing war with mini toy soldiers and get outside in the fresh air for some proper exercise.

But, alas, we did not have this book. Instead, we had panic, powerlessness, and confusion, and we were forced to rely on a medicine that, despite the shiny scalpels and the long Latin names, is deeply flawed. Far too much of the medicine we see and experience, whether at the local doctor's surgery or clinic or in a hospital bed, is not how we would want it to be if we were the people in charge.

I get to see one specific part of the medical process: The end part. People usually come to see me at the tail end of a long medical journey. They have seen a doctor, a specialist, a surgeon, a physiotherapist, and a chiropractor. They have had a blood test, a urine test, an X-ray, an ultra-sound, a CT scan, and an MRI. They have travelled great distances for a second opinion with another doctor, another specialist, and then had a new round of X-rays, ultrasounds, CTs, and MRIs. They have tried every medication the doctors have thrown at them—antibiotics, anti-inflammatories, pain killers, sleeping tablets, and valium. And then, and only then, do they finally step over my clinic threshold and want me to fix them as I am their last hope before a desperate operation to remove some important part of their anatomy.

It would, of course, be ideal if everyone could get timely professional help from someone who knows how to treat them using the best of Chinese medicine, but many people do not have the means or the opportunity. This lack of access does not have to be such a major disadvantage if you are privy to some natural wisdom of the ancients—knowledge that was collected thousands of years ago, firmly anchored to a natural scientific view-point, and based on an acute observation of the world around us; knowledge that is founded on practice, testing, and refining and that has matured like a fine wine in a dusty cellar. A fraction of this raw ecological knowledge is included in this book.

The techniques and advice I have included in this book are all things I tell my patients and encourage them to do away from the clinic. We all need to do what we can to keep our bodies working properly, and there are a variety of things all of us can do at home to prevent disease and ill health and help our bodies to thrive. This book, therefore, contains valuable information that can give you some of the tools to try and rebalance your body yourself.

Essentially, this book will help you return some sense of control to your life, so that your health destiny does not have to be totally in the hands of a white-coated, pill-toting medical industry. The knowledge of the ancients is more relevant today than it has ever been, and when used correctly can transform your life.

I do not just mean physically. What I am really introducing you to is a whole new approach to tackling how you see your body, your health, and your world.

If you can understand how nature is an integral part of how we are and how we should be living our lives, the changes that manifest can be profound on many levels. It can change your life.

How to Use This Book

This book is not designed to replace a health practitioner; Chinese medicine can be extremely complex, and diagnosing even more so.

However, with due care and attention, the pages of this book can provide valuable help, as they are designed to empower you with information about how the body works and what to do to help it thrive. Divided into six parts, this book explains the core principles of Chinese Medicine along with self-care suggestions.

PART ONE aims to explore how we thrive in terms of ancient Chinese medicine and includes explanations of how your body functions. As well as trying to make the world of Chinese medicine more accessible and understandable for people without any specialized knowledge, this part is designed for people to look at the natural world around them and see how it affects their body.

PART TWO looks at visible signs of when the body is not thriving. These signs should be seen in conjunction with the patterns of imbalance or health conditions later in the book, not in isolation. For example, a bluish nose tip does not have to mean intestinal pain if you do not have any; or if, on close examination, you look yellowish, you do not automatically have jaundice. These are just clues that should be added to other clues, which together should help to find the cause for a body not thriving.

PART THREE explains the therapies that can be used to treat the patterns that can cause illness. They have been separated into four categories:

Food Therapy: This is one of the most important categories when treating yourself. We all have to eat, so why not eat foods that will prevent ill health rather than cause it?

Manual Therapy: Touch, whether done by yourself or another person, has a special healing quality about it. Knowing which places to touch, scrape, press, and manipulate can direct this healing where it is needed most.

Exercise Therapy: Along with diet, these stretching exercises are essential for the prevention of ill health. They do not take up much time, are repetitive, and can be done by almost anyone.

Lifestyle Therapy: Old habits can die hard but sometimes it is these habits that are contributing to ill health, and it may be time to kill them off for good.

You do not have to do every one of these therapies at the same time. They are there to give you a choice, as sometimes a therapy may be inappropriate or impractical to do. A combination of three or four done regularly can make all the difference when trying to rebalance your body within.

PART FOUR helps you to locate the various areas suggested in the book: On the body, hand, foot, and ear. These areas can sometimes be tricky to find, but the key is to follow the description and find an area that feels a little sore when pressed. This may be exactly where described, or it may be a short distance away.

PART FIVE introduces the most common patterns in your body and explains how to treat them. These patterns are independent of any disease or illness, and even someone who appears fit and healthy will have some kind of imbalance pattern. Ensuring these do not become too extreme is one of the keys in remaining strong and healthy.

PART SIX lists common ailments. I have chosen these based on how frequently I see them at my clinic. I could have included many conditions in this book but did not, purely because I do not see them often.

The hypochondriacs amongst us may read through the list of symptoms and believe that they have all of them. Indeed, most of us have several basic imbalances going on at the same time, and fixing them can mean a mixture of treatment choices. Symptoms often fit into several patterns, so in order to narrow down your choices, decide which seem to be the key symptoms and which seem to be secondary. The key symptoms are the ones that bother you the most and if you were to go to the doctor to explain your problems, these would be first on the list.

Like life, medicine is about trial and error. As long as you listen to your body and do not force it to do anything on the basis of a fad diet or a random magazine article, little harm should come.

Mistakes can sometimes be made and the wrong diet followed. This could then lead to a worsening of whatever condition is present. But as long as you recognize that a mistake has been made and do not go on doggedly following the same damaging diet, things can usually be reversed and the right diet found.

Take salads, for example. If you have a tendency for heat in the stomach system, a *yin* imbalance or live in a hot climate, the coolness of a salad can be really beneficial. If, however, you have a tendency for cold, a *yang* imbalance, and are tired and run down, a salad would be somewhere near the bottom of the diet list. Salads are indeed healthy, but not for all of us, all of the time.

Ultimately, a large dose of common sense is my prescription for using this book. Use your head, and do not continue to do things that could be harmful to your body. If something feels wrong, it probably is wrong. If it feels right, then it is probably doing some good. Either way, stay in control, and try to weave through the obstacles that life throws at you with a little self-help.

A note about the language of the book. It is customary in some books about Chinese medicine in the West to capitalize the first letter of many of the terms used to distinguish when the writer is referencing the Chinese concept or the Western concept of what is being referred to. Hence you might see both the Liver and the liver, or Heat and heat. The first edition of this book followed this convention in this way.

However, in this edition, I am not, and as you read the pages of the book, you will see why. The distinction between Chinese and Western concepts is an artificial one, as the ancient Chinese writers of the *Huangdi neijing* were referring to exactly the same bodies we know and the same nature we see. We just have to look at the natural world to understand. So when you see me refer to cold, it is the same cold you feel on a winter's day that is in your knee causing pain. It is not necessary to distinguish the meaning with capitalization because the meaning is the same. It is the natural world.

PART 1

What Allows Us
to Thrive?

Within the framework of Chinese medicine and the natural world this system inhabits, there are concepts, ideas, and instructions that will help you on the journey to understanding yourself and your body. In this first section, we look at some of these core principles and what they mean for your past, present, and future health and vitality.

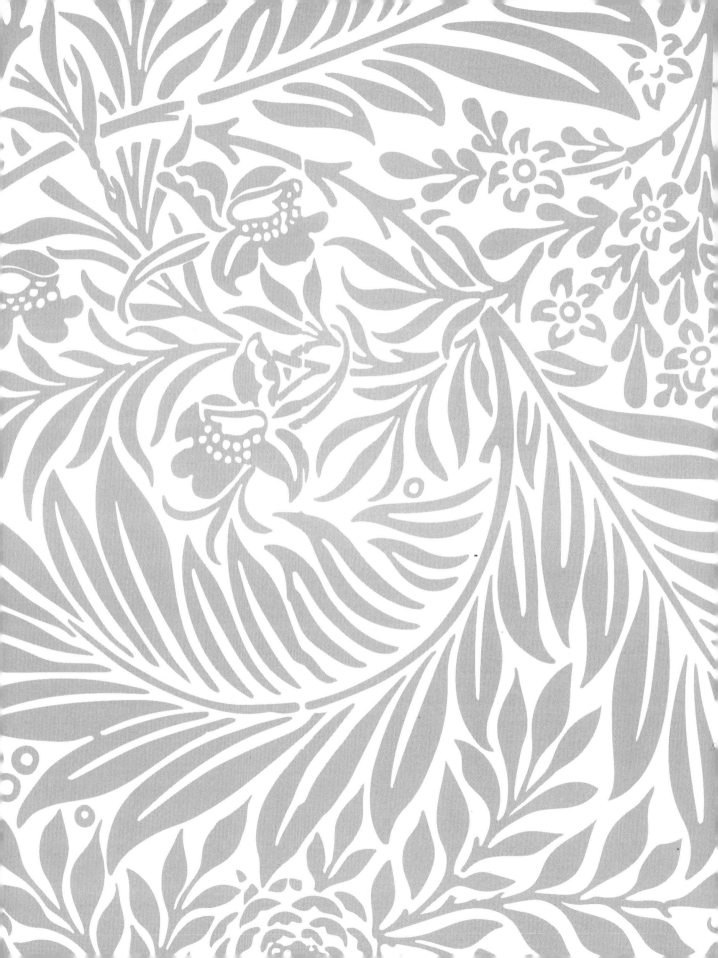

1

When the Breath
Is Moving

A great deal can be gleaned from Chinese medicine about what makes us thrive. In fact, when you delve into ancient texts, you discover that this premise underlies everything, and it is what gives us the basic understanding we need of how to keep in good health. The obvious place to start in any explanation of how to thrive with Chinese medicine is to introduce you to the missing natural links. They are conspicuously absent in most discussions of Chinese medicine, yet have been sitting in texts written thousands of years ago. What they contain is something so complex yet so simple, they can be applied to literally everything. This makes them accessible to everyone, no matter their background or knowledge base.

You may come to this book knowing a little about Chinese medicine, and you may be familiar with some of the terms that have been popularized in the West, such as *qi, yin, yang,* meridians, and so on. But for many people these terms can sound so foreign, so alien to everything they have grown up understanding about life, and seem to be concepts that do not fit in comfortably with their world view.

The problem is that these words do not have any real-world meaning for how many people interact with their environment. To some, *qi* is that weird thing they might hear people talk about in their yoga group or associate with a bunch of people shouting and punching the air at the local martial arts hall.

When something does not have meaning, it can be discarded, or worse still, it can be derided. But it does not have to be like that. This all stems from a fundamental misunderstanding of what these terms mean, and how they relate to your life. And trust me on this, they most certainly relate to your life in more ways than you can imagine.

So while you may be aware of some of the terms of Chinese medicine, perhaps what you did not know is that they are all connected in a web of ideas, not in some abstract, mystical martial art, but in real, tangible things like the plants in your garden, the trees in the park, and the water in a stream.

The ancient Chinese writers of the classic text upon which all of Chinese medicine is based—the *Huangdi neijing*, a collection of writings over two thousand years old—were not documenting an invented approach to how the body works and how to fix it; they were showing us how the principles that govern the natural world around us equally govern the world within us, too.

So this is where we begin—with the natural world and an applied approach to some of the ideas within *Neijing* Nature-Based Medicine.[1] If you can glean the basic principles of how your rose bush grows from a seed to blossom, or how spring water meanders down the hillside, then you can unlock the very secrets of how your body functions, both in sickness and in health.

The universe is not the first place you might think of in order to understand the human body.

It is, however, where you can find the key concept, essential to grasp if you are to comprehend the underlying structure of our bodies and learn how we can thrive.

So let me take you there—to a place of space, matter, and time; a place where stars are born and galaxies multiply; a place filled with cosmic rays and magnetic fields, where light illuminates darkness.

Instead of pointing your attention to things, I want you to focus on motions. In fact, this is what Chinese medicine is, if you really take it down to its bones: It is looking at, sensing, and feeling the patterns and motions of the universe, and applying them to us and everything around us.

But surely you cannot actually feel the patterns and motions of the universe, can you? Here we are on our planet, and all those galaxies and stars in the sky seem a very long distance away. This was one of the beliefs before March 13, 1989, when the entire province of Quebec, Canada was plunged into a power blackout for 12 hours. A powerful geomagnetic event from the sun not only knocked the Quebec power grid offline but sent NASA's TDRS-1 communication satellite out of control and abnormalities in hydrogen readings in the Space Shuttle *Discovery*.[2]

Now, of course, the potential of sun bursts or solar flares, whose explosive releases of energy and high-speed electrons and protons have the capacity to interfere with life on Earth, is better understood. There even now exists an organization called the Space Weather Prediction Center, which forecasts geomagnetic storms and any other events coming from space. But how about if I told you that we can feel movements in space, not just from our sun, our solar system, and our galaxy? We can actually feel the base pattern of the universe.

In 2007, there was a dramatic discovery of mysterious radio waves coming from a dwarf galaxy three billion light years away from Earth. Despite only lasting milliseconds, these pulses, which could

clearly be detected on Earth, had the power of hundreds of millions of suns. It caused quite a stir at the time, with talk of extraterrestrial contact and researchers at the Harvard-Smithsonian Center for Astrophysics even considering a possible intelligent agent behind it as recently as 2017.[3]

It was not until 2020, however, that a consistent pattern began to be detected when these waves appeared. They became known as Fast Radio Bursts (FRB), and they actually follow a 157-day pattern of bursting for 90 days and then calming for 67 days on a constantly repeating cycle.[4] Far from being aliens trying to send us inexplicable messages, these pulses are dramatically showing us a motion that is happening all over the universe, including all around us, and from which the ancient Chinese developed the principles around which they built their medicine.

It is nothing more than a simple pattern of expansion and contraction. During the 157-day cycle of the FRB, evidently there is an active, expansive phase, when the pulses are firing at a rapid rate and the sensitive equipment detecting it on Earth is vibrating as much as the excited astronomers; this is followed by a passive, contractive phase, when a period of calmness appears and nothing is lighting up the display panels. We cannot see it, of course, as it is too far away,

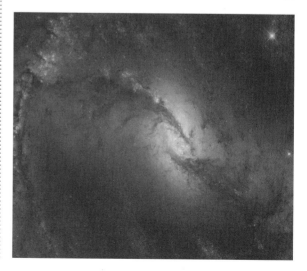

but these pulses allow us to do something that normally is not possible—they allow us to feel it. Even if we were not able to feel this motion happening in another part of the universe, we could still see it happening. Stars are born inside vast clouds of rotating dust called nebulas, floating within galaxies. What happens with the formation of a star is that the nebula cloud begins to contract and divides into smaller circular clumps, called protostars.

When the temperature of the protostars reaches 10 million degrees centigrade, nuclear fusion causes a giant explosion that results in a star. If the conditions are right in the night sky, you can see a nebula with your naked eye in the easily located Orion constellation, which looks like Orion the Hunter firing his bow. Below Orion's Belt in the northern hemisphere (and above Orion's Belt in the southern hemisphere) are what appear to be three stars in a line, collectively known as Orion's Sword. The middle "star" of the sword isn't actually a star at all but Orion Nebula, a giant cloud of glowing star-forming hydrogen gas.

What we are doing is exactly what the ancient Chinese were doing when they looked up to the stars to try to make sense of the world. They saw this motion of expansion and contraction and recognized its importance in how our world works on Earth. Instead of a mechanical name describing the actions involved, we can give it a name that should feel much more familiar to you and your daily life: "Breath motion".[5]

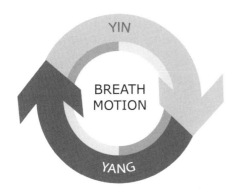

It is the very same breath motion you are doing now: Breathe in, and you have one part of the motion; breathe out, and you have another. Believe it or not, the same constant motion is happening right now in the deepest parts of our universe. The ancient Chinese gave each part a name you may have heard before: The expansion motion of the breath, they called *yang*, and the contracting motion they called *yin*, both being equal parts of the same universal breath motion.

Knowing this simple explanation should allow you to approach the terms *yin* and *yang* in a fresh way. I could give you long lists describing *yin* and *yang*, as this is how I learnt it at school, but using the context of breath, we have something that cuts through all the language and gives us a visible, instinctive idea of what the ancient Chinese were really talking about.

Go ahead and breathe in. Notice the air coming into your lungs and then gradually filling. Notice also how, when they inflate completely, a natural motion seamlessly switches from an inwards motion to an outwards motion, expelling the air, so when your lungs are full, the breathing-out process has already begun. As you breathe out, note how all the air is released, but as you near the final part of exhalation, your lungs are almost spring-loaded to switch immediately back to breathing in again. And then the cycle, of course, repeats itself.

The process happening in your lungs follows the same principle as star formation in a nebular dust cloud, and as it is the universal pattern of all things, it can be seen everywhere. And I mean everywhere. Allow me to give you an image of breath motion from my time as a fisherman working the deck of a Japanese flying fish boat in the East China Sea.

The fisherman phase of my life was based on the premise that in order to truly understand the concepts of nature, you first have to truly live them. So, against my better judgement, I joined up as a crewmember for six months and battled all the elements that nature and the captain could throw at me. I worked on the *Shigemaru,* one of the oldest vessels of the Yakushima flying fish fleet, and we would go off at an ungodly hour of the morning and find a spot a few miles off the space centre at Tanegashima to lay our nets. I particularly liked that spot, not because there were lots of fish to catch but because I could watch the rockets, standing vertically, being prepped for launch. After an hour of drifting on the Kuroshio current, the nets would then be heaved back in, and the deck would fill with all kinds of flying fish, dolphin fish (not the mammal), dart fish, mackerel, the odd sea horse, and, every now and then, what appeared to be a bouncing, spiky ball.

This was a puffer fish, a perfectly rounded ball with two large eyes and a pinched mouth. It is known as *fugu* in Japan, a fish so ugly that it is actually very cute, and so dangerous that, second only to the golden poison frog of the Amazon rainforest, it is the most poisonous vertebrate in the world.

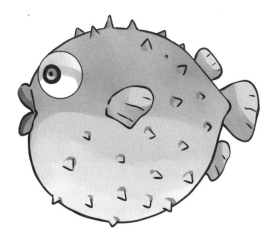

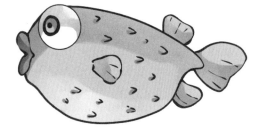

The reason that *fugu* is helpful to understand the *yin/yang* breath is that it does not always look like this. It is normally small, blue, smooth, and rather unassuming (if you discount the mounted bug eyes). The motion of what happens is plain to see from the dramatic changes on the outside, and for all intents and purposes, you could easily believe that it switches between just two states— one seemingly aggressive, bloated, and spiky and the other calm, short, and flat.

It is, however, what is inside that makes the *fugu* fascinating. When our slow-moving spiked friend is relaxed and mulling around in the depths, darting here and there at the sight of microscopic food, it has the appearance of the *yin* motion of breath. When it expands, however, with all the heat and energy required to pump water into its stomach and bend its spine into an almost impossible shape, it appears more of the *yang* motion.

After expanding, the sheer concentration of energy it needed to enlarge itself has all been used up. So when it is sitting on the deck waiting for one of us to find it and throw it right back into the ocean, while the outside is looking *yang*, in fact it is predominately *yin* inside. When it is inert and blue, all that potential for ballooning itself is still sitting there like a coiled spring, so the *yang* motion is inside, despite the more *yin* state on the outside. Even when lying lifeless on the deck in the most *yin* of states, it has enough neurotoxin to kill 30 people.

So while we have the simple breath motion of expansion and contraction that the *fugu* shows us so well, what happens inside is a continuation of breath motion on many levels. Rather than one motion happening all over the body, if we had to visualize what happens, it would look more like the cogs of a grandfather clock, all moving in different directions in a complicated symmetry to ensure that the clock keeps perfect time.

This idea is essential in trying to figure out how the human body functions, as it is not only one thing or the other. As with the *fugu*, there is a lot going on under the surface.

In terms of the body as a whole, the ideal is to have the breath motion smoothly moving, just like you are breathing with your lungs right now. In this way both *yin* and *yang* motions can be balanced. The reality of this perfect state is that the very act of living normally limits this for only short periods. Perhaps if you were able to remove all stress from your life and live a simple happy existence, it may be more permanent but, of course, this is not the reality for most of us.

The norm is that the motion becomes impaired, and the balance of your body swings more towards one or the other. On a simple level, if the *yang* motion is weak, there may be symptoms of cold-ness and tiredness, and, if *yin* is weak, signs of heat and agitation.

If *yang* is too strong, there may be signs of heat rising upwards to the head, and if *yin* is too strong, signs of coldness and water retention.

As the imbalance between the motions becomes more pronounced, either through a weakness or overflow pattern, the signs of one of them predominate.

The same patterns of *yin/yang* breath motion exist when we venture deeper within the body. Blood vessels and circulation systems all have their own breath motion, which may or may not be contributing to the balance of the whole body.

For example, an exhausted person may suffer from lower back pain due to an impairment of *yang* in the kidney system. They may also have head-aches in their temples from too much stress at

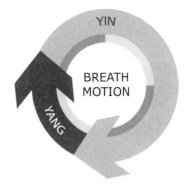

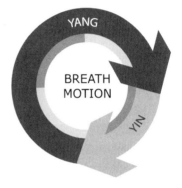

work causing impairment of *yin* in the liver. In this way both *yin* and *yang* motions can be imbalanced at the same time within different parts of the body.

The application of breath motion means that it would be possible to follow this pattern all the way down to a microscopic cellular level and still find the same *yin/yang* breath motion imbalances in individual cells.

The body is, therefore, in a constant state of *yin/yang* balance on many different levels, from one moment to the next. As the balances become more skewed one way or the other, physical signs often appear that give us clues about where the breath impairments are, and also how severe they may be.

When the Natural Circulation Is Maximized

We take for granted the shape of things. A tree looks like a tree because that is what a tree looks like. A river looks like a river. A flower looks like a flower. A cloud looks like a cloud. They all have a distinct shape that we grew up almost instinctively recognizing, and we can assign categories to the shapes we know. But how did these shapes come about? Why those shapes? Why not a different shape? And why are we shaped like we are? We have a head at the top, and four limbs at the corners of a body. Why not some other shape?

To answer this, we have to return to the breath pattern in the universe and look at what is holding it all together. When there is a continual expansion and contraction motion, there has to be something tangible to expand and contract in between, right? There has to be something holding it all in place. For an astrophysicist, this would be something called "ordinary matter", or "baryonic matter", which is believed to be the material we are made of, but there are other materials, too, such as "dark matter" and "dark energy", which are much less understood.

Fascinatingly, the ancient Chinese had an understanding of the binding aspects of the universe well over two thousand years ago. They theorized that the motion of expansion and contraction that constitute breath were held together by something called *qi* (chee). This may sound like we have stepped into the realm of quantum physics,

but *qi* was basically thought of as the fabric of space–time continuum.[6]

In physics, this is a theory that space and time are interwoven in a single continuum that combines multiple dimensions. It does this by combining the three dimensions of space (length, width, and height) with that of a fourth dimension: Time. If you imagine this concept as a piece of fabric, like a sheet hanging outside on a washing line, time gives you the place where you might touch the material; the idea is that if you were to push your finger into the material, it would create a distortion in the sheet and a curvature of space-time around it.

It is this fabric we come to when we want to understand *qi*. In deep space, *qi* is the fabric, the raw material behind the birth of stars, the appearance of new galaxies, and planets being formed. But the further we move from deep space, the more the patterns of motion change, and so does *qi*. This means that in some dimensional environments, *qi* can be immaterial and almost vapour-like, but in others it can be material and totally solid. *Qi* is basically at the mercy of the motion forces around it.

From its Chinese character, it is not automatically evident that *qi* has this deep universal meaning. It looks like this 氣 and represents steam rising above boiling rice. But like most Chinese characters, they are more than what they seem. When motions around *qi* go through different environments, form is created, and this is essentially the idea behind our planet. *Qi* forms the building blocks of every single thing on Earth, no matter the object, no matter the size. The motions on our planet are more complicated than that of deep space, and as you will discover in the other sections, many factors interplay to mould *qi* into the solid forms we are now familiar with.

The same *qi* is essentially stardust floating in space. In truth, we are actually made from the same stuff. We are stardust, and once our time on this planet comes to an end, we will return to stardust.

The shapes formed in this moulding process are not random and make sense. The basic principle is that the circulation pattern within those shapes is maximized for the environment they inhabit, so the fact that we are solid human beings who look like we do, and not like intelligent floating clouds, is down to the manipulation of *qi* in the particular environment on our unique planet. If we had evolved on another planet, perhaps we would look very different.

There is another important aspect to the motions that affect us and influenced how we developed: The growth patterns of nature. The ancient Chinese observed the natural world as it is—not some wild chaotic place but governed by rules and principles that are consistent throughout.

Look at a tree, and follow the branches towards the leaves. Look down from a high vantage point on a river system flowing towards the ocean. Watch a fork of lightning flashing down to the earth. Look at a close-up image of the blood vessels in your eyes. They follow the same shape—not a similar pattern but exactly the same shape. This is because they are following universal growth patterns of nature, which are also clearly present inside our bodies.

Most of my memories of school days were utterly miserable. Worse, I knew they were miserable at the time, much like going to the cinema and realizing within the first few minutes the movie is going to be awful but, unable to get up and leave, you just have to sit through it. So I never thought that the painful years I spent in school studying the industrial revolution in my modern British history class would help me understand the shape of all things, but it did.

The bit of the industrial revolution that stuck with me was the invention in the 18th century of something called the "flying shuttle". This was a simple weaving machine that allowed more fabric to be produced using a wooden bobbin to weave yarn at a much faster speed. Rather than the machine, however, it is the process of weaving that illuminates the natural world.

Weaving works with two threads. One is called the warp, the longitudinal thread that is fixed in

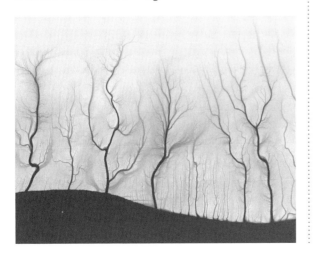

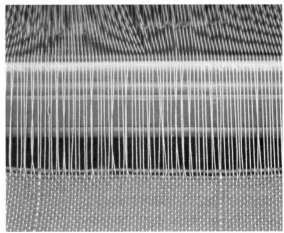

place in the frame and kept stretched as tight as possible. The other thread is the weft, the transverse horizontal thread that is pulled through and inserted over and under the warp. It is the use of both that allows for the formation of a strong piece of fabric or cloth. There are many variations, but this is the basic pattern of weaving.

It is also the basic pattern of growth of everything around us. The warp is the longitudinal growth seen in the trunk of a tree and the main waterway of a river, while the weft is the latitudinal growth seen in the branches of the tree and the tributaries of the river.

The ancient Chinese called the longitudinal *jing* and the latitudinal *luo*, and were able to break down how nature and the human body act in sync by applying these simple principles of growth.[7]

You just have to go outside and find a tree (or plant) to see how these patterns repeat themselves as it grows. The main stem or trunk has a strong longitudinal force pushing upwards, and then this gives way to a latitudinal force as the branches grow outwards. An individual branch has both forces acting on it as it grows straight, and then splits again. The same forces continue this growth pattern until it reaches maturity and stops.

This longitudinal–latitudinal circulation pattern is *yin/yang* breath motion in action, and the same process has formed our bodies. Our main blood vessels coming to and from the heart are the *jing* vessels and are usually long, straight arteries and veins. The many smaller vessels branching from these arteries and veins all over the body are the *luo* vessels. These are within your connective tissue structures. You just have to look at any images of the blood vessel system within the body, and you cannot help but think of trees and rivers.

But what exactly is being circulated around in this system? Is it the mysterious energetic *qi* about which I was taught when I went to Chinese medicine school? Or is it something altogether more down to earth—more tangible, more magical?

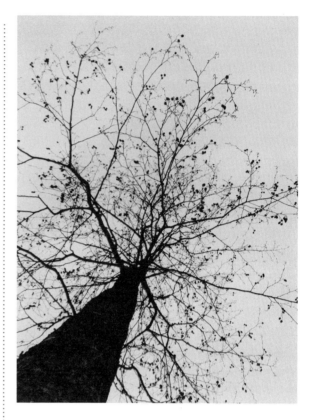

Let me turn your attention to fireflies (also known as glow worms or lightning bugs). I have come across fireflies only a few times in my life. Once was in late spring, around the banks of Miyanoura River on Yakushima in Japan, where they were dancing around the forest like stars in a miniature universe. It is no wonder that Miyazaki, director of the ever-popular Ghibli anime movies, spent time on the island in pre-production research, and I often recognize real places in his imagined worlds.

I have seen them more often in my current home in the mountains behind Barcelona. I am lucky enough to live deep within the protected natural park, which, despite being within the Barcelona city limits, is a place of roaming wild boars, tangled forests, and often complete and utter silence. It is here, in the dusk of early summer, that we often see fireflies. They appear out of the forest on our terrace or on the crumbling path across the valley, and their neon glow is almost in sync with the beep of the midwife toad mating call.

The light of the firefly is created by a process called bioluminescence, which is produced by specific biochemical reactions on the underside of the firefly's abdomen. To a firefly, it is just another way to attract a mate. They are not alone in the natural world in producing this chemical reaction. It is common amongst some species of fungi, bacteria, algae, squid, jellyfish, worms, crustaceans, and fish.

It may sound a little far-fetched at first, but our bodies actually emit light, too—not the same kind of light that happens in bioluminescence or occurs with thermal radiation, which you might see with an infrared device. In fact, it is not a light we can normally perceive at all, but we know it is there because it can, and has been, measured with the right sensitive equipment.

We glow because of something called "biophotons", which are light particles that constantly radiate from the body surface of all living organisms without any external stimulus causing them to glow.[8] They can be detected by a photomultiplier device, which converts photons into an electrical signal that can then be measured.

Studies show that this weak light emission, which is a thousand times weaker than the bioluminescence of a firefly, has a responsiveness that suggests it is not there to attract mates. In plants, it appears to actively interact with its environment. A plant will emit this light depending upon its current state of health and hydration.

The proximity of other parts of the plant causes biophotons to become more active through a dynamic feedback mechanism.[9] The signals in this mechanism show the biophoton-emitting units actually work cooperatively through a process called "quantum coherence".[10] Biophotons are thought to be the result of a whole other intelligent system of communication within and between cells in your body.[11]

Further studies on the emission of biophotons are even more illuminating, in that they are thought to vary according to the location in your body, along with circadian and seasonal rhythms. For example, they are emitted more in summer and less in winter (not connected with any temperature changes). They are emitted less during the day and more at night (not depending on either temperature or light changes). The palms of your hands emit double the amount of photons compared to your back. And your limbs and head have a much higher emission rate than your abdomen and chest.[12]

While researchers admit that the reason these patterns are present within biophoton emission is puzzling, there is something within Chinese medicine to help them figure it all out. For this, we have to look into *Neijing* Nature-Based Medicine and draw out the concept of something called *shenming*.

As with *qi*, we have to go into the world of space–time to understand *shenming*, but unlike *qi*, it is actually outside the rules that govern our universe, and stands apart as the prerequisite for all life. It appears when particular circumstances cause *yin* and *yang* to suddenly interact and merge, and the subsequent spark that this generates is nothing less than life itself.[13]

It is the kind of wondrous explosive event that forms a star in a nebula, or starts the heartbeat of a new human being for the very first time. This is actually how the ancient Chinese saw it. They used the same Chinese character (神明) for the heavens in the night sky and the *shenming* force of light within your body. In effect, what they were saying is that the light of the stars is quite literally within you.

So if we return to biophoton emission with the knowledge of *shenming*, then not only are we made of the stuff of the universe (*qi*), we have the light of the stars (*shenming*) running through our bodies. *Shenming* was described by the ancient Chinese as an organizing force that circulates in the blood of your river systems to restore and repair your body wherever needed.[14] It is basically the template of how you should be.

Shenming is, therefore, the basic circulation pattern of the body that will allow you to flourish. The mesh that holds it together is *qi*, the fabric of space–time. The force of circulation that allows it to grow and function is the expansive and contractive motion of breath (*yin* and *yang*), which guides the longitudinal (up/down), and transverse (sideways) growth patterns (*jingluo*), and the organizing and repairing force of light within your blood (*shenming*) to create a healthy, thriving human body.

3

When the Qualities of Nature Are Balanced

The closer the *yin/yang* breath motion gets to us, the more change it goes through, much like a sound wave changes length and frequency as it hits different mediums. When it interacts with our specific environment on Earth, the ancient Chinese categorized its effect on the natural world into five clear qualities of natural motion, or circulation patterns, known as *wuxing*.

You might know these as the "five elements" or "five phases": Earth (soil), metal, water, wood (plants), and fire. It was noted that these moving and transforming qualities interact with each other within the body, just as they do in the natural world, and form an intricate relationship in maintaining good health and allowing us to thrive.

The image shows the natural motion of the qualities, which flows in a clockwise direction, much like a spinning pinwheel when you blow on it. This is the harmonious movement of nature in balance and is known as *zheng* motion. When this motion becomes impaired, a transverse motion called *heng* (which is represented by the arrows in the middle) creates a different cycle, which causes the qualities to impair each other in a web of imbalance. These are the motions that lie behind the weakness and overflow patterns later in the book.

The following is a summary of how to see these qualities, and how your body may react when one of them is impaired. This information can be of great help in understanding some of our tendencies and where they come from.

WOOD

It is springtime. Life is springing back after the harsh winter months, plants are coming up through the ground, all the animals, insects, birds, and other creatures are noisily making themselves heard, and a strong breeze is blowing through firmly rooted trees, swaying to and fro.

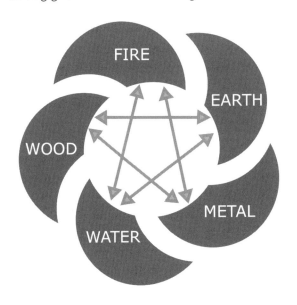

- **Storage system:** Liver and gallbladder
- **Direction:** East
- **Tissue plane:** Connective tissue
- **Colour:** Blue/green
- **Sound:** Shouting
- **Emotion:** Anger

- **Odour:** Rancid
- **Season:** Spring
- **Climate:** Wind
- **Flavour:** Sour
- **Fluid:** Tears
- **Orifice:** Eyes
- **Sense:** Sight
- **Residue:** Nails
- **Grain/Pulse:** Barley and rye

When the wood quality is balanced, it is about new things emerging. It allows you to be calm, rooted and demonstrate good decision-making and leadership skills.

When the wood quality is imbalanced, you can become frustrated, angry, impatient, aggressive, explosive, depressed, moody, unable to structure daily life appropriately, and prone to headaches, eye problems, and stagnation.

A tendency to any of these characteristics or symptoms could mean that the balance of wood holds an important place in allowing you to thrive.

FIRE

Imagine it is the height of summer. The sun is at its peak in the southern sky, meadows of green grass are dotted with daisies lapping up the sun's rays, and the warmth is enhanced by the sound of children splashing each other in a gentle stream.

- **Storage system:** Heart, heart ruler, small intestine, and triple burner
- **Direction:** South
- **Tissue plane:** Rivers
- **Colour:** Red
- **Sound:** Laughing
- **Emotion:** Joy
- **Odour:** Scorched
- **Season:** Summer
- **Climate:** Heat
- **Flavour:** Bitter

- **Fluid:** Sweat
- **Orifice:** Tongue
- **Sense:** Taste
- **Residue:** Hair
- **Grain/Pulse:** Corn and millet

When the fire quality is balanced, you are open-minded, genuinely friendly, enthusiastic, humble, have clarity of thought, and solve problems.

When the fire quality is imbalanced, you can suffer from depression, mood swings, memory problems, confusion, have a pale or red complexion, and be inappropriately open and vulnerable.

A predominance of these characteristics or symptoms could mean that the balance of fire holds the key to you thriving.

EARTH

The summer is drawing to an end, and harvest time is in full swing. It is later in the afternoon, and the air is full of the sweet smell of the last blooms of the season. Distant rumbling rain clouds bring periodic deluges, which the soil will gratefully lap up.

- **Storage system:** Pancreas and stomach
- **Direction:** Centre
- **Tissue plane:** Flesh
- **Colour:** Yellow
- **Sound:** Singing
- **Emotion:** Deliberation
- **Odour:** Fragrant
- **Season:** Late summer
- **Climate:** Damp
- **Flavour:** Sweet
- **Fluid:** Saliva
- **Orifice:** Mouth
- **Sense:** Touch
- **Residue:** Fat
- **Grain/Pulse:** Wheat

WHEN THE QUALITIES OF NATURE ARE BALANCED

When the earth quality is balanced, you can have a strong appetite, smooth digestion, strong arm and leg muscles, and be responsible, stable, creative, and imaginative.

When the earth quality is imbalanced, you can have a poor appetite and digestion, stuck feelings, put on weight, be tired or overly concerned, and worried.

If these characteristics feel more familiar to you, the balance of earth might hold an important place in allowing you to thrive.

METAL

The sun is setting in the west, and there is a slight chill in the crisp autumn evening. The leaves on the trees have changed their colours and begun to fall. The summer has left, and there is a general preparation for the winter to come.

- **Storage system**: Lung and large intestine
- **Direction**: West
- **Tissue plane**: Skin
- **Colour**: White
- **Sound**: Weeping
- **Emotion**: Grief
- **Odour**: Rotten
- **Season**: Autumn/fall
- **Climate**: Dryness
- **Flavour**: Pungent
- **Fluid**: Nasal mucous
- **Orifice**: Nose
- **Sense**: Smell
- **Residue**: Body hair
- **Grain/Pulse**: Rice

When the metal quality is balanced, you can be principled, consistent, ordered, good at prioritizing, and have well-conditioned skin and hair.

When the metal quality is imbalanced, you are more likely to be confused, dissatisfied, disordered,

have dull skin and hair, and unable to let things go or have an inappropriate view of your own worth.

Should any of these symptoms or characteristics ring true, the balance of metal may be the one that holds the key to your health.

WATER

The darkness of winter has arrived, and a cold wind is blowing from the north. Most of the forest creatures are less active and have found refuge beneath the earth to preserve and restore themselves, listening for the first signs of the coming spring.

- **Storage system**: Kidney and bladder
- **Direction**: North
- **Tissue plane**: Bone
- **Colour**: Black
- **Sound**: Groaning
- **Emotion**: Fear
- **Odour**: Putrid
- **Season**: Winter
- **Climate**: Cold
- **Flavour**: Salty
- **Fluid**: Sputum
- **Orifice**: Ears
- **Sense**: Hearing
- **Residue**: Teeth
- **Grain/Pulse**: Beans

When the water quality is balanced, you can be calm, consistent, wise, easygoing, and flexible. When the water quality is imbalanced, you can become fearful and insecure, take inappropriate risks, and have problems with hearing and issues with joints, bones, teeth, and the urinary and reproductive systems.

A tendency for these characteristics or symptoms suggests that the balance of water may hold sway inside and be the one that helps you to thrive.

4

When the Storage Systems Are Balanced

The storage systems were listed in the qualities of nature in the previous section and most have familiar names of the organs in your body (lung, large intestine, stomach, pancreas, and so on). It would be easy to think that those organs, the ones you studied in biology class, and these storage systems from Chinese medicine, are one and the same. But the ancient Chinese had different ideas, and although they incorporate these anatomical organs within storage systems, they are, in fact, the moulding of the qualities of nature into a different form of *qi*.

As the motions of the universe pass through our atmosphere to our planet and into our bodies, they create moving forces around *qi* (the fabric) to form solid structural patterns. This is how our bodies were shaped and also how the storage systems inside them were formed.

For example, let us look at how your liver storage system was modelled. We start in the star constellation of the eastern direction, and as the motion of the universe (*yin/yang* breath) moves towards us from there, it moulds *qi* and forms the wind in our atmosphere. This wind then has its own unique moulding motion, and as the breath continues down to us, it manifests something completely different: The wood quality. This process is repeated with the wood quality motion, which has yet another unique motion, creating the structure of your liver system. In this way, you can see the close connection with all the manifestations of breath, which is core to the understanding of how the ancient Chinese saw our relationships with nature and the universe.

Exactly the same pattern applies to the other storage systems. Your heart system manifests from the southern direction (heat and fire quality); your pancreas system from the centre direction (damp and earth); your lung system from the western direction (dryness and metal); and your kidney system from the northern direction (cold and water). These core structures, which were made tangible and moulded from *qi,* are known as the *zang* storage regions.

The five *zang* storage systems are completely different ecosystems to each other in your body, and they provide the root from which the qualities of nature and river systems are anchored. They are storage regions, not the organs most are named after, and their function is to store *jing*, the life force of breath motion. For this reason, when mentioning these *zang* regions, I use the term "system"—for example, the "liver system" or "stomach system"—to ensure clarity of meaning in what I am referring to.

Lung Storage System

The lung system is formed from metal and is symmetrical on both sides of your body. Every breath your physical lungs take is like the hours of a day, or the seasons of the year. It is a complete cycle of breath motion.

WHEN THE STORAGE SYSTEMS ARE BALANCED

The lung system helps you to:
- regulate your breathing and the passage of life force, from your lungs downwards to the rest of the body;
- provide the force of blood circulation around your body;
- ensure your skin is nourished with enough moisture and blood;
- generate grief to allow you to let go and move on with your life.

Common symptoms of an impaired lung system: Respiratory disorders like asthma, coughs and shortness of breath; skin problems like eczema and dry skin; tiredness; and hand, arm, and shoulder pain.

Pancreas Storage System

The pancreas system is formed from the earth quality and is centred in your body. It is so intertwined with the stomach in all its functions that the stomach and the pancreas are essentially extensions of one another. It is located behind the stomach, and plays a major role in digestion by producing enzymes to break down food and hormones to regulate your blood.

The pancreas system helps you to:
- extract nutrients (the five flavours) from digested food and transport them to your four limbs;
- store body fluids as fat and release it when needed;
- keep your blood in your blood vessels to prevent bruising;
- bring colour to your lips;
- help you think clearly.

Common symptoms of an impaired pancreas system: Tiredness, weak limbs and muscle atrophy, dizziness, pale lips, numb limbs, a heavy feeling, headaches, low appetite, over-worrying.

Heart Storage System

The heart system is formed from the fire quality and is located where it is for a reason. It is the place in your body where *shenming* originates. If you recall from chapter 2, *shenming* is the light that circulates within the blood river systems and organizes and gives coherence to them.

If we draw a longitudinal line and latitudinal line on your body, the place they meet is your heart, so this is where *yin* and *yang* intersect, and the spark of life ignites.[15]

The heart system helps you to;
- control blood, *shenming,* and the blood vessels throughout your body;
- give rhythm and coherence to the complex interactions within your body;
- affect your complexion by controlling the blood supply to your face.

Common symptoms of an impaired heart system: A pale complexion, anxiety, palpitations, sweating easily, tiredness, poor memory, disturbing dreams, insomnia, agitation, and rash behaviour.

NOTE The heart ruler, which is featured throughout this book, is missing in the *zang* storage regions, as it is such an integral part of the heart system that it is included within it. There are some specific actions, however, which can be more attributed to the heart ruler, such as calming your stomach.

Kidney Storage System

The kidney system is formed from the water quality, and is symmetrical on both sides of your body in the area below your ribs in your mid back. More than any of the storage systems, the kidney is the one that acts like your battery power. If it is fully charged, you are raring to go, but if it is depleted, you will inevitably be exhausted.

The kidney system helps you to:
- store your energy reserves;
- produce marrow and keep your bones strong;
- keep your hearing in good condition;
- maintain the strength and colour of your hair;
- regulate your sexual organs and the uterus.

Common symptoms of an impaired kidney system: Urinary problems, hearing loss and ear infections, knee and lower back problems, problems with teeth, respiratory problems (especially difficulty inhaling), and an excess of sexual energy.

Liver Storage System

The liver system is formed from the wood quality, and is actually symmetrical on both sides of your body, if we include your spleen as its pair on the other side.[16] It mirrors many of the functions of your physical liver, such as filtering blood, regulating blood clotting, storing iron, and detoxifying foreign substances.

The liver system helps you to:
- move and store blood;
- ensure that circulation smoothly flows around the body;
- nourish your tendons so as to prevent weakness and cramp.

Common symptoms of an impaired liver system: Headaches (especially at your temples and behind your eyes), neck and shoulder pain, bloating, eye problems, depression, irritability, nausea, gas, a lump in your throat, problems in swallowing, brittle nails, and painful, irregular periods.

These five *zang* systems should mutually benefit from their interrelationships with each other, and if the motion of breath is moving freely between them, you will be thriving. When these interrelationships break down, however, weakness or overflow patterns start appearing.

The *Fu* Systems

In addition to these five storage systems, which are all *yin*, there are other systems that, together, make up the core systems that run your body. But these are not root storage systems of the *zang*, instead they all act in some digestive, draining manner downwards, away from them, and are called *fu*.

Fu systems are the large intestine, stomach, small intestine, triple burner, bladder, and gallbladder. As they are all actively processing rather than storing, they can be regarded as *yang*.

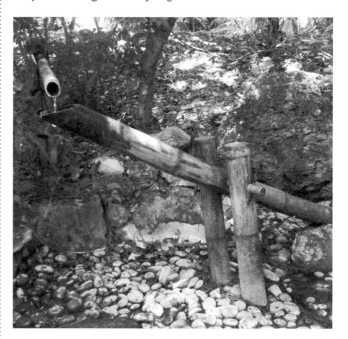

In order to understand the difference between the five *zang* regions and the six *fu* regions, let us look at bamboo *sozu* water containers, which can be found in temples, shrines, and natural places throughout Japan.

Sozu are a particular type of *shishi-odoshi*, which are devices used to scare away wild animals, and they consist of a weighted bamboo container held on a pivot that swings downwards with gravity when filled up with water. What scares animals is the sharp tapping noise it makes after it releases the water and strikes a rock placed beneath it.

The *sozu* container helps us see the nature of the *fu* regions, because neither is designed to hold what fills it. The *sozu* fills with cool water from a stream and immediately releases it below. When it swings back up, it is completely empty, ready to be filled again. And this is the essential structure of the *fu* systems. They are connected with the drainage of the *zang*. The *zang* are the stream feeding the *fu*, and the *fu* are the *sozu* container transforming and moving what is passed to them.

So what do the *fu* regions do exactly?

Stomach: The stomach system is essentially the overseeing system of the *fu*. Along with the pancreas system, it receives the food you eat, and through a process of fermentation with digestive juices and enzymes, it extracts the nutrition your body needs via the five flavours (these are listed in the qualities of nature in the previous section).

The stomach system helps you to:
- break down food into the five flavours and send its nutritive life-force to the rest of the body and the four limbs;
- ensure sufficient fluid levels in your body;
- maintain a downwards motion with circulation (this is the action of peristalsis, the involuntary wave-like muscular action, which governs the digestive tract).

Common symptoms of an impaired stomach system: Anxiety, worry, depression, eye problems, nosebleeds, swelling of the neck, facial pain, weak legs and arms, abdominal pain, diarrhoea, lack of appetite and taste, thirst.

Small Intestine: The small intestine system is where the digestion really gets going. The food comes in via the duodenum and gets broken down with the help of digestive enzymes from the pancreas and bile from the bile duct, and the small intestine system deconstructs and extracts.

The small intestine system helps to:
- process food from your stomach (the "pure" fluids head to the large intestine to be reabsorbed, and the "impure" fluids are sent to the bladder to be excreted);
- help you think clearly by separating out your thought processes.

Common symptoms of an impaired small intestine system: Chest tightness and pain, elbow, arm, shoulder and neck pain, problems with hearing, depression, abdominal pain, bloating, and being unable to understand and work through ideas easily (the reason for some of these may become clearer when you look at the trajectory of the small intestine river system in the next section).

Large Intestine: The large intestine acts like the small intestine by breaking things down, but it then reconstructs them in a different form. By the time the food you eat reaches your large intestine, much of the digestion is already done. So while some of the remaining nutrients from your food are extracted, the work of the large intestine is to transform the leftover digestive waste into your bowel movement.

The large intestine system helps to:
- control the transformation of digestive waste from liquid to solid and transport them out of the body;
- absorb fluid to keep blood volume steady;
- support the lung system so that it controls the pores of your skin.

Common symptoms of an impaired large intestine system: Abdominal pain, diarrhoea, fever, sweating, cold symptoms like a sore throat, skin problems like dry skin, and runny nose.

Triple Burner: The triple burner has a name that follows a different pattern from many of the other organ-named systems, such as stomach or kidney. It is a direct translation of *sanjiao*, the arterial system (the superior mesenteric, the inferior mesenteric, and the celiac arteries) that connects your physical heart with the digestive system.[17]

It does this by acting like a drainage ditch running alongside the digestive tract and extracting warmth and nutrients and sending them up to the heart ruler (the arteries around your heart).

The triple burner system helps to:
- regulate digestion and ensure that fluids and blood are correctly distributed around your body.

Common symptoms of an impaired triple burner system: Hearing problems, including deafness and tinnitus; dizziness; constipation; arm, chest, shoulder, and neck pain; headaches; and eye problems (the reason for many of these may become clearer when you see the trajectory of the triple burner river system in the next section).

Gallbladder: The gallbladder system acts exactly like the bamboo *sozu* in regards to bile, its main contribution to digestion. Bile is a digestive juice that is actually made in your liver system; the liver system is the stream of water filling the gallbladder *sozu*.

When bile is needed to process fat, it is released from the gallbladder into the cystic duct and small intestine. For this reason, it was considered by the ancient Chinese to control what is allowed in and out in more ways than only in digestion.

The gallbladder system helps you to:
- store and excrete bile to assist digestion;
- ensure your tendons are nourished;
- make decisions.

Common symptoms of an impaired gallbladder system: Sciatica, chest pain, neck and shoulder pain, headaches (especially one-sided), an inability to digest fats, dizziness, sighing, and a lack of courage.

Bladder: Your physical bladder expands to store urine and then contracts to empty it through the urethra, but for the ancient Chinese, the bladder system was much more than this, and involved a more metabolic function of fluids. These fluids are more connected to the nourishment of joints, bones, marrow, and the brain.

The bladder system helps to:
- store and release body fluids sent to it by the kidney system;
- stabilize the tissues and organs in the body.

Common symptoms of an impaired bladder system: Lower back pain, sciatica, urinary problems like cystitis, eye problems, and genital and reproductive problems.

In order for your body to thrive, the balance of the five *zang* and six *fu* systems must be maintained. The best way to do that is to understand how their related river systems work.

5

When the River Systems
Flow Freely

Chinese medicine uses the natural world as its reference point. This fact lies behind one of the key misunderstandings of how the body's circulation pathways are organized. You may have come across the word "meridian" to describe the lines that snake over the body like a subway map. This is a mistranslation of the character 脈 (*mai*) by a French diplomat named Soulié de Morant, who introduced an energy idea of Chinese medicine in the 1930s.[18] Unfortunately this was never properly corrected, and to this day it is used widely within the Chinese medicine world.[19]

A more accurate translation would be "blood vessel", or *mai* vessel, and this would make sense, as it is thought that the writers of the original *Huangdi neijing* text had a detailed understanding of the blood vessel system from extensive use of autopsies.[20] The text even describes this explicitly: "Once he has died, he may be dissected to observe his [interior appearance]." And it goes on to explain how to measure and quantify body parts.[21] It is easy to forget, but this was over 2,000 years ago.

If you look at the context of these vessels, it becomes clear that what the ancient Chinese were talking about was something altogether more encompassing and more akin to river watersheds and their complex ecosystems. In fact, the *Huangdi neijing* text correlated each of the systems that you will see in this section to an actual flowing river within China (at least at the time).[22] It is not that they were saying that the vessels in your body are

like rivers, that they appear the same; what they were saying was not a metaphor—they *are* rivers. Because rivers are an expression of *qi* and breath, and moulded from the same motions as we are. Thus, if you observe how river watersheds behave in the natural world, this will allow you to study the action of the same river systems in the human body.

For purposes of clarity, instead of using the terms "*mai* rivers", "channels", or "vessels" to refer to the circulatory system of Chinese medicine, the term "river systems" will be used—the same river systems of headwaters, pools, brooks, streams, marshes, rivers, and deltas you would find flowing down a mountainside on their journey to the sea.

So for the ancient Chinese, these were never mysterious energy meridians of *qi* flowing magically through your body. This simplistic understanding does not do justice to the sheer marvel of what they were explaining. They were describing whole river ecosystems of flowing blood, *qi*, and *shenming*, following demonstrable fascial planes and surrounded by vessels, tissue, fascia, cartilage, muscle, tendon, ligament, and skin, as a flourishing valley frames a river.

And just as river systems act in the natural world, so do they act within our bodies. They can dry up; they can flood; they can get blocked; they can flow too fast or too slow; they can be choppy or calm; they can split; and they can change direction. If you see them as this, it can transform how you perceive and treat your body.

What do you do when a river is obstructed? You find the obstruction and remove it. What do you do when a river runs dry? You try to reconnect it with the water circulation and build up the water supply. What do you do when the water breaches the river banks? You drain the excess water and restore the integrity of the river.

And so, in this way, by looking at real things in the natural world, you can understand how the same principles can be applied to the circulation system inside your body. As you might have guessed, nothing about Chinese medicine is random. It adheres to the same principles throughout. So these river systems are organized according to breath motion and the maximization of circulation patterns.

To understand this better, we need to look at the circulation structure of a tree. This is because a tree has its own circulatory, or vascular, system, which transports water and minerals up and down its length, and as it follows the patterns of the natural world, it has valuable insights into how the ancient Chinese saw the circulation system of our bodies.

Let us start by looking at a tree that was actually around when these ancient ideas were being formulated. Such a tree perhaps predates even the oldest of Chinese theories of antiquity and is still alive today. I have visited it several times and would have done so more often but for the nine-hour hike to get there and back.

This tree is Jomon-sugi, a Japanese national treasure, which sits deep in the forested mountains of the island of Yakushima in the East China Sea. It is 25m (82ft) tall and has a trunk circumference of 16m (52ft), but the most notable thing about it is its age, estimated to be somewhere between 2,600 and 7,200 years old.

It is difficult to comprehend a living thing that has such a vast lifespan. I was a wood craftsman on Yakushima, and we used to work with a special kind of fallen cypress tree called Yakusugi, which by definition had to be over a thousand years old. Many of these grand old trees had been felled during the Edo period in the 19th century and have been lying on the forest floor intact ever since. But Jomon-sugi was left untouched and is a fountain of life, hosting 13 distinct plant species growing on its branches.

The reason trees like Jomon-sugi have such longevity is that they have an extraordinarily efficient circulation system, which maximizes the benefits of its environment. Distinct types of plant tissue make up its circulation system, which are designed to behave in different ways.

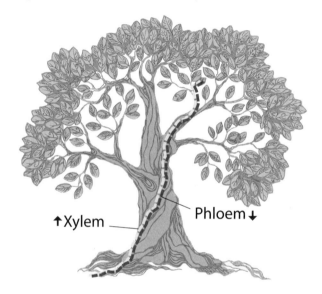

↑Xylem   Phloem↓

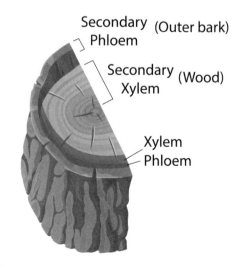

Secondary (Outer bark)
Phloem

Secondary (Wood)
Xylem

Xylem
Phloem

Xylem makes up the innermost tissue layer of the circulatory tissues. It is used mainly for transporting water and other dissolved compounds upwards from the roots. As Yakushima is made up principally of hard granite, many of these roots are visible and above ground, snaking over the undergrowth. The upwards motion rises to the stems and leaves at the upper end of the tree, something that the rhododendron, trochodendron, and mountain ash plants on its branches feed from.

Phloem is the outermost tissue layer just inside the leathery protective bark. It is responsible for transporting food produced from photosynthesis across other branches and stems and all the way down to the roots again.

Although both types of tissue take up a narrow area around the outer part of the inside of the trunk, it is this simple circulatory pattern of the upwards-flowing xylem tissue towards the inside of the tree (*yin*) and the downwards-flowing phloem tissue towards the outside of the tree (*yang*) that gives us the insight we need to make sense of the 12 river systems in the human body.

Let's look at what rivers look like within a human structure. As the tree circulation system is formed by the same patterns of breath motion as we are, there are some similarities.

Like xylem and phloem tissue pathways, human river systems can be neatly divided into *yin* and *yang* according to their location, direction, and depth. They were named according to which of the systems they are associated with, so most match the *zang* and *fu* systems: Lung, large intestine, stomach, pancreas, heart, small intestine, kidney, bladder, heart ruler, triple burner, gallbladder, and liver.

Although these 12 rivers are separately identified, they are all essentially one long current flow, like a river coming all the way down the mountain to the sea, and each one runs seamlessly into the river next on the list. This is the pattern of flow:

The lung river (*yin*) rises to the large intestine river and then falls through both the large intestine and stomach rivers (both *yang*). It then changes flow as it switches to the pancreas river, so that it rises through the pancreas and heart rivers (both *yin*). Change then comes to the flow as it drops again through the small intestine and bladder rivers (both *yang*). It switches direction again as it moves up through the kidney and heart ruler rivers (*yin*), before descending once again via the triple burner and gallbladder rivers (*yang*). It returns to the source, and rises to the lung via the liver river (*yin*) for the flow cycle to start again.

It is common to see the river systems in this order, as it follows the flow of circulation. But let us now look at each part in more detail. The following is a general summary of each river system and some of these common symptoms associated with each individual one.

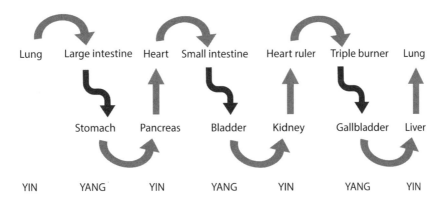

Lung	Large intestine	Heart	Small intestine	Heart ruler	Triple burner	Lung
	Stomach	Pancreas	Bladder	Kidney	Gallbladder	Liver
YIN	YANG	YIN	YANG	YIN	YANG	YIN

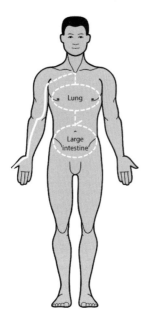

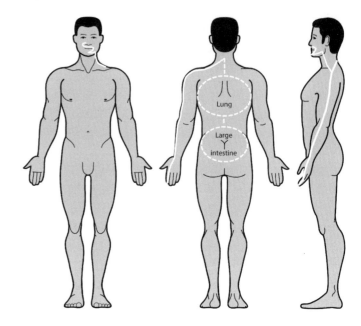

Lung River System

The lung river system begins deep in your mid-digestive system and connects with the large intestine before coming up to the lung area and the esophagus. It then comes out on a more superficial level at the front of your shoulder and roughly follows the brachial artery down your upper arm and the radial artery to your wrist. It then goes through your thenar eminence, the muscle on your palm below your thumb, and up your thumb to finish at the tip (and a branch goes up to the tip of the index finger).

Both the lung and large intestine river systems are within the metal quality, and you can see the deep connection between them here. As the lung river comes down the arm, loosely matching arteries, remember that it is not the artery we are referencing; it is far more than that. The artery is the river at the bottom of the valley, but the river system is the whole valley from top to bottom, including muscles, tendons, connective tissue, small blood vessels, *qi* functions, *shenming,* and so on. The lung river system was considered to be closest to the giant Yellow River in China.

Large Intestine River System

The large intestine river system begins at the tip of your index finger (where the lung river ended) and roughly follows the cephalic vein up the side of your arm towards your shoulder. On a deeper level, it then goes into your lungs and down to your large intestine, and on a more superficial level, it comes up the external jugular vein in your neck, across your jaw to your lower teeth, and ends at the flare of your opposite nostril.

It should come as no surprise, after reading this, that toothache in the lower teeth is often connected to the large intestine river.

NOTE You find a colour depiction of all river systems in the colour insert at the end of the book.

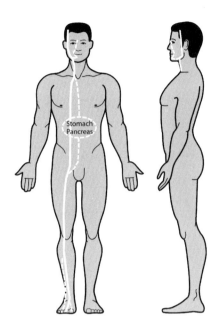

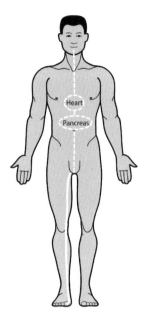

Stomach River System

The stomach river system starts at the bridge of your nose, and goes down to your upper teeth and jaw, and then up to the corner of your forehead. It goes down the front of your chest, through the stomach and pancreas, down the abdomen, and then your thigh, knee, lateral lower leg, and finally reaches the end at either side of the middle toe (and also a branch goes to the tip of the big toe).

This is one of the main river systems because of the sheer amount of your body it transverses. Technically, the large intestine and stomach rivers are two parts of one long river called the *yang-ming*. The large intestine was characterized as the Yangtze River and the stomach as the wide ocean. It should also come as no surprise that toothache in the upper teeth is often connected to the stomach river system.

Pancreas River System

The pancreas river system begins at the tip of your big toe and runs up the inside of your foot and ankle, along the medial marginal vein area, and then along the great saphenous vein up your leg. It continues up through the groin, on a deeper level to the pancreas, stomach, and heart, and finishes at the tongue muscles.

You may have come across this system with a different name, and indeed in some of my previous publications I used the term "spleen". The descriptions of the *Huangdi neijing* text strongly suggest, however, that what is commonly termed "spleen" in English, in translation of the character 脾 *pi,* is actually the pancreas. And the spleen is instead closely connected to the liver system.[23]

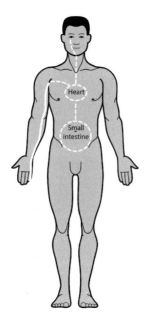

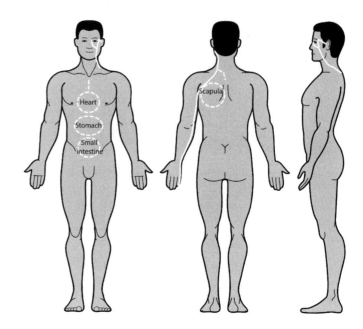

Heart River System

The heart river system begins in your chest and, on a deep level, comes down to the small intestine and up to your eyes, before heading across your lungs to your armpit. Like the lung river system, it follows the brachial artery down your upper arm, but then the ulnar artery on the lower arm to your wrist. It finishes at the end of your little finger.

Small Intestine River System

The small intestine river system begins at the tip of your little finger and heads up the back of your arm, through the scapula (shoulder blade) area to the cheek, via the side of your neck. It reaches either side of your eyes and your ear. It also goes down, on a deep level, through your heart, stomach, and small intestine.

The small intestine river system is one part of the *taiyang* river, which, along with the bladder, has a huge influence over your back, shoulders, and neck, and is often the first port of call in any neck problem.

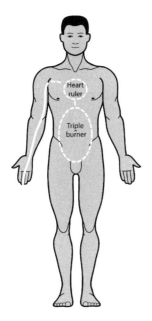

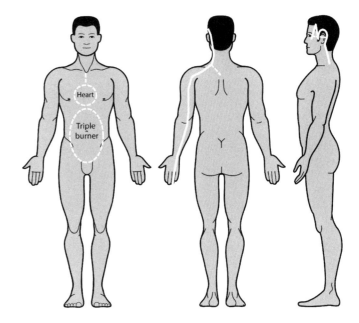

Heart Ruler River System

The heart ruler river system begins in the triple burner area (your digestive tract), and goes up to your heart, before emerging at your armpit, following the brachial artery down your inner arm, with the lung and heart river systems. At your forearm, it travels down the middle, between the palmaris longus and flexor carpi radialis tendons, to your wrist. It ends at the tip of your middle finger (and also branches to the tip of your ring finger).

This is another system that you may know from another name, the "pericardium", which is referring anatomically to a connective tissue structure around your heart. What the ancient Chinese thinkers were describing was more a system of arterial blood vessels around the heart, however, and as the pericardium is a connective tissue structure, it would come more under the influence of wood and the liver than the heart. For this reason, we are using a translation of the Chinese character rather than just repeating the same linguistic error.[24]

Triple Burner River System

The triple burner river system starts at the tip of your ring finger and crosses the outside of your forearm to the tip of the elbow. It then goes up the back of your arm, across your shoulder to the heart ruler area of the heart, and then down to the digestive tract. It also comes up your neck, through your ear area, and ends at your eyes.

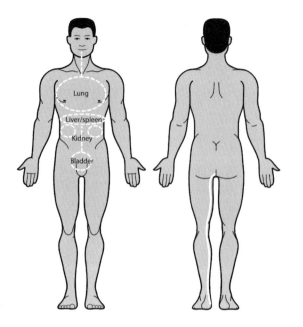

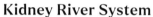

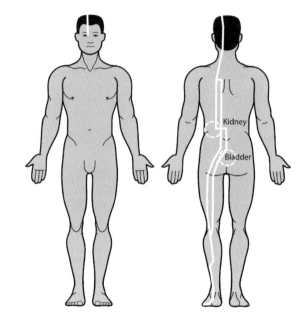

Kidney River System

The kidney river system starts below your little toe at the sole of your foot. It then crosses your sole, comes up the inside of your ankle, then up the inside of your leg to your groin area. It then goes, at a deep level, through your bladder, kidneys, liver, and lungs, until it reaches the veins you can see under your tongue.

Bladder River System

The bladder river system is another of the grand waterways that covers most of your body. It starts at your eye, and goes up over your head, while at the same time going deeper through your brain. It then follows your spine all the way down your back, and passes through your bladder and kidneys. It then goes over your buttocks, and down the midline of the back of your legs. It finishes at the outside of your foot at the little toe.

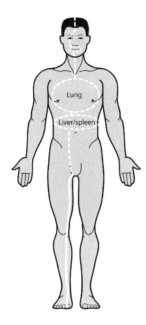

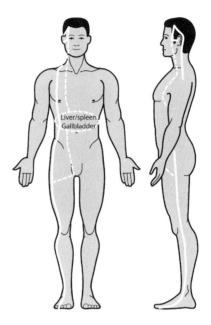

Liver River System

The liver river system begins at your big toe and goes up the dorsal digital vein to your ankle. It comes up the inside of your leg, crosses the pancreas river system, and when it reaches the groin area, it goes to a deeper level and passes through your genitals, liver, gallbladder, lungs, chest area, throat, and finishes at the top of your head. A branch also meets the back of your eye and circles your lips.

Gallbladder River System

The stomach river system spans the whole front of your body, the bladder river system spans the whole back of your body, and the gallbladder river system spans the sides of your body. It begins at your eye, goes up to the corner of your forehead, through your ear, and down your neck and shoulders. It then goes on a deeper level to your chest, liver, and gallbladder, while also coming down the side of your body, the sides of your thigh and lower leg, until it reaches the space between your fourth and fifth toes.

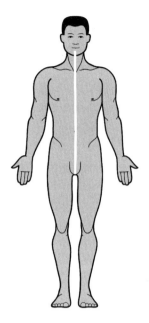
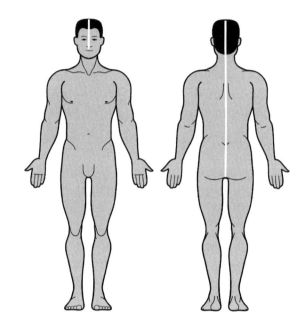

The Reservoirs

In addition to the 12 river systems, there are other waterways that do not behave or look like them. The *ren* and *du* reservoirs are examples of this. They have no directional flow, as they are part of the basic structure of your body formed prenatally. They are both easy to spot on any chart, as the *ren* reservoir goes up from between your legs, along the centre line of the body, over your neck, and into your mouth, and the *du* reservoir goes up the same trajectory but on the back of your body, so up the centre line of the back, over your head, down your nose, finishing above your top lip.

Rather than flowing rivers, it would be better to see these as storage reservoirs of blood and life force. They are both hugely important in treating imbalances, and ill health in general. The *du* reservoir is heavily implicated in back-related problems, and the *ren*, in abdominal, gynaecological, and chest problems.

6

When the Climates Enhance Your Life

Melilla is a Spanish outpost on the North African coast, and for 10 years I had a clinic there that specialized in treating chronic illness. Although few like to admit it, the city is a redundant relic of past colonial times and is more famous for the migrant attempts on its border fence than its distinctive modernist architecture. It sits tightly on the east coast of a Moroccan peninsular that juts into the Mediterranean and sits at the foot of Mount Gourougou, a forested mountain 900 metres high. This geographical location made the city susceptible to particular types of wind that swept across the city and dominated both the climate and every casual conversation.

The wind either blew *levante,* which meant that it came from the east, bringing low clouds and humidity along with heavy swells, murky water, and currents that deposit garbage on the beaches; or it would blow *poniente,* which meant that it came from the west, bringing blue skies, dryness, clear waters, and general happiness to the city. Few residents liked *levante,* and people would often complain of joint pains, even before it arrived, and when *levante* lingered for days, and sometimes weeks, you could sense the change in the city. It affected every aspect of our lives. If the clouds were too low, the airport closed, and all flights in or out were cancelled. If the swells were too high, the ships stopped, both for passengers and goods, and there were times when the shelves of the supermarkets looked bare. Although

admittedly slow to begin with, the pace of the city slowed even more, and people just became less active.

The way we were affected by the easterly and westerly Winds in the Mediterranean is an example of how weather patterns can affect us all. We must, however, understand at a deeper level just how climate and weather can either allow us to thrive and be at the peak of health or do the opposite. To explain this, let us return to space. If you recall, breath motion is the universal expansion–contraction movement that happens everywhere. In the environment of deep space, that motion is uncomplicated and might resemble the simple radio waves of FRB. As it moves further and further away from deep space, and closer to us, it changes, because the environment has changed.

The smooth, simple movements become more complex as it reaches our solar system, where other aspects of the breath movement become evident. The motion of *yin* and *yang* pulling *qi* (the fabric) then develops into a more circular movement around a fixed pivot. The ancient Chinese saw this as the movement of the star constellations around the North Star. We are lucky enough to live in an area where you can see the stars at night, and I often watch the movement of the stars and planets in the night sky. I am always trying to identify constellation systems and individual stars in relation to the North Star, which is sitting there in the blackness in the same spot. For the ancient Chinese this was not the sky, it was the heavens; and those constellations were the five ruling houses that moved with the seasons and influenced life on Earth.

It is with this background that we can start to understand the climates. As the breath motion interacts with our atmosphere, a distinct pattern emerges, which the ancient Chinese organized into climates that are intimately related to those constellations in the night sky. These are the climates that dominate our weather systems and are a fundamental part of the health and wellness of our bodies, too.

The five climates bridge the space between the motions of the heavens (space) and of the Earth, and they are the origins of the qualities of nature. They consist of the following: Dryness (metal), damp (earth), heat (fire), wind (wood) and cold (water).

Let us now look at each climate individually.

DRYNESS

Dryness, like all the other climates in this section, is neither good nor bad; it just is. It is a necessary factor in sustaining life on Earth and is an important and equal balance to the other climates. It is a natural accompaniment to autumn, or fall, and you may notice it from mid-September to mid-November. If you have ever been in a very dry climate, you can directly feel it through the reaction of your body. For example, living or working in a centrally heated building, you may notice how dry it feels from your skin or lips. Should you be anywhere near a desert, this is even more the case.

You may feel quite comfortable in a dry environment, as it balances excess fluids, and if your body has a tendency to accumulate fluid, there can be a welcome draining action. In excess, however, it can have a direct effect on how your lung system functions and how your skin behaves, potentially causing impairments in both.

Dryness can often be seen in symptoms connected to your skin, mouth, bowel movements, and urination, which are usually the result of dryness that comes from the inside, not the outside.

Apart from your lung system, the stomach is the key system here. The stomach system is the origin of all fluids in the body. A sure way to dry up this fluid is to have bad eating habits, such as eating in a hurry, eating late at night, or rushing back to work immediately after a meal.

If you do this frequently enough for long enough, moisture in the stomach system tends to evaporate, leading to dryness and a whole host of associated problems.

DAMP

Damp is the obvious counterweight to dryness, and its action is one of moistening and lubricating. It is associated with the latter end of summer, from early August to mid-September. Our weather in the mountains of Barcelona can be very dry during the summer months, and you can clearly see nature thrive after a spell of rain, with new shoots appearing out of the ground and a deeper green colour to the leaves in the forest.

When there is an excess of damp, however, there is a tendency for saturation. This is exactly what happens when too much rain falls in a short time period, and it can cause flooding and turn solid ground into marsh. This is when damp can cause issues both in the natural world and inside our bodies.

Wearing wet clothes, living in a damp house, sitting on damp grass, wading through water, going to bed with wet hair— all of these activities can introduce damp into your body. Once inside, it is extremely difficult to remove. It is slow, sticky, and heavy, and is notorious for its lingering, hard-to-budge quality.

The usual way that dampness enters the body is via the legs, and it makes it up to the pelvic area.

In women, this could mean in the genital system and the beginning of unpleasant discharges, or it could be the intestines, causing bowel problems or urinary "infections" in the bladder.

Damp can get almost anywhere, and there are generally tell-tale symptoms to indicate that it has. A feeling of heaviness in your arms, legs, or head is a classic symptom, and it can feel as if someone has wrapped you in a giant piece of cotton wool. The reason for this is that the damp is weighing down the motion of *yang* and preventing it from rising to the head to clear the brain. The cotton wool feeling is the damp getting between you and your brain and often leads to a lack of concentration and clarity of thought.

HEAT

Most people can recognize that there are certain heat climates that feel comfortably hot, while others feel stifling and your body does not react well to them. Where I live now, in the forest above Barcelona, the summers are hot, dry, and relatively sweat-free, and they are nothing like the summers we perspired our way through in subtropical Yakushima in the East China Sea, or the year-round sauna heat of Bangkok, Thailand.

The Chinese classification of climates reflects this difference by separating the heat associated with early summer, in April and May, from that of midsummer, from May to July. The former heat is known as *imperial fire*, and allows nature to open up and grow outwards; the latter is *ministerial fire*, and is a mixture of damp and heat that together warm and moisten as nature reaches its growth peak.

Both types of heat gives us the warmth we need to expand and grow, but too much is going to create dryness and, like a drought, it will parch the river beds, blow away the topsoil, and very little can then grow. This can happen anywhere in the body, but with the damp-heat associated with ministerial fire, the digestive system can often be

impaired, specifically the stomach and pancreas systems.

Rather than coming from the environment around you, heat can often be generated from within. This is usually as a result of long-standing obstructions in circulation, often a direct result of wind, cold, or damp being trapped in your body, which is known as a "climate pattern".

WIND

As I noted in the introduction to this section, wind has a particular ability to get under people's skin, both figuratively and literally. Many languages have names for different winds, and the *Huangdi neijing* describes eight winds based on their directional component.[25]

In the natural world, wind allows things to move, and it plays a fundamental role in everything from plant reproduction cycles to migration patterns. It is present just about at any time of year, of course, but in the lunar calendar, it is usually associated with early springtime, from January to March.

Its effect on the body is normally easily demonstrated. For example, on windy days many people have a strange inability to concentrate. Teachers often complain about the behaviour of their students when the wind blows hard, as they are often over-excitable and unable to sit still.

People are most vulnerable where the skin is normally exposed, and the typical area for wind to enter is through your neck. Many of the named areas located around the neck have "wind" in their names, such as Palace of Wind (Du-16) and Wind Pool (Gb-20).

The reason for this is that wind penetrates the body through the skin. The body has a natural defence system underneath the skin, known as *wei qi*. There are many types of *qi* within the body, and the term is used to refer to functional systems that have a clear purpose. *Wei qi* acts as the first line of defence against the natural environment, and will intelligently react to any threat and attempt to expel it. Sometimes, either the climate is too strong or the ability of the body to reinforce *wei qi* is too weak, and wind quite literally comes in and lodges just beneath the skin.

It is no coincidence that in Japanese a common cold is called *kaze*, as this is the word for wind in Japanese.[26] The first sign of wind entering your body could be a chilly feeling and a strong desire to avoid actually going outside in the wind. Your lung is the system most in control of *wei qi* so, if there is wind interfering with its flow, the normal pushing down function that the lung performs gets blocked.

This inability to maintain a downwards direction causes the opposite action, and you find yourself sneezing or coughing, and as the lung system cannot send fluids down, so your nose starts to run as well.

To know what wind does when it enters the body, we only need to look at the natural world and see how wind normally behaves on a day-to-day basis. A still day rarely stays that way for long. Wind often appears out of nowhere and blows the clouds. Changes are fast—a gentle breeze can turn into a gust in seconds and then go back to being perfectly still. By its very nature it is inconsistent and intermittent.

In the body, we can therefore expect wind to bring on symptoms fast, and for them to change just as quickly and move around from place to place. Indeed, it is not uncommon to have a roaming ache that may begin as a sore shoulder and end up as a backache. Wind also affects the top part of the body, causing stiffness, and the skin, tending to cause itching.

The sore neck so often accompanying exposure to wind is connected to how deep the wind travels in the body. As it enters your body through the skin, it reaches the rivers closest to the surface of the skin. This is the small intestine river and the bladder river (together known as the *taiyang*, the most superficial of all rivers). As the wind begins to

wreak havoc with the smooth flow of circulation along these rivers, pain and stiffness appear.

COLD

Cold acts as the counterweight to the wide expansive action of heat and allows the action of contraction. This is essential to ensure that the physical shape and structure remain intact and is normally associated with the winter months, from November to January.

Of all the climates, it is the one most associated with painful obstruction patterns that stay within your body and cause chronic discomfort. Indeed, most back pain has an element of cold embedded in the tissue, as do many gynaecological disorders. This is because it is so effortless for cold to enter the body.

Cold can come from above, via wind entering your nose or mouth. Usually this results in a runny nose, sneezing, an itchy throat, and a stiff neck, which are clear signs of wind in the lung system. When cold is also present, there is a tendency to shiver and be unable to sweat, because the skin pores have contracted due to the cold.

Walking barefoot, sitting on a cold step, or not wearing appropriate clothing allow cold to penetrate the body's normal defences, and it finds its way into the circulation of the *luo mai*, the system of streams and tributaries within your connective tissue structures. If it then finds an area of tissue that has been cut off from circulation, it can attach itself there, and the circulation is unable to remove it.

The most common places cold can attach itself are in the hands and feet, arms, knees, lower back, and shoulders. Of these, it can often be found in the joints. When cold is present, it contracts body tissues and causes pain. This commonly consists of stiff, aching joints that get worse in cold weather, in particular when it is wet and cold.

7

When Emotions Flow Smoothly

One of the most important aspects of the five qualities of nature when it comes to our health is our emotions: What we feel can actually make us ill.

The ancient Chinese did not view emotions in the same light as most people today see them. In the previous chapters, I wrote about the breath motion of the universe—how it changes as it reaches the environment around us, and how it then creates the climates in our atmosphere, which in turn creates the qualities of nature and the river systems. Emotions are a further expression of this same motion.

This is key to understanding emotions and how they interact with our bodies. Emotions are not in your head. They are not cells firing within your brain. They are patterns of nature, just like wind or heat or cold, and they move with the motion of breath. This makes them neither good nor bad. They just are. They exist in a smooth, cyclical motion, irrespective of how you feel about them.

Emotions have certain effects in certain regions in your body, and when the cycle of emotions is moving without restriction, they allow you to function in life. When this motion is impaired, however, there tends to be obstruction.

This obstruction is similar to that of climate patterns, in that an actual physiological obstruction exists within the tissue in a particular location. If you experience trauma, for example, the trauma is in the tissue and stays in the tissue

memory. Your brain will reference it, but it is not in your head. It is in the local tissue associated with the trauma.

This different approach to how emotions impact our bodies has implications for the treatment of common disorders associated with the mind, such as anxiety and depression. If you could remove the obstruction in your body that is causing the impairment of the smooth flow of emotions, then it is quite possible to reverse the symptoms of these normally mind-based disorders.

It is common for people to complain of a condition that began soon after a strong emotional issue, such as a skin condition soon after the death of a loved one; intestinal problems after a much loved only daughter left home for university; a stiff neck and shoulder after a particularly stressful, frustrating week at work. The connection between these events and resultant health problems is rarely acknowledged or, if it is, can often be dismissed as coincidence, since it cannot easily be explained in conventional terms.

For many people, it seems easier to treat the eczema with steroid cream than to see it as a representation of grief. The grief has impaired the motion in metal and within its two systems, the lung and large intestine. The imbalance in the lung system has spilled out into the skin, which, as you may recall, is connected to the lung by its quality of nature. One of the key parts of eczema treatment would be to strengthen the metal quality, so that the grief can then be worked through and the skin can improve.

Likewise, a few pills may take away a mother's anxiety and worry for a while, but the root of her anxiety problem is a weakened earth quality, and strengthening her stomach and pancreas systems through diet and treatment is preferable to the damage that might be caused to the stomach lining by medication.

A stiff neck and shoulders can also be medicated or injected to provide temporary relief. However, unless there is an acknowledgement that frustration at work is causing obstruction in the neck and shoulder rivers due to an impaired liver system, and the appropriate treatment given, the problem may never really go away.

For many people, emotions come and go, and there are no long-standing emotional issues. For others, though, especially when one of the qualities is weaker than the others, the emotion can be harder to let go of.

The longer an emotion remains unresolved in your body, the greater the potential for internal disruption and ill health. The problem is that, by this time, any connection between the health condition and the emotion that caused it can all too easily be forgotten.

What follows is a short summary of key emotions and how they can affect your body.

ANGER: Frustration, Irritability, and Resentment

If you think about where anger is placed within the qualities of nature, it sits firmly within wood. And if you recall the nature of wood, it is very much about rising, opening, and expanding. It is when the sun comes up. It is springtime. It is when the flowers break out of their winter dormancy.

This is where anger fits in. It allows us to move and grow, and to cut through any obstacles that appear in life.

When we get angry, we often "erupt", "burst", "blow a fuse", "go through the roof", or "see red". These common words and phrases describe the dramatic rising motion that can quite literally bring heat up to the face and head.

Angry emotions can suddenly stop the smooth flow of circulation throughout the body, but all things being well, normal functioning is resumed soon afterwards. It is rather like taking the Underground in London or the Subway in New York: Sometimes the train has to temporarily stop between stations. Of course, the way things go, this only ever seems to happen when your very life depends on rushing across the city to make an appointment on time. The windows show only the dirty, black walls of the tunnel, and your eyes dart from window to door to window to insurance advert to window to the nearest passenger in a desperate attempt to will the train along. A short while later it creaks off again, and the journey continues with a slight but all-important delay.

When you finally step onto the platform, en route to your destination, the frustration dies down and emotions return to normal; that is, until you squeeze onto the escalators and try to elbow your way through chattering tourists who do not know their left from their right. Doing this once in a while is going to cause stress and frustration but only on a temporary basis. Doing this day in, day out, every week, means potential long-standing emotional problems.

What sometimes happens is that the emotion of anger or frustration does not totally disappear. It can linger, especially if it is repressed and part of long-running emotional issues, and can easily "fester" inside. This is because, if there is an obstruction pattern in your body, it quite literally gets stuck. This is not a metaphor. There really is something within the connective tissue that is blocking how the circulation pathways pass through it. And what happens is the same as what happens to a river: There is a buildup behind it, and the pressure and subsequent overflow or counterflow will eventually cause physical pain or discomfort or emotional stagnation.

> *Common related conditions include:* Mood swings, depression, timidity, overcontrolling, inflexibility, and physical symptoms such as irritable bowel syndrome (IBS), internal growths, uterine fibroids, and other intestinal conditions.

ANXIETY: Over-thinking and Fretfulness

The act of deliberation allows us to judge and weigh up the quality and value of the things around us. It allows for a measured and moderate assessment of situations and the ability to take in all viewpoints and opinions.

Deliberation becomes pathological when it becomes excessive. When you are particularly worried, for example, you can feel a tightening feeling in your stomach, which is often described as being "tied in knots". Physiologically this makes sense as worry-type emotions are associated with the earth quality and the two associated systems, the stomach and pancreas. The feeling, therefore, is quite literally in the stomach area and represents an impairment in the smooth breath motion of the stomach system.

These systems are responsible for digestion and extracting the nutrients we need from the five flavours of the food we eat. An impairment in the stomach and pancreas systems can also make someone more susceptible to worrying, and then a vicious circle can develop, whereby continued worrying weakens them.

> *Common related conditions include:* Ulcers, nausea, digestive problems, constipation, diarrhoea, frontal headaches, and a tendency towards repetitive thinking, a lack of clarity, and obsessiveness.

GRIEF: Sadness, Loss, Regret, and Separation

If we look at where grief is placed in the qualities of nature, it is within metal. This means that it is connected to the releasing quality of the western direction. It is the sunset of the day or the autumn of the year, a time of letting go and allowing the breath to go on. We need to do this on a regular basis in order to continue on through life.

The sudden experience of grief and loss can cause temporary breathlessness and a struggle to "catch your breath". This is often felt because the emotion of grief goes directly to the lung system (which is metal), where it causes dispersion and obstruction. Grief does not have to be due to events like the death of a loved one and can be felt in less obvious situations, such as when something changes in your life. It can also come from looking back on how things used to be with some regret.

If the emotion is expressed and worked through, grief can strengthen your lung system and your general health, but when it is repressed it can do the opposite.

The paired system of the lung within the metal quality is that of the large intestine, hence there are often intestinal symptoms connected with this emotion.

> *Common related conditions include:* Lung congestion, asthma, recurrent lung infections or colds, skin conditions, and intestinal problems such as IBS and colitis. There may also be a tendency to be detached, critical, arrogant, and stubborn.

SHOCK: Fright and Distress

Shock can seem to almost freeze time. When shocked we cannot speak, cannot think, and cannot move. It is only when the emotion sinks in that time appears to start up again and the body responds.

This physiological response is because shock quite literally scatters *qi*. This means the fabric that is usually holding you together and ensuring that everything is in its place suddenly loosens. Stamp your feet near a flock of feeding pigeons and they fly off in all directions to temporary safety. When they think you are no longer a threat, they will fly back and continue their pecking at the scattered breadcrumbs on the ground. The same thing happens to *qi* after a shock. It shoots off in all directions, and normal functioning is resumed only when it returns to its natural ordered state some time later.

Sometimes this ordered state is not the same as it was before, and an impairment can develop. This could result in a general feeling that things have never been the same since. Shock can take many forms, from a difficult birth or an accident to a marriage breakup, and the heart is the main system affected. The sudden loss of circulatory force around your body affects the heart system and can lead to a weakening of the *yin* motion of the heart and a weakness in the circulation of blood around your body.

Common related conditions include: Chronic pain, sleep disturbances, chronic fatigue syndrome, and fibromyalgia.

FEAR: Panic, Anxiety, and Apprehension

Fear is part of the water quality. It is also part of an essential natural response to dangerous situations. I think we may all agree, a little fear is a healthy thing to have. If not, danger would be lurking around every corner as you would not be able to make a sensible risk assessment of any situation. We perceive a danger, recognize it and respond to it, usually by reducing the threat in some way.

When we feel fear, the kidney system induces a rapid downwards motion. For this reason, it can sometimes feel as if our insides have sunk, and there is an urgent need to visit the toilet.

Weakness in the kidney system can often feed or be the cause of some fears and anxieties. Any strong imbalance can lead to a state of general fear and anxiety, where the actual threat is undefined.

Common related conditions include: On a mental level, symptoms such as panic attacks, paranoia, suspicion, phobias, and a sense of anxiety about life; on a physical level, symptoms like backache and urinary problems.

JOY: Mania, Overexcitement, and Vulnerability

Joy is placed firmly within the fire quality and is very much about love, laughter, and enjoyment. When we feel these, the storage system most affected is the heart.

The heart system slackens with these emotions, and we can then experience the normal range of happy feelings, often to the benefit of our core and the release of stagnation in the body. This is because the motions of *yin* and *yang* become temporarily balanced with joy.

This can affect not only our own happiness but those around us. According to a heart study in the US, feelings of joy increase the likelihood of partners, siblings, and neighbours being happy by up to one-third. The study also found that the relationship between people's happiness can extend much further—up to three degrees of separation, in fact (to the friend of one's friends' friend), and that people who are surrounded by many happy people are themselves likely to become happy in the future.[27]

When, however, an imbalance in the heart system develops, people can find it very difficult to deal with feelings of joy and happiness. Sometimes their reactions are inappropriate—too much at the wrong time or in the wrong place, or even a total absence of happiness. An insatiable desire for joy, pursued relentlessly through work or play, can put a great deal of stress on the heart system and can sometimes be the cause of this imbalance.

The heart and the mind are part of the same continuum, hence an excess in the heart can disturb your mind. For this reason, many of the symptoms connected to imbalances in the heart and the effects of joy come under familiar psychological names.

Common related conditions include:
Palpitations, insomnia, manic behaviour, heart problems, and a tendency to be defensive, overly sensitive, paranoid, and uncommunicative.

8

When Obstructions Are Minimized

Most people are born with an aptitude for something. Some realize it straight away, but for others it can take a lifetime to find out what it is, if they ever do. This is not something you learnt to do and practised over and over. It is something you are just good at, as if it is in your DNA.

For me, it was seeing concepts. I realized that I could see things other people cannot—I do not mean imaginary friends or ghosts, but an ability to go into something grand and complex and see the various individual parts within my head.

It is like going into a large library, seeing all the bookshelves around you, pulling out books, and being able to file where that information fits within the other books and how that book fits into the library structure. It is not exactly a superhero skill, but it comes in useful when it comes to analyzing the complex world around us, seeing patterns, and visioning potential. It also helps with writing books.

What you are good or bad at in life is often heavily influenced by your physical constitution. This is how you are. It is how you were born and how you initially developed in this world. All constitutions, no matter who or where you are, are flawed in some way, with some parts of the constitution being strong and some parts being weak. This could be due to your family line, and I am sure that you are well aware that it is common for people to share similar strengths and weaknesses inherited from their parents or grandparents.

Or it could be due to how, when, and where you were born. If there were complications in the pregnancy or how you were developing, but equally, where you were when you took that first gasp of air, something imprinted itself in the core of your body. Or perhaps it is a result of your early life and how you processed emotional changes, or your lifestyle or diet or particular restrictions in your life.

These are the factors that can shape your constitution, and this gives us the general background to any illness pattern and the imbalances that lie behind it.

These general tendencies to having strong or weak aspects of your physical constitution are not what make you ill. You can live a long and happy life with your flawed constitution without much going wrong with your body, and many people do. The thing that creates ill health and disturbs the functioning of the body the most is something called an "obstruction pattern".

Your constitution can make some obstruction patterns more likely in some places over time, but an obstruction can appear anywhere. The obstruction will impair the *yin/yang* breath motion through tissue and, like a tree falling into a river, it will affect how the circulation passes through or around it.

If the obstruction is due to some external trauma or is superficially located in the body, then you can see it in the form of a lump or scar or skin-type feature or perhaps feel it in the form of muscle tension or soreness. But often the obstruction is hidden away, sometimes deep within the tissue structures, and you might not know that it is even there. If you do feel symptoms, then it could easily be in a different place, much like a blockage in a river can be felt from its effects on the flow downstream or upstream.

The causes of an obstruction pattern are often climate patterns, which we looked at earlier. These environmental motions are all around us. We can sense them easily, and they come to visit inside our bodies, too.

Most people have a general sense of this when, on a really cold day, you can literally feel the cold in your bones. Or you sit too long in the sun, and the heat stays with you all night. Or the wet weather makes your joints hurt. These are examples of the climates interacting with your body. As noted earlier, perhaps the most evident is wind, which lies behind a common cold. It is often a container for heat, cold, or dampness, and as a result leads to varying symptoms.

It would be perfectly normal for those climates to pass into your body, breach its surface-based protective barriers (*wei qi*), and then for your body to react to what it regards as an external invasion and expel the climate. This is what would happen in a healthy situation, when the climate and body are in a balanced state. But what often happens is either your body has an impairment that prevents it from expelling the climate, or the climate is just too strong, and it sinks deeper and remains.

It is able to remain because somewhere along the circulation river pathways, there will be an area that has lost its connection to the flow. This is known as a "backwater", and although it was once a tributary or inlet connected to the river, over time, it has become disconnected from the main current of water. When the climate stumbles across this area of disconnection, it attaches itself there, and with no circulation or breath motion

running through, the body is unable to expel it.[28]

This is a common pattern that explains how climates can cause an obstruction pattern, but it is not just natural climates that can get trapped in these backwaters. Anything that is not indigenous to your body has the potential to fix itself within tissue, including the medications we take, the pesticides and hormones in our food, and the pollution in the air we breathe. Any one of these can, and will, become lodged within your tissue indefinitely, given the right circumstances.

The obstruction pattern does not have to be generated from an external cause. Impairments in the river systems can create their own endogenous heat, damp, and cold, but one of the most common causes is emotional.

As we looked at in the emotions section, emotions are more than a brain-based phenomenon. They will physically obstruct tissue when they become pathological. This is especially true when the emotion you are feeling is overwhelming or long-standing. It will become tightly trapped within the layers of tissue until you are able to remove it. It is not uncommon to treat certain areas of the body, and for people to sometimes feel a traumatic emotion again or have a long-buried memory reappear suddenly.

These types of blockages are happening all the time and are all part of living. The older you get, the more you potentially will accumulate, and your body has a very efficient way of sealing off any areas of potential harm. The ideal is to minimize the effect of obstructions and wherever possible remove any areas that may be obstructed. This means a regular maintenance regime ensuring that the river systems circulate well, and whenever there are obvious signs of obstruction, such as pain or discomfort, especially musculoskeletal, to address them and prevent ill health before it happens.

9

When You Respect
Your Digestion

How you eat has a great impact on health. Food that has been gulped down, or eaten when under stress at work or while engrossed in front of a screen, is often not processed in the way it should be. Our eating habits directly affect the digestion process and the ability of the body to extract the energy it needs from the food.

If those eating habits are good, the whole process is optimized and runs like a well-oiled machine. If they are bad, no matter how beneficial your diet may be, it will get caught up in a slow, sluggish process, which will either add to or cause a series of blockages and imbalances and ultimately ill health.

The following are general guidelines for maintaining good eating habits.

Enjoy Your Food

Eating should be a pleasurable experience, not only in how it tastes but how it affects your senses. In the Far East, professional and home chefs take great pains to ensure that food is presented in an appealing way, based on the knowledge that digestion begins with your eyes, your nose, your ears, and the texture of the food.

Staying present while you eat is a very important concept, one that is connected to this idea of appreciating your food. At the risk of stating the obvious, in order to really enjoy your food, you have to be aware of the fact that you are eating. It is easy to be distracted by a whole variety of things during meal times, from a television programme to screaming children, but, unless you realize and acknowledge what you are actually doing, eating can become just another routine, similar to other daily tasks, such as driving a car. Few people have to think much when behind a wheel. The body generally does it all automatically. Sometimes you can drive for many miles thinking or daydreaming before suddenly realizing where you are and what you are doing.

Focusing on the eating experience—the tastes, the colours, the sounds, the smells, the textures, and fellow diners—if only for a short time, can remove automatic eating behaviour from the dinner table and help strengthen your digestive system.

This idea of enjoyment of food is also relevant when it comes to restrictive diets that force people to eat certain types of food they may or may not like, all in the hope of losing weight. In situations like this, it is sometimes important to also eat personally enjoyable food and, when eating, to really appreciate it. This can often provide nourishment for the spirit as well as the body.

Chew Well

Chewing breaks down the food so that your stomach system has to use less energy in the digestive process. It can also serve to relax your body and ease stress at meal times. The actual chewing action is essential for some types of food to break down. Whole grains, for example, do not reach their optimal nutritional state unless broken down with saliva in the mouth first.

I am fortunate to have a father-in-law who is the epitome of good chewing. He is always the last to leave the table and, when everyone else just has pools of sauce where the food once was, he is invariably still crunching on his pre-meal fermented pickles!

This camel-like ability to chew would not be practical for most of us, so unless you share the same ancestral genes, ideally food should be chewed for long enough to put down any eating implements during each mouthful.

Chewing well is especially important for anyone wanting to lose weight, as the more you chew the less you end up eating. According to research in China, those who chew food 40 times consume about 12 percent less calories than those who chew the same food only 15 times.[29]

Observe Regular Eating Habits

The natural cycle of the body usually requires several meals a day at regular intervals (for most people this means three main meals), and this is important to maintain strength in the digestive system.

Regularly missing meal times can cause a range of problems:

- Neglect breakfast, and the pancreas system can become impaired. Traditionally this was the main meal of the day and served to fuel the body to go out and work. If the pancreas system becomes weak, digestion slows down and damp can accumulate. What this means in real terms is that if you miss breakfast, or any meal for that matter, you are more likely to put on more weight at the times when you do choose to eat. For anyone wanting to lose weight, avoiding breakfast is, therefore, somewhat self-defeating.

- Neglect lunch, and heat can develop in the stomach system, as it prepares for food but none is delivered. The heat can impair the stomach lining, moisture levels, and weaken the motion of *yin*. This can result in a burning, uncomfortable sensation in your stomach, constant hunger, thirst, and weak gums.
- Neglect dinner, and the *yin* motion of your stomach weakens further, causing a lack of appetite, stomach discomfort, and a dry mouth.
- Eating between meals and snacking can cause stagnation and allow damp to accumulate. This is another cause of weight gain, as well as pain and discomfort, wind, and bloating.
- Frequent changes of diet, such as when travelling or dieting, can also impair the stomach system.

Regulate the Speed of Eating and Drinking

Eating too quickly can damage the stomach and pancreas systems and put a burden on the process of digestion. It can lead to stagnation and the production of damp. This is confirmed by Japanese research which studied the habit of eating quickly at meal times. It concluded that people who eat quickly are three times more likely to become overweight than those who eat at a normal speed.[30]

Drinking too much can flood your stomach and should be avoided during meal times so as not to put a strain on the stomach and pancreas systems. Meal times should be accompanied by sipping rather than gulping.

Eat Without Distractions

Avoid eating during an emotionally charged situation, an argument, a discussion, or in front of the television or a computer screen, while working or studying, or generally when stressed. All of these activities can injure digestion.

If stressed, the circulation patterns can become blocked, and the delicate relationship among your liver, pancreas, and stomach systems can become impaired. This can cause indigestion, stomach pain and bloating.

Eat with the Seasons

We live in a time when you can eat any food at any time of the year, regardless of seasonality. While the technology that allows this may be convenient in many areas of your life, the actual availability of foods outside of the season you are in is not so beneficial and can affect your body negatively. This is because your body is attuned to the environment you are in, whether you are aware of it or not. The *yin/yang* breath motion applies to a whole year, and each season is a different aspect of breath. In order to thrive and be healthy, your body should stay in sync with the seasonal breath motion as much as possible.

Regulate the Quantity of Food

Overeating is such a part of everyday life that most of us do not even realize how often it happens. The extreme symptoms of overeating, including indigestion, bloating, and wind, are no longer extreme. In fact, they are now so commonplace that people put up with them on a daily basis without realizing that it is not their body at fault but their eating habits.

Eating too much at once can cause food to stagnate, as there is literally not enough room to pass it all through. This can cause pain and discomfort in your stomach, bad breath, bloating, constipation, and tiredness. Damp and heat can also develop in the stomach system, as the stagnation starts to build up counterflow heat and accumulate fluids. This can cause frontal headaches; nausea; a sense of heaviness, pain, and discomfort in your stomach; and diarrhoea. The ideal time to stop eating is before you feel full. This usually means when your stomach is around two-thirds full.

Be Cautious with Diets

Weight-loss diets that require undereating also can weaken the stomach system by generating heat and damaging the *yin* motion. Following this type of diet will probably shed fat, but the effect on the stomach and pancreas systems often means that, once you are off the diet, it returns. Diets that require eating a lot of one type of food can also create a stomach or pancreas imbalance and often lead to the accumulation of damp/phlegm.

Be Cautious with the Combination of Foods

Combining too many different types, flavours, and qualities of food in a short space of time can prove too much for a weakened stomach system to process, and lead to stagnation, or damp accumulation. In this case, it is best to keep meals simple.

Fruit can be very moistening for the body, easy for your stomach to digest, and can help to keep bowel movements regular. If eaten during meal times, however, in combination with other foods, many of these benefits get diluted. To receive the greatest benefits from fruit, it should be eaten alone outside of main meals, if possible.

Eat a Balanced Diet

Studies show that many of the features of a traditional Mediterranean diet contribute substantially to a long life. These include moderate consumption of alcohol, low consumption of meat and meat products, and high consumption of vegetables, fruits and nuts, olive oil, and legumes.[31]

The Mediterranean diet promotes dietary habits that have much in common with those considered beneficial for strengthening the stomach and pancreas systems in Chinese medicine. If the two main digestive systems are processing food efficiently, the whole body will benefit.

Even as far back as the time of the *Huangdi neijing* text, it was clear on the importance of a balanced diet in allowing your body to thrive. A Chinese medicine–based diet is based on the core principles that it recommends:

- Grains to provide nourishment.
- Fruits to provide support.
- Livestock to provide enrichment.
- Vegetables to provide filling.

A diet of this type would "serve to supplement the essence, and to enrich the *qi*".[32]

Within these principles of balance, an ideal diet in Chinese medicine is one that includes all of the five flavours (see Food Therapy for more information on the flavours). We are all, however, individuals, with different bodies, impairments, preoccupations, and lives, so the exact combination of flavours and temperatures is going to vary from person to person. What may be healthy for one person can make another sick. People with a General Weakness, for instance, can easily feel bloated with dairy produce, but those with *Yin* Weakness can thrive from its moisturizing effect.

For most people, a balanced diet based on the original principles of Chinese medicine may consist of the following:

UP TO 40 PERCENT: Whole grains, such as rice, millet, barley, wheat, oats, corn, rye, quinoa, and amaranth.

UP TO 30 PERCENT: Fresh seasonal fruits and vegetables.

20 PERCENT: Legumes, seeds, or nuts, including beans, lentils, sunflower seeds, almonds, and walnuts.

10 PERCENT OR LESS: Animal proteins, including dairy foods, meat, fish, poultry, and eggs.

As much food as possible should be of the highest quality and organically grown, as commercial animal products may contain growth hormones, antibiotics, and steroids, none of which we want to enter our bodies with any great frequency. This is the base of a balanced diet and should be adjusted according to individual needs.

Vegetarians

As animal products should ideally be no more than 10 percent of a normal healthy diet, vegetarians should not be overly concerned that they lack the nutritional benefits of meat. Legumes, grains, and nuts can more than compensate when eaten regularly. It is important, however, to avoid relying on concentrated foods like nuts and seeds and to focus more on eating grains.

A common problem is that because meat generally has a warming quality, without it, there can sometimes be a lack of balance. Many vegetarians eat a lot of cold-natured, raw foods like salads, which can weaken overall digestion, and certainly the *yang* motion. This can be redressed with the addition of warming foods, such as ginger, cinnamon, and other spices.

It is also common for vegetarians to develop a weakness in their blood circulation, not because they are not eating meat but because of the combinations and the quality of the food that they do eat. To redress this, see Blood Circulation Weakness for more details on diet.

Food Allergies

Some people suffer reactions to certain types of foods, such as nuts. If this is the case with you, please listen to your body rather than strictly following a diet or list of foods. If you have an "allergic" reaction after eating what should be beneficial foods, then those foods are probably not beneficial for you, and you should find alternatives. Remember, common sense is the key. Your body has a wisdom of its own.

10

When You Live
According to Your Path

We used to see some people in our chronic illness clinic who were in the wrong place for them to thrive. Living in Melilla was not normal. It was quite literally like living in a big cage. If you climbed high enough up the mountain you could see Algeria, and on one side were the clear waters of the Mediterranean sea and on the rest were razor-topped fences up to 10 metres high. This is the political frontier between Europe and Africa, and the area you could move around in without crossing the international border into Morocco was 12 square kilometres. For many people that was their world.

Some were happy to be there, but others found it a daily nightmare, especially the patients who married into local families and were originally from outside the city, or some local people who dreamed of another life far from the dust and sweat. These were the patients who were not going to get better. It would not matter what therapy they had, there was something so deep, so consuming, so existential that it was always going to obstruct the treatment. These people were essentially not on their path in life.

This is not about anything predestined. It is just about finding the right place for you as a unique individual. You are a beautiful flower, and you need to be planted in the right kind of soil in which to bloom. If it is the wrong soil, it can be very difficult to thrive, and you are more likely to suffer from impairments to your growth. This is because the breath motion is not harmonious, and in each cycle something is pulling it (and you) off sync.

The only way for some of those patients to control their symptoms was to leave, but then they had to balance the potential harm with the real or perceived difficulties of moving out of the safe bubble they lived in. It was not easy, but if they found their way into an environment that suited them better, their bodies would no longer complain in the same way, because when you are on the right path for you, the breath moves through your tissues with ease.

Sometimes, it is just as difficult to change your lifestyle, but a very useful approach is to see *yin/ yang* breath motion in the right context. Breath motion can be at the level of a single cell in the human body. It can be the force of circulation along a whole river system. It can be the daily cycle of night and day. And it can be the seasons over the year. The same force is applied no matter what it is applied to.

And this goes for your life. Your whole life is a single breath motion. You are born in the east, at the dawn of your life, and as you grow, you go through the stages of life, as the sun goes across the sky and the year goes through its seasons. Spring turns to summer and then the autumn of your life brings the winter, the sun of the day begins to set, and the time comes for you to return majestically to stardust, and rejoin the universe you are part of.

As your life is a breath motion, it would make a great deal of sense that in order to lead a life that enhances who you are and who you can be, you should follow that motion. The ancient Chinese were very explicit about this:

"*Yin* [*qi*], *yang* [*qi*], and the four seasons, they constitute the end and the beginning of the myriad beings, they are the basis of death and life. Opposing them results in catastrophe and harms life. If one follows them, severe diseases will not emerge. This is called 'to achieve the Way.'"[33]

Achieving the "Way" was to live in harmony with *yin* and *yang* and the four seasons, and the text of the *Huangdi neijing* gave us clear instructions about how wise sages were able to live over 100 years. They moderated their diet, had consistent routines, were economical with their time, and took care of themselves physically and emotionally.[34] What they did not do—and clearly the ancient Chinese were referring to a situation that is just as familiar in the 21st century as then—is drink too much alcohol and stray too far from a life of moderation.[35] Indeed, a recent study in the US reported that more than half of the deaths from chronic conditions like cancer and heart disease in women could have been avoided if they had exercised, not smoked, and eaten a healthy diet, low in red meat and fats.[36]

So if you want your lifestyle to be more in tune with the breath motion, the seasons, and the natural world, how exactly do you do it? Let us now look at the lifetime, seasonal, and daily patterns that might help us in our goal of finding the right path.

Lifetime Patterns

Your body was designed to mature in a certain way, and there are markers that guide you through the breath motion of your life. These vary according to your sex but have a similar circular pattern. They provide a snapshot of where you might be and what might be happening in your body at key stages in life and reproduction. The *Huangdi neijing* described them as the "eight benefits" and the "seven injuries", and in understanding our life patterns, they looked at Nature's cycle of evolution and the patterns of nature (heaven, human, and Earth). The life of a female was separated into periods of seven years and that of males into periods of eight years.[37]

We start with the first part of the breath motion, when we are growing and developing. These are the "eight benefits". Think of this as the spring and summer of your life.

The four benefits for females are the following:

1. At 7 years old, your kidney system becomes abundant in life force, and your reproductive system starts to develop, your teeth change, and your hair grows stronger.
2. At 14 years old, your menstruation appears as the *ren* (Sea of *Yin*), and the *chong* (Sea of Blood) reservoirs fill up and prosper.
3. At 21 years old, your kidney system becomes balanced and your teeth fully developed.
4. At 28 years old, your vital energy and blood is substantial, your four limbs are strong, and your body is at its optimal condition.

The four benefits for males are the following:

1. At 8 years old, your kidney system is full, your hair strengthens, and your teeth emerge.
2. At 16 years old, your kidney system surges with vital energy, which allows your reproductive system to function.
3. At 24 years old, your kidney system has developed, your extremities are strong, and your teeth have formed.
4. At 32 years old, your body has developed into its best condition, and your musculo-skeletal structure is firm and strong.

After these ages, life goes into the next stage of breath motion and gradually moves from autumn to winter. These are the "seven injuries".

The three injuries for females are:
1. At 35 years old, the strength of your kidney system starts to decline. The energy of the *yangming* river system (stomach and large intestine) becomes less forceful, your face starts to show wrinkles, and your hair can start to fall out.
2. At 42 years old, the three upper *yang* rivers (large intestine, small intestine, and triple burner) weaken their flow, your face starts to show further aging, and your hair starts to whiten. As fertility energy declines, it can become more difficult to conceive.
3. At 49 years old, the *ren* and *chong* reservoirs lose their storage capacity, your menstruation stops, you have less strength, your body shape changes, and you can no longer naturally conceive.

The four injuries for males are:
1. At 40 years old, your kidney system declines, your hair weakens and falls out, and your teeth start to decay.
2. At 48 years old, your kidney system declines even more in combination with the force of *yang*, your complexion changes, and your hair starts to whiten.
3. At 56 years old, your liver system declines, causing your tendons to become more rigid, and your body loses its flexibility.
4. At 64 years old, your essence has been depleted, your bones are more fragile, your teeth can fall out, and your body is weak.

These markers of the stages of life that the ancient Chinese identified give us a clue about how we should follow the breath motion. Of course, the stage markers are not fixed to the ages that are given, and we are all individuals with unique bodies that may or may not follow these precise patterns; however, they give a general guide to how we go through life, and if you were to behave in a way that goes against these cycles, then there would be obvious impacts on the health of your body. For example, this has implications for when to conceive for both men and women, and also how to approach the subject of aging of the face. Despite what society seems to scream at us, aging is perfectly natural and beautiful.

Seasonal Patterns

One of the most obvious emanations of breath motion in the natural world is the change in the seasons. If you live in an area of the world that has clear seasonal changes, you might already recognize how your lifestyle and behaviour changes with the season. You put on less or more clothes, you sit outside or inside, and you are more or less active. But following seasonal patterns includes all aspects of your life, including the food you eat, the exercise you do, your behaviour, and your emotions.

While this was once straightforward, it has been complicated by the effects of climate change. Our world and our bodies have been synched to respond to the regularity of seasons. Each season has its own special climate, light, temperature, and weather patterns that repeat yearly. It does not matter whether it is the seasons of the northern hemisphere or the heat of the tropics, there are consistent and regular changes in the yearly rhythm that follow the breath cycle of that environment. With climate change, however, the smooth motion of the seasonal breath has been impaired, and weather systems that did follow a regular pattern have started to change. This has a direct impact on all living things, including us.

You may have noticed this yourself—the seasons are not the same as they were within this generation. For example, in spring, things are no longer in sync. In parts of Europe, a mismatch of almost two weeks has developed since the 1970s between the time when caterpillars are most abundant and the breeding dates of great tits.[38]

In summer, the weather systems have stagnated. There are fewer summer cyclones and there is an interruption of the jetstream in summertime, both of which cause frequent lingering heat waves and air pollution.[39]

The clear demarcations of seasons, no matter which season, are out of balance. Instead of smooth gradual motions, there are sudden sharp changes that throw our carefully balanced ecosystems offline. This inconsistency is going to have an increasingly major impact in our ability to follow the seasonal breath pattern and so maintain our good health and thrive.

Nevertheless, here is a short summary of how you can follow the seasonal breath motion as much as is possible within this context:

SPRING: This corresponds to the wood quality of nature. It is a time of growth and involves an upwards and outwards motion and the start of new beginnings. It is a time to be active and outside, doing gentle exercise like yoga, tai chi, walking, hiking, and swimming. It is about reinvention and seeing people and situations in a new light.

SUMMER: This corresponds to the fire quality of nature. It is a time of blossoming, flourishing, and cultivating the *yang* motion of breath. It is a time for activity, fun, and to live your passion, whatever it may be. The days are drawn out and more active, so late nights and early starts are much more tolerable than the rest of the year.

LATE SUMMER: This corresponds to the earth quality of nature and the idea of transformation. It is a time of gathering and slowing down. The last of the summer warmth still lingers, and it is harvest time, a time to enjoy the fruits of your labour. Within this is the idea of nourishing yourself and others. Listening and attending to the needs of others, and them to you.

AUTUMN/FALL: This corresponds to the metal quality of nature and has the idea of harvesting, sorting, and preparing for the winter. Like many trees and plants that shed their leaves, it also has the idea of not holding on to things and letting go of old attachments and emotional baggage. It is a time for rummaging through the possessions you have collected throughout the year and clearing out the junk. It is important not to put on too many layers as temperatures begin to drop in autumn/fall. Ideally the body should gradually adapt to the change.

WINTER: This corresponds to the water quality of nature and the idea of storage and containment. Like the rest of nature during the winter months, the focus is on slowing down, rest, and conserving energy. It is a time for reflection and thoughtfulness, and for being more aware of your senses, dreams, and goals in life. Shorter days also mean going to bed earlier than in the rest of the year.

Daily Patterns

The day/night breath motion is one of the most immediate places you can make lifestyle changes, if needed. The breath motion is a continual cycle from sunrise throughout the day to nightfall, and throughout the night. In general, the balance of how you lead your daily life can all too often become either too *yang*-based or too *yin*-based and, therefore, a potential cause of impairment in the breath.

Yang-Based Activities

Working long hours, being stressed, eating late in the evening, sleeping in the early hours, rushing from place to place and doing too much.

Yin-Based Activities

Seated at a desk for most of the day, using an electronic device, playing computer games, surfing the Internet, driving instead of walking and snacking.

A useful indicator about your daily lifestyle is the tidal rhythm clock. This is following the same pattern of circulation of the rivers as they flow through the body in one full cycle in a complete day. This was observed carefully by the ancient Chinese, who noted the effects on the body in particular time frames.

If you are able to follow the patterns of the tidal clock when the force of your body is concentrated in particular systems at particular times, then you are more likely to be following the breath motion of the day.

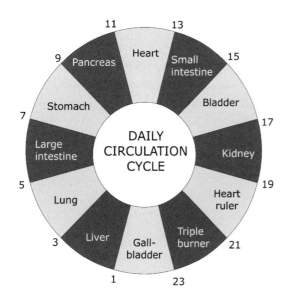

Lung System: 03:00–05:00

The lung system controls your breathing, the force of blood around your body, your skin and its ability to sweat, and the strength of the defensive shield that surrounds you (*wei qi*) and protects you from climate patterns. During this time, it needs to recharge itself to protect your body for the coming day. For monks, the early-morning hours are a time of reflection and prayer, and they traditionally meditate at this time, as the lung system is thought to be most connected with the heavens.

As the lung system controls breathing, some lung patterns and coughs can worsen at this time. Also, an impairment in the lung system could feature if regularly waking early, although this is more likely to be connected to feelings of grief or detachment, the emotions that can affect the lung system the most.

Large Intestine System: 05:00–07:00

The large intestine system is in charge of transforming digestive waste from fluid to solid and transporting it out of the body. As the focus of your circulation is concentrated here at this time, logic dictates that it is the best time to open your bowels. Like the lung system, the large intestine can also be affected by grief, detachment, and a general feeling of being stuck in life. This can often manifest in a physical form as constipation or as a more general malaise at this time of day.

Stomach System: 07:00–09:00

The stomach system is at its most efficient at this time, so it is the optimal time to eat and digest food. This is one of the reasons why breakfast is such an important meal. If there is an impairment here, there may be a lack of appetite or difficulty in waking or getting out of bed.

WHEN YOU LIVE ACCORDING TO YOUR PATH

Pancreas System: 09:00–11:00
Breakfast is processed by the pancreas system at this time, and it sends freshly extracted nutrients into circulation around the body. This allows much better concentration and clarity of thought, so this period is by far the best time to study.

Heart System: 11:00–13:00
The heart system is like an engine room that powers the mechanics of the rest of the body. For this reason, lunch time is not a good time for strenuous exercise that may push that engine too far. This is especially so for those with any history of heart problems, as circulation and heart-related conditions often appear more pronounced at this time.

Small Intestine System: 13:00–15:00
The food that enters the small intestine system via the stomach is broken down, separated, and absorbed during this time. This idea of separation in the small intestine allows you to think clearly, make judgements, and gives you powers of discernment. The ability to see with clarity before an important decision is heightened in this time period.

Bladder System: 15:00–17:00
The bladder system has a stabilizing effect on the nervous supply to all of the tissues and organs of the body during this time. This means that it is usually the least productive time of day and thus, a good time to rest.

Kidney System: 17:00–19:00
The kidney system stores the energy reserves you draw on during the day. During the early evening hours, the kidney system replenishes what has been used, and it is a good time to continue to relax and allow it to do so.

NOTE The two water systems above are squeezed between the four fire systems: the heart and small intestine before and the heart ruler and triple burner after them. For this reason, they act as water does in nature and dampen the fire around them by soothing and calming the body.

Heart Ruler System: 19:00–21:00
Your body becomes more active again at this time, and the heart ruler is associated with greater mental functioning and increased brain activity. This is, therefore, a good time to try to come up with ideas and solutions.

Triple Burner System: 21:00–23:00
The triple burner system extracts warmth for the digestive process and sends it up to the heart ruler and heart systems. Fevers and body temperature have a tendency to stabilize at this time, as heat is redistributed. If you are slightly under the weather or recovering from an illness, this is a very beneficial time to go to bed.

Gallbladder System: 23:00–1:00
The gallbladder system secretes bile to help digest fats and oils, and along with the liver system ensures that circulation flows smoothly around the body. If there is an imbalance here, sometimes it is difficult to switch off and fall asleep. This time has the additional quality of helping us sort through problems and reach decisions. This is why sometimes we wake up in the morning with the solution to something that the night before seemed quite intractable.

Liver System: 1:00 –3:00
During this time, the liver system is very busy filtering and replenishing blood, and your body needs to rest while it detoxifies the excesses of the previous day. Sleep-related problems during this time period suggest a liver system impairment. As this system is easily affected by strong emotions like anger, frustration, and resentment, and stress in general, this imbalance is quite often due to emotional factors.

The closer your lifestyle is to breath motion in all of its manifestations, the greater the chance you can thrive. If you can live in a place where you are happy, work at something you enjoy, be with people who enhance you, live according to your stage in life, follow the seasonal patterns, adjust your daily habits, and eat for balance, then you are closer to finding your path through life which maximizes *yin/yang* breath and allows you to live up to your potential.

In this way, you can bloom like the beautiful flower you are.

PART 2

What Are the Signs of Not Thriving?

Making sense of the many things which may appear in your body is not an easy task. There are, however, certain ways in how the body behaves and the signs and signals that it shows which can be loosely categorized into meaningful imbalance patterns. In this section we look at what the body may show you and what this may mean which can help in understanding and treating it when things go wrong.

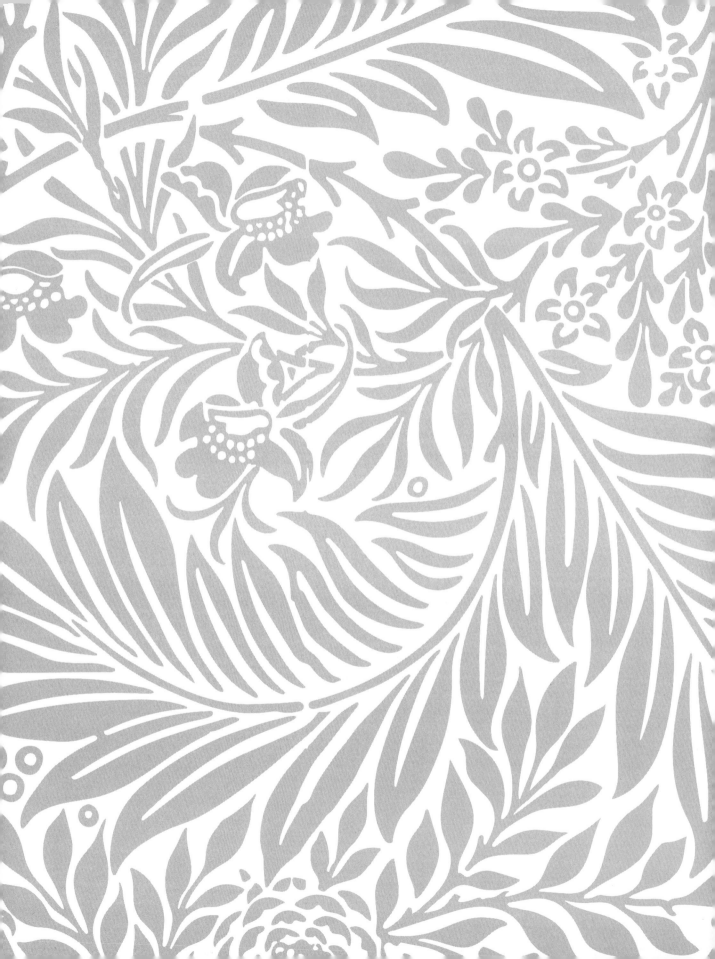

11

Physical Characteristics to Look Out For

You can tell a lot by "reading the body". The following are some physical characteristics to look out for that suggest certain patterns of imbalance might be present in your body.

The Body in General

The ancient Chinese described specific body shapes connected to how your body develops in terms of *yin/yang* breath motion and the qualities of nature.

For example, particular body shapes are attached to a natural quality:

METAL shape consists of a pale complexion, square face, small head, shoulders and upper back, and a tight abdomen.

EARTH shape is a more yellowish complexion, round face, larger head, strong shoulders and back, large abdomen, and well-developed thigh and calf muscles.

FIRE shape has a red complexion, pointed face, small head, well-developed back and shoulder, buttock, and abdomen muscles, and small hands and feet.

WOOD shape consists of a greenish complexion, small head, long face, wide shoulders, tall, straight body, and small hands and feet.

WATER shape is a darker complexion, large head and wide chin, narrow shoulders, a large abdomen and tall spine.

While these types of body shapes make a great deal of sense in how the qualities of nature and storage systems react within your body, the reality is that many people have a combination of features, some of which are constitutional and some acquired.

Someone who is overweight, for example, normally has an accumulation of damp and phlegm, no matter their constitution. If there are any health problems, the obvious place to start would, of course, be to reduce the sources of damp and phlegm, which may mean anything from dietary to environmental changes.

People who remain very thin, despite eating well, can often have an impairment in *yin* motion, which burns up the fluids that would normally help increase weight.

Those who persistently under-dress in cold weather—shorts or a T-shirt instead of a fleece and woolly hat—probably have a pattern of heat or weakness of *yin*. This makes their bodies feel warm, despite the low temperatures.

Those who over-dress in the heat probably have the opposite pattern. If cold or weakness of *yang* is predominant in the body, you can feel chilly whatever the weather.

Habitual posture can reveal a lot about how someone feels or where problems may lie. Someone who is usually hunched over their desk at work can often have weakness in their chest (heart and lung systems), perhaps owing to some unresolved emotional issue.

Hair

Hair, or the lack of it, can often give us clues about the state of your circulation:

GOING GREY EARLY can look rather distinguished on some but, in fact, it reveals a weakness in the kidney system. This is because the kidney system stores the energy reserves you were born with and uses these, along with enriched blood, to maintain your bones, teeth, and hair.

BALDNESS can also mean a weakened kidney system but often depends on where the baldness is located. If, for example, it is on the upper forehead and upper part of the temples, a common site for hair loss, it is considered the realm of the stomach and large intestine systems as this is the area where the *yangming* materializes (the stomach and large intestine together is the *yangming*). If there is excessive heat in either of these systems, the greater the likelihood of a receding hairline in this area.

The simple logic to this is that, whereas the body grows hair in particular areas to protect from the cold, it will lose hair in areas it needs to cool down.

DULL, LIFELESS HAIR means that the circulation is not getting to the skin and nourishing the roots. It suggests a weakness of the kidney and lung systems.

DRY, BRITTLE HAIR AND DANDRUFF can mean blood and *yin* weakness. The roots are not being nourished, and the low heat from the *yin* being too weak to be able to balance *yang* burns up body fluids and the moisture in your skin and hair.

Complexion

Your face is an obvious place to look for an imbalance, and this can often be found in its colouring. In general, your face is the flowering of the heart system, but like all flowers, it can have multiple tones and shades, which lie superficially or hidden underneath. When seen in natural light, red, yellow, green, white, and black hues that stand out from your normal shade can sometimes be seen clearly.

These colours can generally signify the following:

RED can mean heat.

YELLOW can mean an impaired pancreas or stomach system and/or the accumulation of damp. It might also be accompanied by puffiness.

GREEN is often a liver system imbalance.

WHITE can be a weakness in blood circulation or *yang*.

BLUE may be a sign of cold and stagnation.

BLACK can mean a kidney system imbalance or perhaps cold and pain.

Nose

The colour of your nose can sometimes be quite revealing:

GREEN or **BLUE** could accompany abdominal pain.

YELLOW signifies the presence of damp and heat somewhere in the body.

WHITE/PALE can mean a weakness of blood circulation.

RED suggests heat in the lung and pancreas systems.

Eyes

Different colours found in the whites of your eyes and around the eyes themselves may reveal several health conditions:

REDNESS in the whites of the eyes suggests heat in the heart system.

YELLOW in the whites of the eyes suggests an accumulation of damp and heat somewhere in the body.

BLUISH TINGE to the whites of the eyes can mean an imbalanced liver system.

RED, SWOLLEN EYES normally mean the liver system is overflowing and rising up, or wind and heat has entered the body.

DARK RINGS OR SWELLING UNDER THE EYES suggest a weakened kidney and stomach system.

SWOLLEN EYELIDS can mean a weakness in the pancreas or stomach systems.

Ears

Ear characteristics are also useful in diagnosing body patterns:

SWOLLEN EARS signify a climate pattern – wind, damp, heat, or cold has entered the ear and is blocking how it functions.

THIN EARS suggest a weakness in the body and blood circulation.

DRY & RED INSIDE EARS could be connected to an impairment in the gallbladder or triple burner river systems as the middle of your ear is where these river systems (together called *shaoyang*) materialize.

STICKY WAX IN EARS is often a sign of damp and heat, especially when profuse.

Mouth, Lips, and Lower Face

Your lips are the flowering of your centre digestive systems, the stomach and pancreas.

PALE LIPS can mean a weakness in blood circulation, as there is not enough nutritive blood to give the lips a full colour.

OVERLY RED, DRY LIPS often mean heat in the stomach system. Your lips reflect the state of the stomach system, as they are an expression of the earth quality of nature. When there is heat and therefore less moisture in the system, this then manifests with redness and dryness of the lips.

BLUE OR PURPLE LIPS mean stagnation of blood circulation. This can accompany serious conditions like a cardiac arrest, and appropriate measures should be taken then.

OPEN MOUTH can often signify a weakness. This is rather like leaving the door open because nobody has the strength to get up and shut it.

DOUBLE CHIN suggests a weakness in the kidney system, as the area under your jaw is where the *shaoyin* (heart and kidney river systems together) materializes.

Teeth and Gums

WEAK TEETH can mean a weakness in the kidney system. The kidney system controls the strength of your teeth and bones by producing marrow from its reserves of life force, or *jing*.

DRY, GREY TEETH suggest a weakened kidney system. Heat from an overactive *yang* has dried up body fluids both in the kidney system, causing discolouration, and in your mouth to make them dry.

PALE GUMS normally mean weak blood circulation. There is not enough enriched blood in the body to reach them to make them a healthy pink.

BLEEDING GUMS suggest heat in the stomach system. The state of the stomach directly affects the strength of the gums and, when the heat rises, the gums can no longer contain blood within the connective tissue.

Hands

In general, the state of your nails is a materialization of wood and the liver and gallbladder systems, as this is the area of the body that opens like flower petals on a plant to show us the quality of nature within.

PALE, BRITTLE NAILS suggest weak blood circulation. Not enough nutritive blood can reach the nail beds to strengthen them.

BLUE TINGE TO YOUR NAILS may mean stagnation in the river system and perhaps an obstruction pattern that is restricting circulation.

TINY BLUISH OR RED BLOOD VESSELS The thenar eminence (the fleshy muscle on the palm below the thumb) can sometimes have tiny bluish or red blood vessels. This usually signifies cold (blue) or heat (red) in the stomach system.

BLOOD VESSEL ON THE INDEX FINGER The lateral side of the index finger of an infant under three years old can be used to diagnose the severity of an illness. Sometimes there is a visible blood vessel along this finger, and the length of this blood vessel stretching from the knuckle indicates how deep a pattern of disease has reached. The creases at the finger joints are referred to as "gates". The first gate is "Wind Gate", and if the blood vessel extends out of this, it suggests a climate pattern. If the vessel continues past the next gate, at the first finger joint, it has gone through "*Qi* Gate" and is now much deeper into the body. If it is still visible and goes past the second joint, it has gone through "Life Gate", and the illness has become very serious.

Skin

DRY SKIN conditions are often caused by a weakness in blood circulation.

VISIBLE SMALL BLOOD VESSELS and capillaries anywhere on the body are areas telling you about the river system below them. They suggest an obstruction within the connective tissue circulation and imply that the closest river system may have impairments in that area. If the vessels appear dark or purple, then it suggests that this is a long-term stagnation pattern, not unlike a blocked stream that later runs into the river.

ACNE conditions are usually caused by damp/phlegm and heat rising within the stomach and large intestine river systems.

Taste

BITTER TASTE in the mouth is usually caused by heat, often rising up from the liver and gallbladder systems.

SWEET TASTE in the mouth can often be caused by damp and heat in the pancreas or stomach systems.

SOUR TASTE can signify an accumulation of heat in the liver and stomach systems.

LACK OF TASTE is usually due to the dysfunction of the digestive systems – the stomach or pancreas.

Voice

WEAK VOICE suggests a cold pattern or weakness of *yang*.

FORCEFUL VOICE suggests a heat pattern often coming from agitation from within.

SHOUTING OR CLIPPED voice, as if someone is annoyed or angry, indicates an imbalance in wood.

LAUGHING voice suggests an imbalance in fire.

SINGING voice, which goes up and down as if singing, indicates earth.

WHIMPERING, WEEPING voice, which sounds as if the person is about to burst into tears, is metal.

GROANING OR MOANING tone suggests an imbalance in water.

SIGHING A LOT probably means a stagnation pattern due to emotional stress that causes muscles and tendons to tighten.
   Your body then tries to release pent-up emotion by expanding your chest muscles and sighing.

Odours

The following apply to breath, urine, stools, vomit, sweat, and any discharges:

STRONG ODOURS are due to heat.

LACK OF ODOUR, when there should be one, is a sign of cold.

BAD BREATH often means that there is heat in the stomach system. This can often be due to poor dietary habits and overeating, which can literally cause stagnation of food in the stomach.

SWEET SMELL is linked to an imbalance in the stomach or pancreas systems and can sometimes be connected to diabetes.

URINE-LIKE SMELL is associated with a kidney system problem.

Tongue

The tongue can reveal some very useful indicators about what is happening in the body. I grew up noticing that my tongue sometimes had a coating with random circular bare patches and sometimes a coating on just one side. I knew that it had to mean something but, in the dark days before the Internet, information was so much more difficult to find.

If someone had told me that it was not just disorganized tongue fur but my body informing me to stop damaging my liver or gallbladder systems, I would have perhaps listened and gone to bed earlier or done a bit more exercise.

An analysis of the tongue is very much a part of Chinese herbal medicine and has traditionally been divided into areas corresponding to the key systems in the body.

FRONT: The chest systems – the heart and lung.

MIDDLE: The digestive systems – the stomach and pancreas.

SIDES: The circulatory systems – the liver and gallbladder.

BACK: The lower systems – the large and small intestines, kidney, and bladder.

Marks, discolourations and spots on particular areas of the tongue can give you information about the corresponding system.

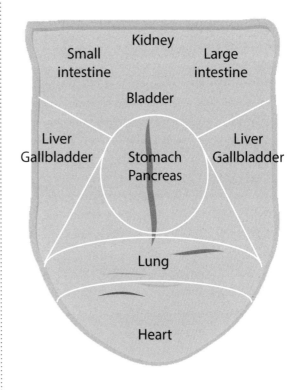

A line or groove in the middle of your tongue, for example, indicates that body fluids have been impaired in the stomach and pancreas area, which usually signifies that the *yin* motion of the stomach system is weakened. This is commonly caused by an improper diet, and if it continues over a long period of time can lead to heat in the stomach system and digestive complaints. This could then cause a correspondingly deeper groove in the midline of the tongue.

When examining your tongue, keep in mind the following observations:

- Look at the tongue in clear daylight, otherwise, the variations in artificial light can make you believe you have all kinds of imaginary disorders.
- Some types of food and drink, such as coffee, beetroot, gum, and lollipops, can change the colour of the tongue coating.

Some common features of imbalance seen on the tongue are as follows:

NORMAL HEALTHY TONGUE: This is not an easy one to qualify, but in Chinese herbal medicine, a normal healthy tongue is considered to be pale red with a thin, white coating. It should be neither thin nor swollen, it should be moist but not wet and should not tremble when stuck out.

PALE TONGUE often means weakness, especially of the *yang* motion, and means that there is not enough nutritive energy to bring the blood circulation up to the tongue. It would usually be accompanied by General Weakness symptoms.

RED tongue often means weakness in *yin* motion. Heat rises from agitated *yang* motion (which is not being balanced by *yin*), dries up moisture on the tongue and removes its coating.

THICK WHITE COATING on the tongue suggests the presence of cold inside the body.

THICK YELLOW COATING suggests the presence of heat inside the body.

PALE SIDES usually mean a weakness in blood circulation. The liver system helps in circulating and storing blood, so when this is impaired, it is logical that paleness appears on this area of the tongue (liver and gallbladder area).

SWOLLEN TONGUE can mean that too many body fluids have expanded your tongue and usually reflects the amount of damp accumulated in the body.

TEETH MARKS AT THE SIDES OF THE TONGUE can mean a weak pancreas system and also the buildup of damp as a byproduct of this. The tongue has expanded so much that the only available space is being squeezed into the gaps of the teeth.

PURPLE TONGUE suggests an obstruction pattern and can sometimes be a warning sign of a serious condition.

CRACKS ON YOUR TONGUE appear because of a lack of moisture and body fluids and usually signify a *yin* weakness.

PATCHES IN THE TONGUE COATING can also mean a *yin* weakness, which allows the *yang* motion to overact and send up heat, which burns off the moisture on the tongue. This can be caused by some medications, in particular antibiotics.

MOUTH ULCERS signify heat rising upwards from the body. If they are under the tongue, the heat could be from the pancreas or kidney systems; if the ulcers are actually on the tongue, it could be from the heart; or if they are on the gums, it may be heat in the stomach system.

PART 3

How Can You Treat Yourself?

In the following chapters there are lists of patterns and corresponding manual therapies, areas of treatment, dietary and lifestyle changes, and exercises. These are quite specific and may not be fully understood without a clear explanation of the details of each therapy. In this section, therefore, each therapy is explained and illustrated so as to provide a useful resource to refer back to in the later sections.

12

Food Therapy

Most people are familiar with the idea that foods can be broken down into separate categories according to what they contain. For example, food can contain various combinations of protein, carbohydrates, fats, minerals, and vitamins.

If in doubt, the food can be tested scientifically with simple chemical solutions to see in which category it lies. This is how we know, for example, that potatoes are carbohydrates, meat is protein, and folic acid is a vitamin. They have been broken down, analyzed, and clearly categorized.

If you eat any of those foods, your body then contains more of that category than it had previously. So, for example, after lunching on a steak, your body very probably has more proteins and fats than it did beforehand.

This way of looking at the body and food is to see both in terms of their chemical constituencies. The body needs protein, carbohydrates, and fats to create its calorific energy, so in order to maintain our stores of energy, the appropriate requirement of calories should be consumed every day. Again this can be measured and quantified down to the last ounce.

There is, however, something missing from this mechanical picture of the body and nutrition. This is that the relationship is much more than the nuts and bolts of nutritional theory.

There is no simple chemical test to see how the body actually reacts to the food it consumes.

During the digestive process, when food is transformed into energy, different food will cause different reactions within the body's circulation structure.

In a laboratory, a carbohydrate is a carbohydrate, but when that carbohydrate arrives in the warmth of the stomach, along with a cocktail of other foods, it will do something to the body around it that could be completely unrelated to the fact that it is a carbohydrate. It could heat things up or cool things down, speed them up or slow them down, or even strengthen or weaken a storage system.

It is here, *after* the food has reached the stomach, *not before*, that the ancient Chinese began their classification of food.

They developed a theory that all food can be categorized according to the five flavours and temperature. It is defined by the effect the food has on the body after digesting it, not by the actual taste or temperature the food is eaten at. Let us start with the temperature of food.

Temperature

An awareness of temperature can be of great benefit to understanding how food fits in with the overall picture of maintaining health and balance in the body.

For example, for someone who is suffering from heat rising to the head, as is often the case with migraines, menopausal hot flushes, or trigeminal neuralgia, consuming food classified as hot or warm, like coffee and rich meat, can easily exacerbate the problem.

At the other end of the spectrum, someone who feels exhausted, chilly, and with a sore lower back, should avoid eating too many cold foods, such as salad and uncooked fruit.

With just a little of this knowledge, changes can be made to eating habits which can keep us healthy or even have the power to transform long-standing medical conditions.

The following is a list of foods and their temperatures, but it is not exhaustive nor is it exclusive. Sometimes foods can be in more than one category at the same time, so for some foods I have simplified this by keeping them in just one.

Inevitably, there will be some individual differences with this list and others that may be found on Chinese food classification and should be seen as a set of guidelines rather than rules.

Foods That Cool Down the Body

Cold-Natured Foods

Cold foods cool down the body with an inwards and downwards motion. They will also slow digestion and the circulation flow around the body.

Too many cold foods can weaken digestion and cause weight gain. For anyone with a *yang* weakness or cold pattern, too many of these foods can worsen the pattern.

FRUIT: Bananas, cranberries, grapefruit, persimmons, limes, melons, mangos, tomatoes, and watermelons

VEGETABLES: Bean sprouts, cucumbers, lettuce, and seaweed

HERBS AND SPICES: Salt

LEGUMES, SEEDS, AND NUTS: Tofu, mung beans, and bamboo shoots

MEAT, FISH, AND SEAFOOD: Crab, clams, and octopus

DRINKS: Iced beverages in general, milkshakes, and yogurt drinks

OTHER: Ice cream or ice lollies (popsicles), cottage cheese, spreads, and yogurt

Cool-Natured Foods

Cool foods also have a cooling effect on the body but less so than cold-natured foods, and they can also help strengthen blood circulation.

Too many cool foods may weaken digestion and *yang*. Any long-standing cold pattern may also worsen.

FRUIT: Apples, avocado, blackcurrants, lemons, pears, prunes, mandarins, oranges, strawberries, tangerines, kiwi, and mulberries

VEGETABLES: Artichokes, aubergines (eggplants), broccoli, cauliflower, chicory, button mushrooms, radishes, rhubarb, spinach, and watercress

HERBS AND SPICES: Marjoram, peppermint, and nettle

LEGUMES, SEEDS, AND NUTS: Almonds and soya beans

MEAT, FISH, AND SEAFOOD: Oysters, pork, rabbit, frog, and snails

DRINKS: Beer, cow's milk, soya milk, almond milk, coconut milk, green tea, chamomile tea, oolong tea, and mint tea

GRAINS: Barley, millet, buckwheat, wheat, and wheat bran

OTHER: Cheese (the harder the cheese, the less cooling it is), sesame oil, soy sauce, and miso soup

Foods That Warm the Body

Warm-Natured Foods

Warm foods create warmth in the body by moving circulation upwards and outwards from the centre. They also strengthen your core and replenish your energy reserves.

For anyone with a *yin* weakness or heat pattern, too many of these foods will exacerbate the heat.

FRUIT: Coconuts, dates, pomegranates, peaches, raspberries, blackberries, tomatoes (cooked), hawthorn fruit, and nectarines

VEGETABLES: Asparagus, onions, garlic, kale, leeks, parsnips, green peppers, squash, and fennel

HERBS AND SPICES: Basil, cardamom, caraway, chives, coriander, fresh ginger, parsley, sage, turmeric, cumin, cloves, nutmeg, oregano, thyme, and rosemary

LEGUMES, SEEDS, AND NUTS: Almonds, black-eyed peas, chestnuts, sunflower seeds, sesame seeds, walnuts, and pine nuts

MEAT, FISH, AND SEAFOOD: Chicken, turkey, mutton, ham, venison, lobster, mussels, anchovies, prawns, shrimps, eel, and most freshwater fish

DRINKS: Coffee, black tea, jasmine tea, Pu'er tea, wine, and goat's milk

GRAINS: Oats, quinoa, and glutinous rice

OTHER: Chocolate, cocoa, egg yolk, brown sugar, vinegar, and butter

Hot-Natured Foods

Hot foods speed up the *yang* motion of circulation in your body, and they encourage a rising and outwards movement.

Anyone with a heat or *yin* weakness pattern should be very cautious with these foods as they are likely to increase the heat and worsen the pattern.

HERBS AND SPICES: Black and white pepper, chillies, cayenne pepper, cinnamon, dried ginger, Tabasco sauce, mustard, and horseradish

MEAT, FISH, AND SEAFOOD: Lamb, smoked fish, and trout

DRINKS: Whisky and strong alcohol

OTHER: Peanut butter

Foods without Heating or Cooling Qualities

Neutral foods are those that have no particular leaning towards hot or cold. They tend to strengthen and encourage circulation to move freely around the body.

FRUIT: Apricots, cherries, figs, grapes, pineapples, and plums

VEGETABLES: Green beans, beetroot, cabbage, carrots, celery, corn, olives, peas, potatoes, pumpkins, turnips, Brussels sprouts, and sweet potatoes

HERBS AND SPICES: Rosehip and coriander

LEGUMES, SEEDS, AND NUTS: Aduki beans, chickpeas (garbanzos), lentils, and kidney beans

MEAT, FISH, AND SEAFOOD: Whitefish, beef, duck, pigeon, salmon, mackerel, sardines, and abalone

DRINKS: Water

GRAINS: Buckwheat, rice, and rye

OTHER: Honey, olive oil, peanut oil, raisins, white sugar, and eggs

Temperatures and Cooking Styles

The temperature of food can also be heavily influenced by how it is cooked. Fruit can be very cooling when eaten raw but by cooking lightly before eating, it loses this cooling quality. Bananas, for example, become less cooling when baked or when eaten with cinnamon or brandy added. The same is true for other foods, such as some types of tea, which increase their warming quality with the addition of cardamom or ginger. Note, however, that cold foods cannot actually be made into hot foods by cooking—only less cool or less cold.

The following are the effects on temperature of different cooking styles:

COOL: Juiced or raw food tends to be cooling.

NEUTRAL: Steaming or boiling are neutral and normally have no effect either way.
WARM: Stir-frying, stewing, and baking create warmth.
HOT: Barbecuing, grilling, roasting, and deep-frying can be very heating.

The logic of this information is simple yet unfortunately seems not to be widely known. For example, for someone suffering from migraines, with a red face and a hot head, it would not be a great idea to have a barbecue. Equally, someone who is weak and pale should probably not eat raw salads every day.

The Flavours of Food

In addition to hot and cold, all foods can be classified according to their flavour. As each flavour corresponds to a quality of nature, and each quality corresponds to a system, food can be directly related to impairments within the body. Just to be clear, the meaning here is flavour not taste. When you taste something you are ascertaining its flavour by eating some of it. Taste is something that happens in your mouth; flavour is the quality of the food that affects your sense of taste. It is what creates the joy in eating.

Choosing the right combination of foods can, therefore, help remove an imbalance, and choosing the wrong combination can worsen it.

The following is a list of the flavours and their corresponding foods.

Bitter

The bitter flavour is considered part of fire. This means that it can influence the four fire systems: Heart, small intestine, triple burner, and heart ruler.

It is firming, drying, and cooling, and has the effect of pushing downwards in your body. It helps digestion, helps cool fevers, can help open your bowels, and can help clear away congestion when taken in small amounts.

When large amounts are eaten habitually, however, too much moisture is dried and the *yin* motion can then be impaired. It can also overload your digestive system, causing a swollen sensation in the abdomen.

The following foods are considered bitter:
FRUIT: Grapefruit rind
VEGETABLES: Asparagus, broccoli, celery, lettuce, turnips, radishes, watercress, and bamboo shoots
GRAINS: Hops, corn, millet, and oats
HERBS AND SPICES: Chicory, chamomile, basil, and parsley
LEGUMES, SEEDS, AND NUTS: Alfalfa beans
DRINKS: Beer, tea, and coffee
OTHER: Vinegar

Sweet

The sweet flavour is part of the earth quality and has a strong influence over the stomach and pancreas systems. It is the most common flavour in a standard diet and can be found in almost all naturally grown food, no matter what other flavours they may have.

It is usually warming and helps digestion when taken in small amounts. It also builds up tissues and fluids (*yin*) and is generally strengthening.

Too much sweet food (usually in the form of processed sugary food like chocolate, cookies, and cakes) can have the opposite effect and weakens the stomach and pancreas systems.

When weak, these two main digestive systems begin to crave sweetness, as this is the flavour that will strengthen them. However, this craving is usually fed by more concentrated sugar-based sweet foods, leading to a cyclical destructive cycle.

The more concentrated the sweet food consumed, the weaker the stomach and pancreas systems become, and the weaker they become, the more sweetness they crave.

The following foods are considered sweet:

FRUIT: Apples, apricots, dates, figs, grapes, grapefruit, mandarins, papayas, oranges, peaches, pears, pineapples, plums, raspberries, strawberries, and tomatoes

VEGETABLES: Almost all vegetables, but especially beetroot, cabbage, carrots, celery, cherries, courgettes (zucchini), corn, cucumbers, lettuce, button mushrooms, peas, potatoes, pumpkins, radishes, spinach, and sweet potatoes

GRAINS: Almost all, but especially wheat and barley, oats, malt, and rice

LEGUMES, SEEDS, AND NUTS: Aduki beans, almonds, chestnuts, chickpeas (garbanzos), kidney beans, mung beans, peanuts, walnuts, sunflower seeds, and pine nuts

MEAT: Most meats, but especially beef, chicken, lamb, pork, and rabbit

DRINKS: Milk and wine

OTHER: Cheese, olive oil, butter, honey, and sugar

Pungent

The pungent flavour is in the metal quality and can affect the lung and large intestine systems, in particular.

It has a warming effect and helps move circulation around the body and expel phlegm, especially from your lung system.

If taken in large quantities, pungent foods will dry your lung and stomach systems and create a weakness, especially the *yin* motion. This can lead to flabby muscles and lack of drive or spirit.

The following foods are considered pungent:

VEGETABLES: Cabbage, chillies, garlic, leeks, turnips, onions, radishes, and watercress

HERBS AND SPICES: Black pepper, cayenne pepper, basil, cloves, cinnamon, cumin, peppermint, rosemary, marjoram, nutmeg, and chamomile

GRAINS: Rice

OTHER: Mustard and horseradish

NOTE The degree of pungency can be reduced through cooking.

Salty

The salty flavour is the water quality and can influence the kidney and bladder systems.

It cools and moistens your body, has a downwards motion, acts as a diuretic, and can soften any hard masses.

Too much salty food can worsen dampness, impair *yin,* and weaken the strength of your bones and blood.

The following foods are considered salty:

VEGETABLES: Brined or fermented vegetables, kelp, and seaweed

HERBS AND SPICES: Parsley

GRAINS: Millet

MEAT, FISH, AND SEAFOOD: Crab, duck, ham, lobster, mussels, octopus, oysters, pork, pigeon, and sardines

OTHER: Miso, fermented soy products, umeboshi plums and pickles

Sour

The sour flavour is in the wood quality and can affect the liver and gallbladder more than other systems.

It has a contracting, shrinking effect and controls the release of fluids by closing the pores to stop sweating and constricting the urinary system to stop urination. For this reason, sour foods are often recommended in cases when body fluids are leaking, as in diarrhoea and bleeding.

An excess of sour food can cause your body to contract too much and keep in too much fluid. This can slow down the digestive system and impair the *yin* motion. It also weakens your tendons and ligaments.

The following foods are considered sour:

FRUIT: Apples, apricots, blackberries, blackcurrants, gooseberries, grapes, grapefruit, hawthorn berries, lemons, limes, lychees, mandarins, mangoes, peaches, pears, pineapples, plums, pomegranates, raspberries, sour plums, strawberries, tangerines and tomatoes

VEGETABLES: Green leafy vegetables, olives, and sauerkraut

LEGUMES, SEEDS AND NUTS: Aduki beans

GRAINS: Barley and rye

MEAT, FISH, AND SEAFOOD: Trout

DRINKS: Tea (black and green) and wine

OTHER: Vinegar, pickles, yogurt, and cream cheese

Seasonal Flavour Changes

While eating certain flavours of food will support the qualities of nature and the storage systems associated with them, the change in the seasonal breath should be taken into account in any diet. For example, the associated flavour for spring is sour, as both emanate from the wood quality. This means that during the months of spring, the sour-flavoured foods, which are usually used to support wood, should be reduced so as to regulate any overflow of the wood quality. Instead, mildly sweet foods should be increased to reinforce the earth quality, which is often diminished by wood during this time.[40]

A similar pattern should be followed for the rest of the year. During summer, bitter foods should be reduced to regulate fire, and pungent foods increased to support metal. In late summer, sweet foods should be reduced to regulate earth, and salty foods increased to support water. In autumn, pungent foods should be reduced to regulate metal, and sour foods should be increased to support wood. And in winter, salty foods should be reduced to regulate water, and bitter foods increased to support fire.

In this way, you can adjust your diet to the seasonal breath pattern and help prevent weakness and overflow patterns from taking hold.

Adjusting Diet

When it comes to your body, knowledge is power, but too much knowledge can sometimes be confusing. It is important, therefore, not to get too distracted with the classifications of temperature and flavour.

They are guidelines to empower changes in diet that will improve health and are not designed as restrictive recipe lists.

If, after reading through this book, it is clear that there is an imbalance pattern of heat and cold somewhere inside, the lists can be used to identify any foods in your diet that may be adding to the problem. You can then reduce or remove some of these foods, and by trial and error, adjust your diet appropriately.

Likewise if there is an obvious system impairment, food of a particular flavour can be added or taken away to adjust the diet.

It is never too late to change according to some experts. Even those over 65 years old who change to a low-fat diet high in fruit and vegetables (and accompanied by regular exercise) can decrease their chances of developing chronic conditions, such as hypertension, cancer, and osteoporosis.[41]

An important principle to remember is that too much of anything, no matter how good it is supposed to be for you, can be bad for you.

Be skeptical of the claims made in commercials for yogurts that help your digestion or morning cereals that protect your heart. There may be some truth in their claims if seen in the context of a healthy lifestyle with regular exercise and a carefully adjusted diet, but alone, and seen in terms of the relationship between an impaired pancreas and stomach system and the retention of dampness, they can actually do more harm than good.

13

Manual Therapy

Manual therapy affects the interactions between the internal and external matrix of the body through targeted touch therapy. While just the simple action of touch can be enough to make changes beneath the surface of the skin, it is only with the knowledge of how your body is interconnected that you can treat it in a targeted, efficient, and effective manner.

What follows are the two key manual treatment techniques for self-treatment. One uses your hands as the therapeutic agent and the other uses a tool. They can be done separately or in combination and are powerful in how they can make real changes in your body.

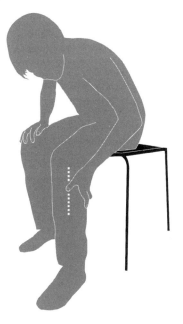

Acupressure

I first seriously started using acupressure techniques after my years in Thailand in the 1990s, and although I became an acupuncturist and studied a great deal about Chinese medicine, the skills I learned in Chiang Mai all those years ago have remained with me and have been a mainstay in the self-care help I give my patients.

Acupressure consists of using your fingers or hands in the application of sustained pressure or manipulation techniques to encourage circulation through the *luomai* rivers and streams (small blood vessels) within the fascial planes of your connective tissue. These small rivers and streams flow into the larger river system (*jingmai*), and so have an impact on how the systems in your body behave. We could go into a great deal more detail both in Chinese medicine or Western anatomy on acupressure, but the idea here is to bring simplicity to something that is often presented with undue complexity.

It is no coincidence that *anma*, the Japanese acupressure therapy that is thought to have developed out of *tuina* and is the forerunner to *shiatsu*, was principally a therapy administered by blind practitioners. It is all about feeling and sensing the body with your hands, and not an academic exercise of points and lists to follow and copy.

While you could press and poke anywhere you like on your body, and maybe you could force some change somewhere, the key to effective treatment with acupressure is reactive areas. These are the areas of tissue that will react to the stimulus of pressure.

A reactive area is one that might have tension, hardness, pressure pain, or soreness. For example, if you are stressed or overworked, your shoulders might be tense, stiff, and hard to the touch all over. If you then press and explore the shoulder area, there will be certain areas that will be the focus of the tension, and they may be more tender. These are the reactive areas. This does not mean that they are the sole focus of acupressure; it just means that you know the focal point for the treatment.

Some of these reactive areas may coincide with the caverns, root regions, and other specified areas on your body, but sometimes they may not. And my approach is to always treat the body according to its three-dimensional matrix structure and not a collection of random acupoints. When done correctly, you create the space for breath motion in the places that need it most, and the body's natural template systems (*zheng qi* and *shenming*) will take care of the rest.

The techniques of acupressure and manipulation in this book have been drawn from Thai massage, Chinese tuina, and Japanese shiatsu. They follow no one tradition exclusively and have been chosen according to practicality and effectiveness and used with the applications of the principles of Chinese medicine to which they all belong. The following is a brief summary of the techniques involved.

Acupressure Techniques

Press

An exploratory press with your thumb or finger to see if there is any tightness or discomfort.

Hard-Press

Press with your thumb with your body weight behind it and keep it in place for several seconds.

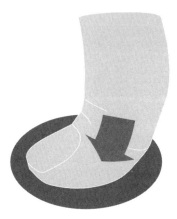

Knead

Press with your thumb while slightly rotating it in a circular motion. Make sure both that your thumb stays in one fixed place and that pressure is maintained.

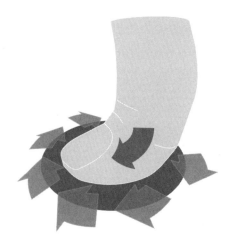

Knuckle-Press

Note that if you are using these manual techniques on yourself there are some areas—on the back, for example—that can be difficult to treat effectively. In this case, it is usually better to use the knuckles of a closed fist to apply pressure instead of your fingers or thumb.

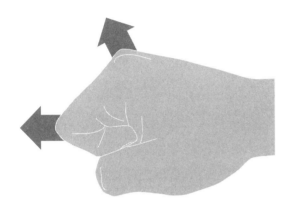

Acupressure Along the River Systems

Thumb-Press

Press in a forwards motion with your thumb(s) and continually moving along a river system or muscle.

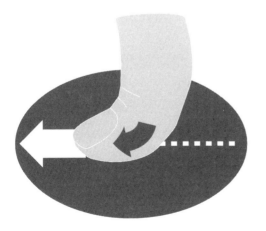

Finger-Press

Press in a forwards motion as above but with the tips of your fingers.

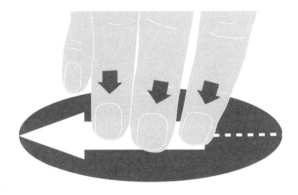

Thumb-Circle

Circle in a forwards motion with firm pressure usually on your face, hands, or feet.

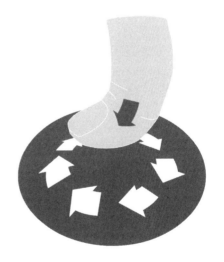

Finger-Circle

Circle in a forwards motion with firm pressure usually on your sternum (breast bone).

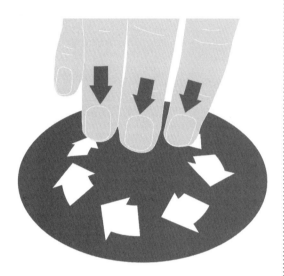

Treating a Large Surface Area

Palm-Circle

Circle with the full palm of your hand so as to cover a wide area, usually on the abdomen.

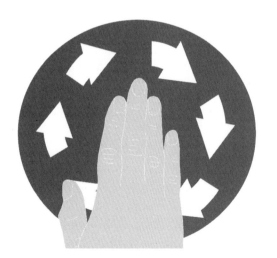

CAUTION: These acupressure manual techniques are generally safe, but caution is needed in the following situations:

- Care should be taken with frail or weak people not to press too strongly or for too long.
- Do not manipulate or press on or around open wounds, varicose veins, tumours, inflamed or infected skin, sites of recent surgery, or areas where a broken bone is suspected.

Gua Sha

The techniques and ideas of Gua sha in this book are those developed by me over 20 years, and many of them are taken from Ecology in Motion (EIM), an approach to using Gua sha based on the ecological principles of ancient Chinese medicine in this book.

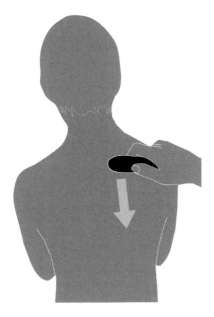

There is unfortunately a great deal of misunderstanding surrounding Gua sha in the West, which has restricted it to a pale shadow of what it should be and has tainted newer developments such as Facial Gua sha. This is partly due to the poor introduction of Gua sha to the western world, but also how it has been molded to fit into the tight confines of modern TCM which only developed in the 1950s and 60s.

This standardization has meant that Chinese medicine has been presented in a certain way as if it has always been like that. But it has not. The diversity and beauty of the flourishing garden of ancient Chinese medical ideas just became more elusive and difficult to find.

So I have learnt that my approach to Gua sha is not the same as others. This is unsurprising, as I did not come to it via a standard route. I was not constrained by the limits that other people set when you learn in a more traditional way. After I first learned about Chinese medicine at college over 20 years ago, it took me many years before I shook off the mindset of a group of people who were reinforcing each other's flawed perceptions. It was a self-perpetuating cycle of misrepresentation.

And so with Gua sha, I went another route. I went off on a tangent, set up my North African clinic, and quietly and consistently created my distinct approach to Gua sha over the following 10 years.

So what is Gua sha? And why have I devoted many years and three books to it? The answer is as elegant as it is simple. It is a manual friction technique on the surface of your skin, usually with a tool, which is used to restore the breath motion to tissue. This alone is the action that will make changes to the biomatrix, improve blood circulation, and resolve climate and obstruction patterns. Because of the simplicity of approach and the fact that no special equipment is needed, Gua sha lends itself perfectly to healthcare on a world scale. Essentially, restoring breath motion to tissue is about creating space, and when you create space, life flourishes.

In conventional medicine, the picture is less elegant, and although the causes of the therapeutic effects of Gua sha are unknown, they are thought to be due to either a reduction in pain-promoting substances, the inhibition of neuronal responses, the effects of counterirritation, the antinociceptive effects of nitric oxide, or the old favourite, placebo effects.

There is one important point about Gua sha that needs to be made clear and which is about the red marks that sometimes appear on the skin during treatment. These are referred to in studies and reports as "petechiae" and "ecchymosis", because the language of these reports is that of conventional medicine. The red or purple dots that appear on the skin are, however, neither. They are *sha*, the heat generated from the restoration of breath to obstruction patterns in your connective tissue.

If there is no obstruction pattern underneath, then no *sha* will appear on the skin. Your body quite literally tells you where it is impaired. For much of this book, *sha* is not necessary (nor sometimes desired) when the goal is improving circulation patterns. It features strongly, however, with all the overflow patterns.

Equipment

Tool

The tool used in scraping should have a rounded edge so that the scraping action will not damage your skin, and be comfortable as it glides over it.

There are a great many choices in the shape and material you can buy, and selling tools is a big business, with equally big marketing claims about what they can supposedly do. But before you get distracted by all those shiny, colourful shapes, the reality is that the tool is the least important part of Gua sha. Let me repeat that. The tool is the least important part. It is your technique, and your technique alone, that is able to make changes in the breath motion within your connective tissue structures.

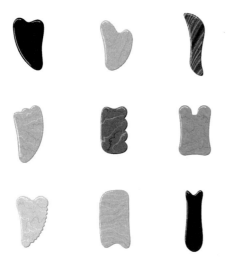

That being said, you can use what you might already have. Whenever I go to a homeware store, I usually end up trying out objects that were not designed for Gua sha on my skin, and I have a whole drawer of plates, saucers, spoons, and jar lids. The object I most recommend is something most people can access easily and inexpensively: A porcelain Chinese soup spoon. And believe it or not, I still use it as my main tool professionally. I do, admittedly, have nice-looking porcelain spoons, but the reality is that they are spoons, and some spoons are rounder than others, so be selective.

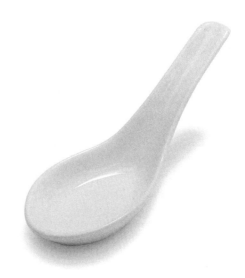

As for buying a tool, the choices are fairly wide. Just choose a tool that fits into your hand comfortably and is an appropriate size and shape for where you intend to use it. Whatever you use, the essential thing is that the edge that scrapes your skin is firm but rounded.

Lubricant

In order to prevent any injury or discomfort, the area you scrape should be lubricated beforehand. Certain areas, such as your head, do not need lubricant as your hair protects the skin, but anywhere the skin is exposed needs to be protected.

As with tools, you can get distracted with an array of different salves, creams, oils, and pastes for Gua sha, and they are hugely beneficial. Remember, though, the lubricant is not the treatment, so you can use any type of oil on your skin that you are comfortable with. Many people use massage oils, such as sweet almond and blended essential oils. In wintertime, Vaporub can be a soothing lubricant.

Gua Sha Techniques

Two simple strokes are enough for you to benefit from treating yourself with Gua sha: Wide-stroke and narrow-stroke. You can use them interchangeably, depending on the best way to treat the body part. These are not specified in the text of the treatment sections, as it is left for you to decide the most appropriate stroke.

Wide-Stroke

This is using the longest part of the tool to scrape in one direction along a river or body part. Each stroke is about the width of your hand. This stroke is usually used on larger surface areas, such as your back and limbs.

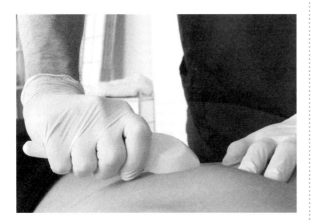

Narrow-Stroke

This is using the thinner end of the tool to scrape in one direction along a river or body part. Each stroke is normally shorter than wide-stroke. This stroke is usually used on smaller surface areas, such as your hands/feet and fingers/toes.

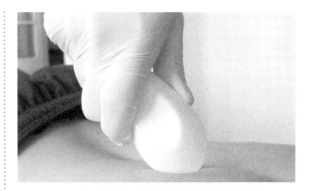

In the text of the treatment sections, there are instructions to sometimes press areas. You can press with a tool, which can make it both easier on your hand and a stronger treatment.

Press

Using the smooth, rounded side of the tool, apply pressure into one fixed area of tissue for no more than 10 seconds.

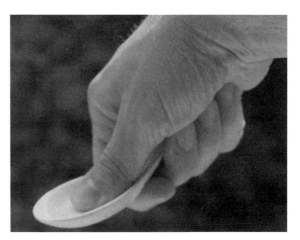

Procedure

- The lubricant should be applied to the area to be treated.
- The tool should be held at the appropriate angle to the skin using your dominant hand.
- Note that the angle of the tool has an impact on the strength of the treatment. An angle of 45° to the skin (++), against the direction of stroke, is stronger than an angle of 90° to

the skin (+), which in turn is stronger than an angle of 45° against (-).

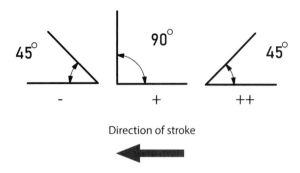

Direction of stroke

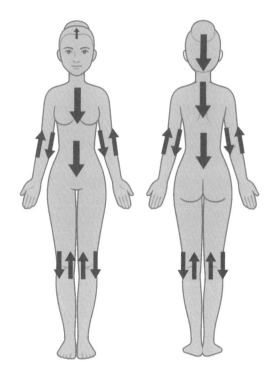

- Scrape gently at first, with a steady increase in pressure until the strokes are firm, short, and brisk, but still within the comfort zone of the receiver.
- Apply slight downward pressure as you scrape, so that the tool is not only on the surface but in contact with the connective tissue below your skin.
- As a general rule, the scraping should be downwards on your head, neck, shoulders, chest, abdomen, and back, but on your arms and legs, the direction is dependent on the direction of the river systems.
- On your arms and legs, if you are scraping a small area, then the direction of scraping is unimportant, as you are not following the river. This is important to remember. So, do not be too concerned about direction when treating areas of tension in the connective tissue, including fascia, and the muscles.
- If, however, you are following part of, or a full, river system trajectory, then follow the direction of flow. The *yin* river systems on the arm flow down the medial side (inside) of your arms and the *yang* river systems flow up the lateral side (outside). This is the direction on your arms. On your legs it is the opposite. The *yang* river systems on the leg flow down the lateral and back of your legs and the *yin* river systems flow up the medial.

- The scraping should be continued with varying pressure, and often the red spots of *sha* will appear. If the skin remains pink from the scraping but shows no *sha* after several strokes, move on.
- Areas where *sha* might appear often feel tense and resistant under the skin. And once they appear, continue around the area to bring out as much as possible, but be aware of your comfort or that of the receiver if treating someone else.
- Any areas with *sha* can be pressed and kneaded afterwards, but often the scraping is treatment enough.
- Avoid exposing the area of treatment to the outside climates—especially wind and cold—until the *sha* has faded.

CAUTION: When scraping, the tool will come into contact with body fluids and skin cells, so there is potential for cross-contamination if different people use the tool. Ideally, other people should have their own specific tools, but they can be disinfected with disinfectant wipes, a bleach solution, or professional cleaning chemicals.

Do not use Gua sha techniques in the following situations:

- With particularly weak, frail people
- On an area with a fresh injury, including swelling, bruising, cuts, and scrapes
- On an area of skin that is sunburnt
- On any existing skin condition, such as a rash or eczema
- On any moles, blemishes, spots, or raised skin features— cover these with a finger, and take care to scrape only the surrounding area
- On breast tissue (unless the treatment is breast-specific)
- On the abdomen of a pregnant woman
- Over existing *sha* marks until they have faded from the skin (this can take three to four days).

Applying the Manual Therapies

There are many ways to treat your body with the acupressure and Gua sha techniques featured here. What follows is how they are applied in this book to guide you in making the most of these powerful treatment techniques.

Treat Locally

Instinct usually tells you to treat pain or discomfort directly. Without thinking, the first thing you do is rub any pain or discomfort with the palm of your hand. And, of course, we can follow the same principle with treatment.

How effective this is depends on whether the local area where you feel the symptoms, and where you are treating, is where the main obstruction pattern is located. The main obstruction pattern is the one causing the symptoms but is not necessarily where the discomfort is. In fact, it often is not.

With headaches, for example, the actual pattern causing the sensations of pain and discomfort in your head is not usually in the head. It may be in your neck or your shoulders or further down in the river systems of your limbs.

So treating the area of discomfort is not as obvious as it might appear in terms of obstruction patterns, but it is a valid treatment strategy that can restore breath motion directly to the impaired tissue.

The important issue with local treatment is the presence of heat or inflammation. If these are present, then it often is not a good idea to treat on, over, or around them. Instead, choose other areas connected to the river systems, either upstream or downstream to the problem.

Treat Distally

For any given problem, the complicated relationships within your body can be broken down into rivers. If an area of tissue is impaired and a particular river system runs through it or close by it, then that system will be involved in some manner. It may be part of the cause of the impairment, or it may be showing the results of having been affected by it.

As the rivers are not static objects but living ecosystems, it should make sense that you can treat one part of that river further upstream or downstream (distally), and the effects can be felt at that tissue area, without any local intervention at all.

Using the interrelationships between river systems, it is possible to apply treatment to one river and for the effect to be on another. This would allow you, for example, to treat your arm in order to treat your leg. There are no magical, invisible connections in this elegant idea. It is simply the application of the principles of the natural world.

Other distal areas, known as "holographic microsystems", can be treated and will impact the river system due to their inbuilt therapeutic action.

The idea behind such microsystems is that embryonic cells hold your body's genetic information and, as the embryo grows, individual parts develop and split off from the same source material. This means that completely separate body parts on different sides of your body were once one. This is how the triple burner came about. It is the main blood vessel system connecting the digestive tract and the heart system, and stems from how your gut developed embryologically.[42]

Microsystems follow the same patterns of breath motion that influence our world. Organizing motions of breath in the universe are based on the principle of self-similarity. It may appear chaotic when you look into the vastness of the night sky, but the universe is perfectly ordered in ever-repeating patterns of fractal scaling, whereby patterns are repeated over and over, on an ever larger scale.[43] There is probably an example of fractal scaling in your garden. A tree is the living embodiment of this fractal scaling, and is the natural motion of the constantly repeating *jing* (longitudinal) and *luo* (latitudinal) growth patterns. Look at the pattern on the leaf, the shape of the twigs, the branches, the trunk, and the roots. Each individual part of the tree is formed in an identical growth pattern to the whole tree.

The ancient Chinese understood this well. There are examples of them applying holographic projections of microsystems on several parts of the body. In the *Huangdi neijing* text, there is a description of body systems and parts projected onto your face, written as if you were walking into the centre of a giant ancient city.[44] Although this description was for diagnostic purposes only, the main principle of the holographic microsystems is that if you treat the local area corresponding to the distal body part, a change can be made.

Use the Microsystems

For the purposes of this book, I have included three microsystems: Hands, feet, and ears. Let us now look at each one in more detail.

Hand Microsystem

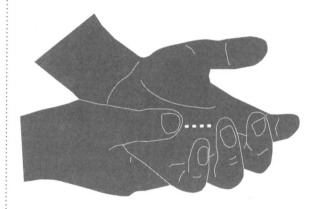

The hand microsystem has only fairly recently been popularized in the treatment of ill health. From the work of William Fitzgerald in the US in the early 20th century to Dr. Yun-Peng Fang in China and Dr. Tae-Woo Yoo in Korea in the 1970s, the hand has proved to be an important microsystem for the treatment of a whole range of illness patterns and diseases.

It is based upon the idea that the hand, like many other parts of the body, contains the same basic information as the whole body itself. It is in essence a mini-version of the whole body and will reflect any imbalances that exist there. So if we know where each individual part of the body is reflected on the hand, we can treat it directly via the hand.

Techniques

Hand Acupressure

The techniques of hand manipulation are almost identical to those for the body: Press, knead, and hard-press to focus on one point and thumb-press and finger- or thumb-circle to follow along a line.

Hand Gua Sha

The techniques of Gua sha on your hand are similar to elsewhere on your body (wide-stroke and narrow-stroke), but the surface area to be treated is smaller, especially around your fingers. Gua sha as a technique is greatly beneficial to your hand, and using a tool can be very useful for self-treatment. The strokes of the tool are short on the hand area, and when applying Gua sha to the fingers, it is important to cover the sides of the fingers, too.

> **CAUTION:** Do not massage, press, or use Gua sha on or around open wounds, growths, nodules, inflamed or infected skin, sites of recent surgery, or areas where a broken bone is suspected.

Hand Circulation Sequence

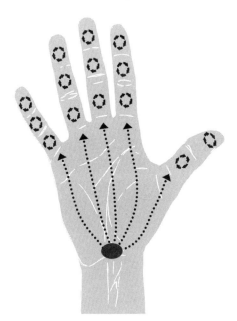

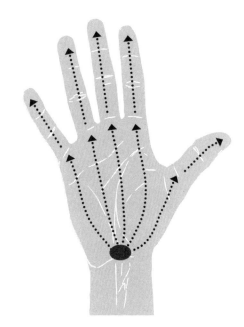

The following circulation sequence covers many of the main areas on the hand, and can be very beneficial both locally to the hand and also generally for the body.

Palm Circulation

Hand Acupressure

- Hard-press at the centre of the wrist crease at the base of the palm.
- Thumb-press from here up to the base of the little finger and then thumb-circle up to the fingertip.
- At the tip pull the finger to stretch it.

Hand Gua Sha

- Press with the tool at the centre of the wrist crease at the base of the palm.
- Scrape with short strokes from here up to the base of the little finger and then scrape over the finger to the fingertip. Pay close attention to the joints.
- Repeat with all five digits.

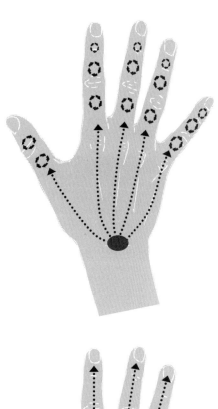

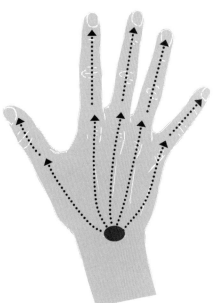

Dorsum Circulation
Hand Acupressure
- Hard-press at the centre of the wrist at the back of the hand.
- Thumb-circle from here all the way up to the base of the little finger and then thumb-circle again up to the fingertip.
- At the tip pull the finger to stretch it.

Hand Gua Sha
- Press with the tool at the centre of the wrist at the back of your hand.
- Scrape with short strokes from here up to the base of the little finger and then scrape over the finger to the fingertip. Pay close attention to the joints.
- Repeat with all five digits.

Foot Microsystem

Although used in ancient times, and thought to be in use in Europe six hundred years ago, the foot microsystem has become well known after the work of William Fitzgerald in the US, who developed a system of zone therapy in the early 20th century that later became known as reflexology.[45]

The basic premise of the foot microsystem is that the shape of the foot resembles the shape of the body, with the head at the toes, the chest at the

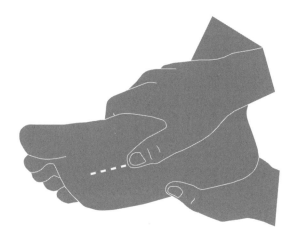

ball of the foot, the spine on the arch of the foot, and the abdomen and main organs in the centre of the foot, with many of the lower positioned organs, such as the bladder and intestine, towards the heel of your foot. This map has been fairly consistently used since then, even in traditional Chinese medicine (TCM), which co-opted it.

Indeed, the holographic map of the body on the foot follows general principles that are shared by all microsystems, and Eunice Ingham, who introduced the first version of this map in the 1930s, perhaps did not realize at the time that she was actually imitating the natural holographic patterns of the universe.

Techniques
Foot Acupressure
The techniques of foot acupressure are almost identical to those for the hand: Press, knead, and hard-press to focus on one area, and thumb-press and finger- or thumb-circle to follow along a line.

Foot Gua Sha
The techniques of Gua sha on your foot are similar to elsewhere on your body. The soles of your feet can usually receive a stronger pressure of the tool than the sides or dorsum (top) of the foot. The strokes of the tool are short in the foot area, and when applying Gua sha to the toes, it is important to cover the sides of the toes, too.

> **CAUTION:** Do not manipulate, press, or scrape on or around open wounds, growths, nodules, inflamed or infected skin, sites of recent surgery, or areas where a broken bone is suspected.

Foot Circulation Sequence

The following sequence covers many of the main areas on the foot and can be very beneficial both locally to the foot and also generally for the whole body.

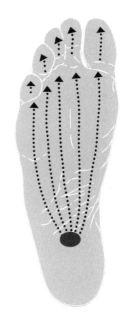

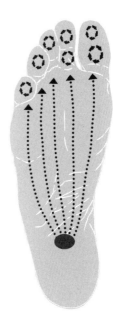

Sole Circulation
Foot Acupressure
- Hard-press at a central point just before the ball of the heel.
- Thumb-press from here up to the base of the little toe and then thumb-circle up to its tip.
- At the tip pull the toe to stretch it.

Foot Gua Sha

- Press with the tool at a central point just before the ball of the heel.
- Scrape with short strokes from here up to the base of the little toe and then scrape over the toe to the tip. Pay close attention to the joints.
- Repeat with all five toes.

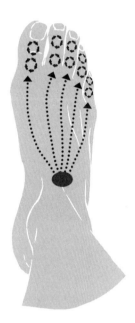

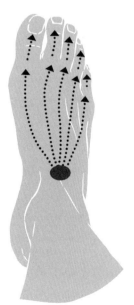

Dorsum Circulation

Foot Acupressure

- Hard-press at the centre of the ankle at the front of the foot.
- Thumb-circle from here down to the base of the little toe and then thumb-circle again up to its tip.
- At the tip pull the toe to stretch it.

Foot Gua Sha

- Press with the tool at the centre of the ankle at the front of the foot.
- Scrape with short strokes from here down to the base of the little toe and then up to its tip. Pay close attention to the joints.
- Repeat with all five toes.

Ear Microsystem

The ancient Chinese knew the importance of the ear in health. After all, the *Huangdi neijing* describes the heart, kidney, lung, pancreas, and stomach river systems all meeting within it.[46] But although there have been simple ear maps for several hundred years in China, it was a French

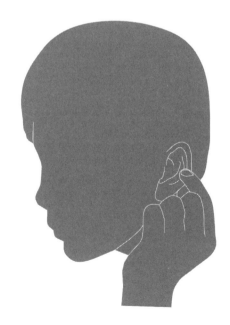

neurologist called Dr. Paul Nogier who comprehensively introduced it in the 1950s. He mapped the ear in terms of treatment and introduced a microsystem whereby the ear can be seen, quite literally, as an upside-down, curled-up foetus. Areas on the body correspond to the represented foetal position of the body part on the ear.

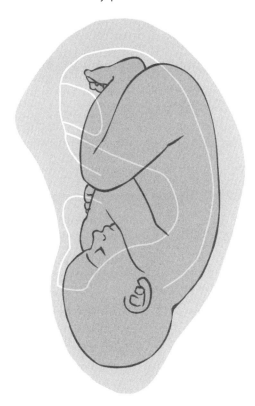

The Chinese combined Nogier's embryo theory with the theories of organs and channels in TCM. The result was two competing and very different maps to treat the same conditions and body parts. But rather than be a source of confusion, Nogier did what the ancient Chinese did and looked to nature for an explanation. In fact, he looked at the moon. He theorized that just as the moon goes through phases and its appearance changes through the month, the same principle could be applied to the ear. Areas on the ear could, therefore, have differing locations depending on changes to the resonant frequency of tissue.

Techniques

- If you have a weakness pattern, it is important not to manipulate your ear for too long as it can stimulate too much circulation, potentially leaving your body weaker.

- It is important to use acupressure only on an area that is tight or uncomfortable under a little pressure. Apart from the Ear Circulation sequence, do not just follow an ear chart and blindly massage according to the instructions given. Feel your own ears and look for the reactive area. This may be exactly on the area being suggested, somewhere nearby, or at a completely different location. This is the reality of the infinitely complex human body and how individualized the pattern can be in each person.

- Use the nail of your index finger to press on the relevant sore areas several times. It is important not to keep your nail static. You should knead the area but stop when there is pain. At the same time, use your thumb to support the back of the ear.

- Apply gentle pressure at first to find the sore areas and then increase pressure with a circular movement until the soreness improves.

- Sometimes a matchstick or other blunt, thin object can be used to apply pressure. Many Chinese medicine suppliers sell metallic ear probes for just such a purpose. For static pressure, you can use vaccaria seeds, plant seeds, or magnetic seeds, which are either bought with an adhesive tape attached, or can be fixed on simply with separate tape.

- The standard TCM approach is to apply pressure on both ears for neurological, cardiovascular, endocrine, genitourinary, and gynaecological disorders; and to apply pressure on only one ear for conditions on one side of the body, such as shoulder, elbow, wrist, finger, hip, knee, tooth, jaw, earache, or tinnitus pain.[47] Most commonly, the seeds are renewed every 1–3 days.

CAUTION: Commonly given TCM cautions about pregnancy warn against ear manipulation if you are pregnant and have a history of miscarriages, and also avoid the uterus point and ovary point.

Ear Circulation Sequence

The following is a general daily ear sequence to maintain health and balance in the body by enhancing circulation. You can do it with your fingers or with a Gua sha tool and follow the same basic pattern using either.

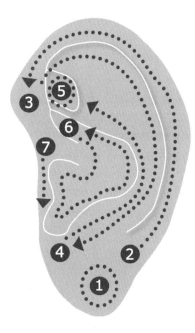

Start by stretching the ear with your fingers:

STRETCH 1: Pinch your ear, and pull the cartilage outwards, away from your body. Pull the bottom half of the ear diagonally downwards and the top of the ear diagonally upwards.

STRETCH 2: Twist your ear with your thumb and finger. The thumb slides up the back of the ear, while simultaneously the finger pushes down. You should feel a slight strain at the bottom of the ear. Repeat several times. Then do the following in one continuous movement.

Acupressure Sequence

STEP 1: Gently massage your ear lobe between your thumb and index finger, the index finger at the front of the ear and the thumb supporting the back.

STEP 2: Knead upwards along the outside of the ear to the top and then follow the bend around to where the ear meets the head. While massaging, gently pull the ear outwards and upwards.

STEP 3: Move slightly inwards, towards the centre of the ear, and knead downwards, following the contour of the ear.

STEP 4: At the bottom of your ear, again move inwards slightly, and knead upwards along the ridge. Follow the contour of the ear, and drop into the dip at the end.

STEP 5: Massage this dip in a circular fashion.

STEP 6: Drop into the central cavity, and again massage in a circular fashion.

STEP 7: Massage downwards along the attachment of your ear, where it meets your cheek.

STEP 8: Search for any sore, tense areas with the nail of your index finger. You may have noticed some in the previous exercise. Knead any of these areas several times.

Gua Sha Sequence

For Gua sha, use your non-dominant hand to stretch and manipulate your ear into optimal positions to use short scraping movements, pressing and circling in a similar way.[48]

STEP 1: With your thumb behind supporting the ear lobe, keep the tool fixed in one place and circle for 10 seconds.

STEP 2: Support the back of your ear with your non-dominant hand, and stretch the ear slightly in order to scrape upwards along the outside of the ear to the top, then follow the bend around to where your ear meets your head.

STEP 3: Move slightly inwards, towards the centre of the ear, and scrape downwards, following the contour of the ear.

STEP 4: At the bottom of your ear, again move inwards slightly, and scrape upwards along the ridge. Follow the contour of the ear, and drop into the dip at the end.

STEP 5: Press and circle within this dip (the triangular fossa) for 10 seconds.

STEP 6: Drop into the central cavity, and again scrape in a circular fashion.

STEP 7: Scrape down the tragus, at the attachment of the ear.

STEP 8: Search for any sore, tense areas with the tool. Knead any of these areas several times.

14

Exercise Therapy

The importance of regular home stretching exercises cannot be overstressed. It is a major part of Eastern cultures to relieve stiffness and tension through exercise before they turn into a source of ill health.

In Japan, collective daily exercise is known as *taiso* and consists of a set routine to simple, repetitive music. This tradition, although gradually dying out in urban areas, was very much alive and kicking in the part of Japan I used to live in. For years, I had to listen to a tortuous piece called "Taiso No. 4" every day at precisely 3 p.m. from crackling loudspeakers spaced so strategically around our island home that there was no escape.

In it, a man literally barks instructions and pert piano chords keep up the rhythm until the whole sequence of swinging and swaying comes to a halt 10 minutes later. As far as the music went, it was rather like an annoying pop song that is repeated endlessly on the radio until it becomes so familiar that, despite yourself, you actually start to like it. As for the exercises—they are simple, repetitive, and invigorating for your health.

The exercises used in this book have been heavily drawn from Japanese stretching exercises (but not that one) and are variations on what are called *sotai* and *makko ho*. There are also some variations of qigong exercises from Chinese traditions.

While there are many levels on which these exercises can be perceived, none of them requires any special body awareness, visualization techniques, or meditative quality in order to be effective. Ideally, follow any advice about breathing, but it is the repetitive actions themselves that are of most benefit.

Stretching the Five Qualities of Nature

The Five Qualities of Nature stretches consist of a set of gentle exercises derived from traditions of *shiatsu* in Japan. Each of the exercises is associated with one of the five qualities and its corresponding systems.

They are based on a set of exercises originally developed by Shizuto Masunaga (1925–1981) and consist of yoga-like stretches to maintain good health. When done together, the sequence of exercises reflects the daily cycle of circulation and can be very beneficial to ensure that this cycle runs as smoothly as possible.

The following exercises consist of *makko ho* stretches and variations thereof, and should be done slowly, mindfully (as in relaxed and without distraction), and without any physical strength or effort. They can be completed all in one go as a daily exercise routine or separately to rebalance a quality or system.

For comfort, you may wish to use a yoga mat and even double up the mat, or perhaps place folded towels or blankets under your body to create a more comfortable surface when kneeling or doing these stretches.

❶ *Metal*

Strengthening the Lung and Large Intestine River Systems

This exercise stretches the lung and large intestine rivers in your fingers, hand, arms, and shoulders.

Stand with your feet shoulders'-width apart, knees slightly bent, and link your thumbs behind your back.

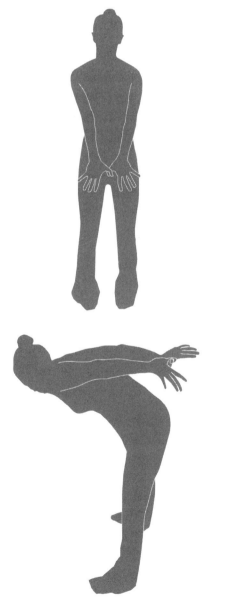

Breathe in and, keeping the thumbs linked, stretch the fingers out. While breathing out, bend your upper body forward, keeping your fingers stretched out but relaxing as much as you can.

Hold the bent position, breathe in and out slowly and deeply three times, and visualize letting go of any tension in your body. As you breathe out the third time, slowly raise your upper body into an upright position. Repeat several times.

❷ *Earth*

Strengthening the Stomach and Pancreas River Systems

This exercise stretches the stomach and pancreas rivers in your chest, throat, and face, and also in your knees, shins, and feet.

Kneel on a comfortable flat surface, and sit on your heels (a supporting pillow or cushion can be used if necessary).

Breathe in, and while breathing out, place both hands facing backwards behind you, and lean backwards.

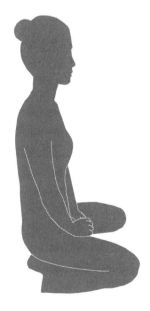

❸ *Fire*

Strengthening the Heart, Heart Ruler, Small Intestine, and Triple Burner River Systems

This exercise stretches the heart, heart ruler, small intestine, and triple burner rivers in your arms and shoulders.

Sit with your legs crossed, right leg over left. Place your left hand on your right knee and your right hand on your left knee so that the right arm is on the outside of the left arm.

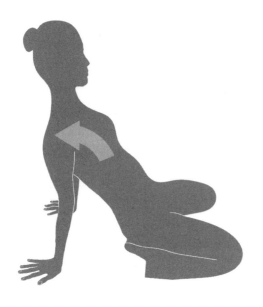

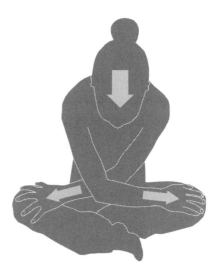

Lean forward, and bring your head towards the floor. If you can, stretch your arms further away from each other to intensify the stretch.

Hold this position while breathing in and out three times, before slowly returning to the original position. Then repeat swapping arms.

❹ *Water*

Strengthening the Kidney and Bladder River Systems

This exercise stretches the kidney and bladder rivers in your back and legs.

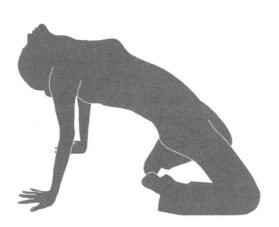

Allow your head to fall back so that you can look behind. If possible, lift the hip area upwards and forwards to arch your body backwards.

Hold the position for a few moments and then return to an upright position.

Sit on the floor with a straight back and your legs straight out in front of you. Raise your arms above your head, and, as you breathe out, bend forward from the hips. Make sure that your knees are kept straight.

⑤ *Wood*
Strengthening the Liver and Gallbladder River Systems

This exercise stretches the liver and gallbladder rivers on the sides of your body and legs.

Sit with a straight back, and spread your legs as wide as possible. Link your fingers, and stretch your arms above your head, palms up.

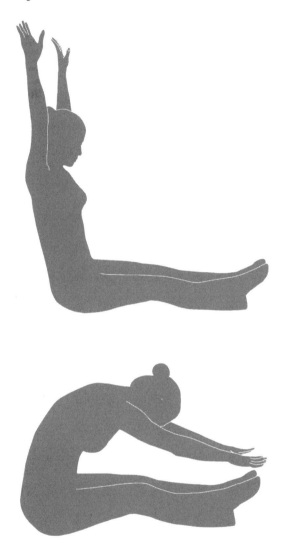

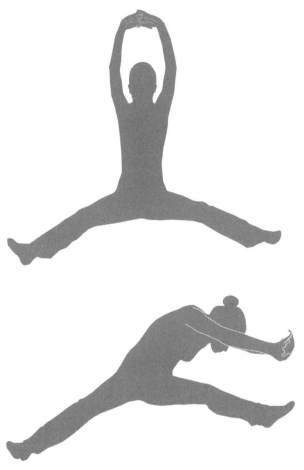

Inhale, then on the exhale, reach as far forward between your legs as you can.

Hold this position while breathing in and out three times, then slowly return to the original position.

Breathe in deeply, and turn to look at your right foot.

Breathe out, and lean your body sideways towards your right, stretching your arms out towards your right foot.

103

Facing your right foot, hold the position while breathing in and out three times, then repeat the sequence on the other side.

End the stretching sequence by leaning forward in the middle, holding and then returning to the original position.

Tips for Completing the Exercises

- These stretches are best done in the morning, preferably before breakfast, and in the evening before going to bed. Be gentle with your body.

- Do not go farther than your body will allow. As soon as you reach resistance, stop. The more you do the exercises, the more flexible you become.
- All of these exercises can be done by people in a weakened condition, as they are natural body movements and only require slow, gentle breathing.
- While some discomfort can be expected when teaching your body to move in ways to which it is unaccustomed, discontinue any of the stretches that cause severe discomfort or pain. Also, be cautious with bending exercise if you are pregnant.

15

Lifestyle Therapy

The key to leading a lifestyle that will enhance your potential is to follow breath motion. This has already been introduced in chapter 10, where we discussed how the ancient Chinese talked about following the "Way". But how exactly do you go about following the Way or breath motion? There are many ways to do this, and here are some examples.

Sleep

Night and day are realizations of the universal breath motion that affect every part of the environment around us. The day starts with an intake of breath at dawn, and as it progresses, it goes through various aspects of the *yang* motion of breath (inhalation), until, at dusk, it switches to exhalation and progresses through the *yin* part of breath throughout the night. At dawn the following day, a new cycle of daily breath motion begins the cycle again.

It should come as no surprise, therefore, that sleep should come during the *yin* motion (night) and our waking hours during *yang* motion (day). Consistently breaking this rule by staying up late or doing night-shift work can create an impairment in the motion of breath in your body and be the cause of a weakness or overflow pattern.

Sleeping is rejuvenating for your body, but too much can weaken the balance in your storage systems. As with all things, sleep should be in moderation, and regular extended periods of sleep should be avoided.

The ideal sleeping time for most is thought to be between seven and eight hours. A sobering study suggests that consistently sleeping for less than six hours can lead to a 12 percent increased chance of dying prematurely, while sleeping for more than nine hours can lead to a 30 percent increased chance of dying prematurely.[49]

Work and Rest

The correct balance between work and rest is essential for the maintenance of good health and to give expression to the potential inside you. Compromising who you are and who you were meant to be is a choice we are often forced to make in order to hold down a job and survive in this world. Of course, life gets in the way, but as an intention, as a goal, as something to strive for, following the Way is just as applicable to your job as it is to your homelife.

The breath motion of the work you do, whether your choice or assigned to you, impacts you and your life. When someone likes their job they feel comfortable, and rather than being the cause of stress, it can actually enhance their life and help the breath motion within their body move smoothly. The exact nature of the job does not matter, as that is down to individual preference; it is the action and motion of doing the work that enhances the breath. Conversely, when you dislike your job or the work you do, and have done for a long time, you are not moving with the breath. You are going against it. What this might mean for your general health should be clearer by now.

Standing

Long periods of standing can have obvious effects on how well your circulation system is able to function without impairments. In an ideal world, our bodies prefer movement. They do not thrive with long periods of inactivity, whether it be sitting or standing. Think in particular about those river systems that start at your feet and go up into your body: The pancreas, liver, and kidney river systems. These river systems tend to be the ones that stagnate the most as a result of standing for long periods on a habitual basis. They are the core zang regions that store our essence and run at a deep level within our bodies.

Standing is thought to be especially harmful to the kidney and bladder systems, which is often connected with the backwards and inwards structural movements needed to keep your body upright. This would explain their close connection to lower back pain.

Sitting

Long periods of sitting can weaken the pancreas and heart systems and can slacken your muscles and lead to stagnant circulation, resulting in aches and pains. Australian researchers who monitored the waist sizes, blood pressure, and cholesterol levels of several thousand people found that prolonged sitting actually leads to larger waist sizes and higher cholesterol levels, even in people who exercised regularly. Their recommendation was that even short breaks in sitting time, which could be as little as standing up for one minute, can help to lower this health risk.[50]

Possible solutions to avoid habitually sitting for too long include using a standing desk (but note the potential issue with standing above), taking frequent stretching or walking breaks (five minutes for every 30 minutes of sitting), balancing sedentary time with physical activity, and using devices and apps that allow you to monitor and control your postural habits.

Screens

As well as the above effects from sitting for too long, extended periods sitting in front of a screen can cause yin and blood circulation weakness. This is because prolonged use of your eyes can impair the smooth running of the heart and liver systems. As noted in chapter 5, in the section on the trajectories of the heart and liver rivers, both channels rise to the level of the eyes, and when strained and overused, disrupt circulation and the effects can be felt farther down the rivers.

Your Mind

Overthinking can cause damage to the heart and pancreas river systems. As discussed in chapter 7, deliberation is one of the emotions associated with the earth quality of nature. When it becomes pathological, this will have a detrimental effect on the earth systems of the stomach and pancreas. This can easily affect the balance of the heart system: too much concentration and thinking can lead to heart palpitations, absent-mindedness, insomnia, dream-disturbed sleep, anorexia, bloating, and loose stools.

It can become a vicious circle, whereby overthinking causes imbalance, and the subsequent imbalance causes more overthinking, worry, and anxiety. This means that if you are in this pattern of emotion, it is important, apart from treating the systems affected, to find ways to enhance the calmness within you.

Physical Activity

Regular exercise is essential to keep circulation flowing smoothly, but too much exercise can impact the liver system and interrupt how it maintains your connective tissue structures or impact the kidney system and cause damage to your joints and bones. People who overexercised as children often have joint or bone conditions causing discomfort and pain well before old age.

If you have not done much physical activity for a while, it is best to start in a warm swimming pool, if possible. This can be a regular swimming-based activity, or it can be an exercise activity in the water. The benefits of this are widely reported. For example, a study that looked at women suffering from rheumatoid arthritis who did water-based exercises noted significant improvements in pain and functional capacity compared to the control group who exercised out of water.[51]

Variety in exercise can also be important. There can be a tendency to do a particular kind of exercise that will create a pattern of movement in the body. In cycling, for example, the pattern of motion is very much in your legs and less so in your upper body. It can be a good idea to vary the way you exercise so that your whole body can benefit from movement. If you were to exercise several times a week, you might think about walking one day, cycling another day, and swimming another, or variations of this.

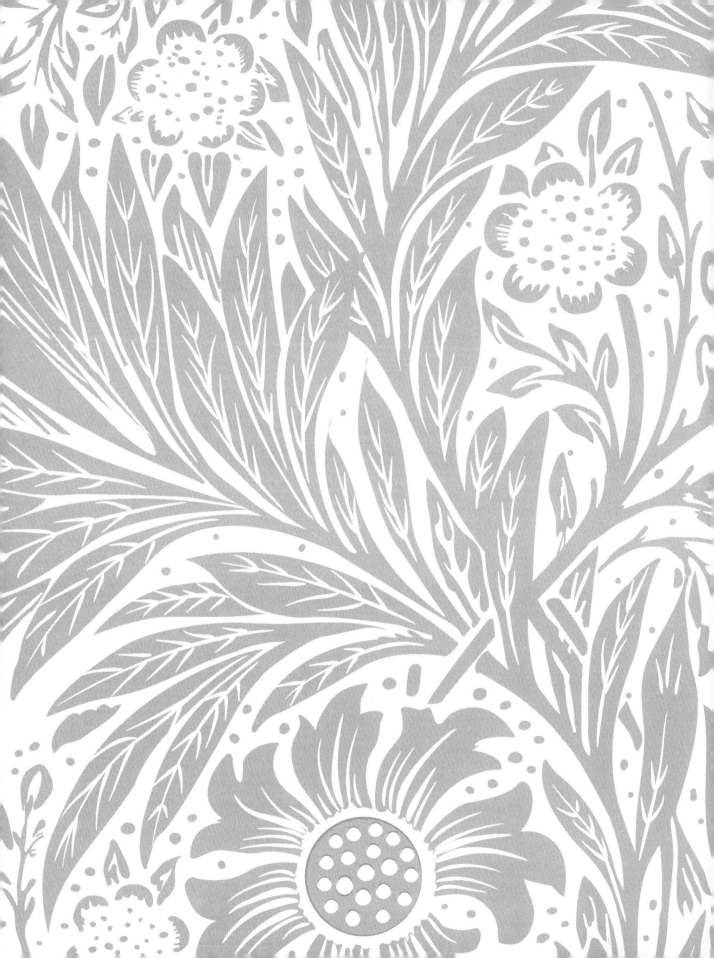

PART 4

How Do You Find Which Areas to Treat?

Knowing where to pressure and scrape can make all the difference to how you treat yourself. In this section, you will find the areas, regions, and zones that can be used to treat the specific imbalance patterns and health conditions listed in the treatment chapters that follow. It serves as a reference point for you to locate suggested areas of the body in the treatment sections.

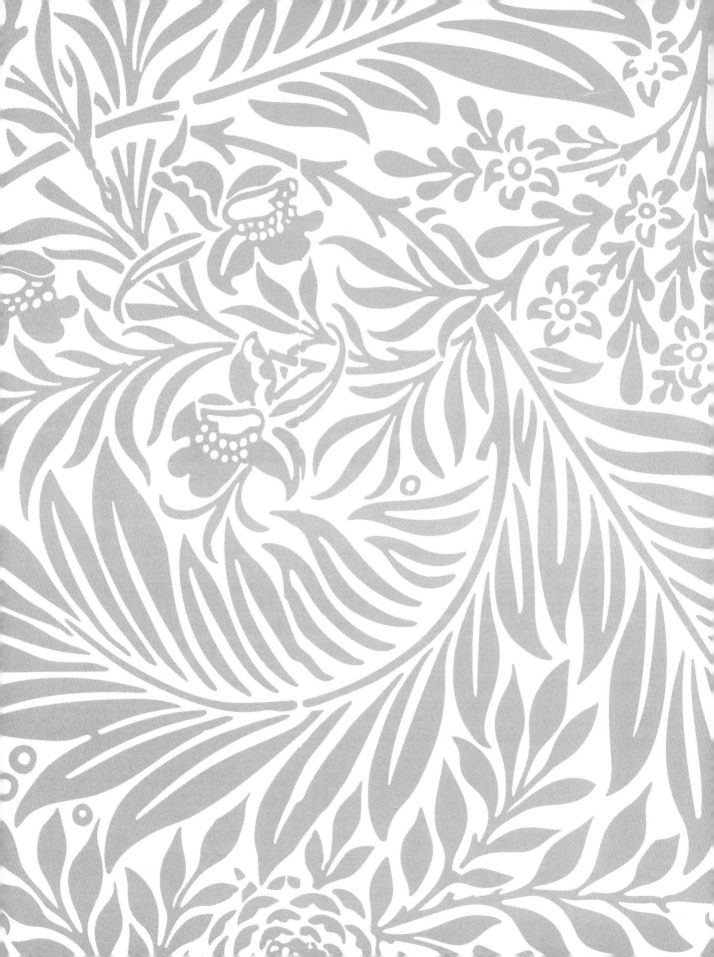

16

Treatment Regions on Your Body

Manual techniques that are applied along the main rivers (larger blood vessels, or *jing*) and in areas where the streams, brooks, creeks, and drainage ditches flow into them (small blood vessels within connective tissue, or *luo*), can make all the difference. Pain and muscular tightness are not isolated and cut off from the rest of your body. They often reflect internal impairments via the river systems.

For example, muscle soreness in the middle of the upper trapezius muscle on your shoulder is often a reflection of disturbance in the bladder or gallbladder river systems, usually due to stress or emotional factors affecting them or a structural pull coming from the fascia in the back area. Loosening any tight muscles and tendons in this area (in effect, restoring breath motion) will usually positively affect the deeper imbalance.

It is for this reason that we start the treatment region section by looking at the river system.

Treat the River System

One of the reasons for mapping out the river systems in chapter 5 is that they are essential for treating the body. If you know where these rivers flow, and in which direction and at which depth, then you have the key to unlock a basic diagnosis and an effective, simple treatment.

The rivers I have detailed are not exactly the same as the maps of "meridians" you might find in a typical modern acupuncture, tuina, or shiatsu school. They are similar, but there are differences in trajectories, starting places, and general understanding of how the system works. This does not mean that their maps are wrong and mine are right; it only means that we are using different sources.

The versions of the river systems in this book are taken directly from the descriptions found in the *Huangdi neijing*, the text that everything else is based on. Although it can sometimes take a little guesswork to determine which anatomical part is being referred to, many of the river descriptions are quite straightforward and relatively easy to decipher.

Identify the River

The reason it is important to know the trajectory of the rivers is that when there is a problem in your body, the first thing you need to do is try to establish which river system is involved. Sometimes this may be obvious, but other times it may require some investigation.

Knowing which of the river systems is connected to any given problem will tell you which one to treat—or at least, which to look at first. Remember that Chinese medicine is not an academic exercise, where you treat by following a strict protocol. It is about responding to the live, three-dimensional person in front of you. This may mean that the river which theoretically should be involved may not be reactive and feeling perfectly fine without any other symptoms or signs of tension or soreness.

If there is tightness or soreness in a different system from the one you had thought you needed to treat, then that is where you should focus your attention. It is important not to be dogmatic and rigid in your thinking. The natural intelligence of your body, or *zheng qi*, knows exactly what needs to be done.

When you have established which river systems might be appropriate to treat, the next step is to think about the rivers that are directly connected to them.

Treat the Parent River

The rivers are all much longer than you might think. The ones we have looked at up until now have actually been split, but if we put them back together, they make up a larger parent river with a different name.

These are the individual halves and their parent river systems:

Parent River	Individual Rivers
Taiyang	Small intestine and bladder
Yangming	Large intestine and stomach
Shaoyang	Triple burner and gallbladder
Shaoyin	Heart and kidney
Taiyin	Lung and pancreas
Jueyin	Heart ruler and liver

Using this information, instead of one river to treat, you now have two, as for all intents and purposes, they both are different stages of the same river.

For example, if you found there to be an impairment in the stomach river system, you could in theory treat it from the large intestine system. They are both parts of the *yangming* river. This then gives you options and allows you to see some of the intricate connections that exist in the body.

Treat the Paired River

In addition to the parent rivers, there is another simple connection to the river systems: The paired river within the qualities of nature. You may recall from chapter 3 that each of the qualities of nature has associated rivers. For metal, it is the lung and large intestine river systems; for earth, it is the stomach and pancreas river systems; and so on—these rivers are paired by their natural quality. Parent rivers stretch across the body and are exclusively *yin* or *yang*. Paired rivers, however, are on the same body part and are a mix of one *yin* river and one *yang* river.

These are the paired river systems with their natural quality:

Natural Quality	Paired River Systems
Metal	Lung (*yin*) and large intestine (*yang*)
Earth	Stomach (*yang*) and pancreas (*yin*)
Fire	Heart (*yin*) and small intestine (*yang*)
Water	Kidney (*yin*) and bladder (*yang*)
Fire	Heart ruler (*yin*) and triple burner (*yang*)
Wood	Gallbladder (*yang*) and liver (*yin*)

So now there are three possibilities to treat for the same impairment. You can treat the river that is affected, you can treat the whole parent river, or you can treat the local paired river. Just with this basic information, you can grasp some of the complexities of how the body works and treatment is approached using the simple natural principles of Chinese medicine.

If, for example, the lung system is affected by a climate, obstruction, or weakness pattern, then in order to help it via the river system, we could treat the lung river directly on your shoulder and down your arm (the local river), the pancreas river coming up your leg (*the taiyang* parent river), and the large intestine river coming up your arm to your shoulder area, neck, and face (the paired river). While you can treat a whole river system from beginning to end, this is only part of how we can understand treatment. Structurally, the body will tell you where along a river is impaired, and you can find this at the reactive areas. Reactive areas are those that are tight or sore along and around the river system.

So instead of following a river blindly, it is important to feel the skin and the tissue beneath it for signs of reactivity, such as tightness or soreness. The reactivity will inform you of where along the river system you should treat.

We are not referring to a detached river flowing in a vacuum. It is a river *system*, which means it is the banks of the river, the ecosystem of the slopes of the land, the forests, the steams, and everything within the valley, all the way to the top of the ridges on either side. Similarly, in the body, the river system is just as all-encompassing, and includes the "ecology" of your blood vessels, muscles, tendons, connective tissue, fascia, and skin. These reactive areas can appear anywhere within your tissue, but other areas have a fixed position along or around river systems. These are the natural formations in your body's ecosystem that allow more direct communication with the circulation of the rivers.

Treat the Caverns, Roots, Junctions, and Sources

Chinese medicine was never designed to be a list of points and protocols to treat medical conditions. It just developed that way. I do not mean in a natural, organic way, but that political choices were made and the effects of standardization and modernization, along with the influence of conventional Western medicine, meant that certain parts of its rich tradition were promoted and others were discarded.[52]

This has had a strong effect on how modern TCM is taught and disseminated, and has meant losing touch with how nature plays such a major part in how we can understand the body. Ecological features such as "body caverns" are a prime example of this.

Treat the Local Caverns

The clinical acupoints that have become the cornerstones of acupuncture and manual therapies such as acupressure were not described as such by the ancient Chinese. They called them *xue*, or "caverns", and they were actually referring to real geological features that can be found dotted around the natural world.

The Minyé sinkhole in the Nakanai Mountains of Papua New Guinea gives us an idea (albeit on a grand scale) of what they were referring to. It is basically a giant dark hole, 350m (1150ft) wide and around 500m (1640ft) deep, located amidst lush green jungle.

Sinkholes naturally occur when water dissolves the surface rock, which is often limestone, and then collapses. And this is what happened with the Minyé sinkhole. The thing that makes this sinkhole special, though, is that at the bottom of the sinkhole, clearly visible from above, is something we normally would not be able to see: A large, gushing underground river.

This is more likely what they meant when ancient Chinese visionaries described caverns in the body: A natural depression through which there is a direct connection with the river system underneath. It is a way to influence the inner circulation system through the natural contours and fissures within the structure of our bodies.

In this book, I have used some of the commonly used abbreviations to refer to these caverns so that they are easier to find.

As many of them are along the trajectories of the river systems, it should offer a sense of which river might be affected. Note that the pancreas (Pa) corresponds to spleen (Sp) and heart ruler (Hr) corresponds to pericardium (P) in standard TCM charts and descriptions.

The following abbreviations for the river systems are used in the location of the caverns in this book:

LU: Lung	**KD:** Kidney
LI: Large intestine	**BL:** Bladder
ST: Stomach	**HR:** Heart ruler
PA: Pancreas	**TB:** Triple burner
HT: Heart	**GB:** Gallbladder
SI: Small intestine	**LV:** Liver

Treat the Root Regions

As these natural depressions, or sinkholes, are not just dips in the surface of the body but have a direct or indirect effect on the river system, their influence can extend beyond the local area of the cavern into other areas of your body. This is the case with the root regions, or *shu*.

There are several categories of *shu*, but an important group for this book are those regions that communicate with the river systems directly. These *shu* can all be found in the extremities of the body, between the fingers and elbows and toes and knees. They are located here because this is where each of the river systems either begins and builds its flow or ends and runs its course. It is thought that these areas are more accessible from the surface level because the river flow is considered more in the interior, above the elbow and above the knee.

The following is a list for your reference:

Arm Root *Shu* Regions

FINGER AREA: Lu-11, Ht-9, Hr-9, Li-1, Si-1, and Tb-1

HAND AREA: Lu-10, Ht-8, Hr-8, Li-2 & 3, Si-2 & 3, and Tb-2 & 3

WRIST AREA: Lu-9, Ht-7, Hr-7, Si-5, and Li-5

LOWER ARM AREA: Lu-8, Ht-4, Hr-5, and Tb-6

ELBOW AREA: Lu-5, Ht-3, Hr-3, Li-11, Si-8, and Tb-10

Leg Root *Shu* Regions

TOE AREA: Pa-1, Kd-1, Lv-1, St-45, Bl-67, and Gb-44

FOOT AREA: Pa-2 & 3, Kd-2, Lv-2 & 3, St-44 & 43, Bl-66 & 65, and Gb-43 & 41

ANKLE AREA: Pa-5, Kd-3, Lv-4, St-41, and Bl-60

LOWER LEG AREA: Kd-7

KNEE AREA: Pa-9, Kd-10, Lv-8, St-36, Bl-40, and Gb-34

Treat the Back *Shu* Regions

The back *shu* regions are mainly used to expel heat, cold, and other climate patterns or pollutants from within your body. Like all *shu* regions, they have a particular resonance deep within the storage systems. They are located on your back, and rather than repeating the narrow points of modern TCM, our focus is on larger regions that more resemble those of the *Huangdi neijing*. This allows you to use a wider area and for you to respond to the body's ecosystem in a much more realistic and practical way in the context of home treatment. The back *shu* regions featured are:

Back *Shu* Regions

LUNG: Connects directly with the lung system.

HEART: Connects directly with the heart and heart ruler systems.

DIAPHRAGM: The diaphragm is that dome-shaped muscle at the bottom of your chest cavity, but it does have a place amongst these *zang* storage regions. All of the rivers in your body pass through it, and it has a major influence on breath and the force of blood circulation.

LIVER: Connects directly with the liver system and gallbladder systems.

PANCREAS: Connects directly with the pancreas system, which, in effect, means the stomach system and whole digestive tract, including the triple burner system.

KIDNEY: Connects directly with the kidney system and also includes the bladder system.

Treat the Water and Heat *Shu* Regions

The water regions are connected with the redistribution of fluids in your body, and particularly in how your lung and kidney systems metabolize water. They are located in specific areas in your body, as seen below, and like all *shu* regions affect the body distally.

Water *Shu* Regions
SACRAL AREA
KIDNEY RIVER: on the mid thigh
KIDNEY RIVER: between Kd-3 and Kd-7 near the ankle

The Heat regions are connected with the redistribution of heat in your body and are located around your head, torso, and legs. When stimulated appropriately, they can cause the heat from certain parts of your body to rapidly dissipate.

Heat *Shu* Regions
HEAD HEAT: Du-20 area
CHEST HEAT: Bl-11, quepen, and lung back *shu*
STOMACH HEAT: St-37 and St-39
LIMB HEAT: Lu-2, Li-15 and Bl-40

Treat the Source and Junction Regions

Other cavern regions can be imaged differently. The junction regions are simply junctions in the river to transport you to other areas, and the *yuan* source regions are more like geysers, bursting up from deep within the earth and affecting the circulation around the surface. This gives these regions a quality that other regions do not have, and the potential to influence the storage systems below. There is some overlap with the root *shu* and *yuan* source regions on the *yin* systems (lung, heart ruler, pancreas, kidney, and liver).

The following is a list for your reference (note that the heart is treated via the heart ruler):

Junction Regions
Lung: Lu-7; large intestine: Li-6; stomach: St-40; pancreas: Pa-4; small intestine: Si-7; kidney: Kd-4; bladder: Bl-58; heart ruler: Hr-6; triple burner: Tb-5; gallbladder: Gb-37; liver: Lv-5

Source Regions
Lung: Lu-9; large intestine: Li-4; stomach: St-42; pancreas: Pa-3; small intestine: Si-4; kidney: Kd-3; bladder: Bl-64; heart ruler: Hr-7; triple burner: Tb-4; gallbladder: Gb-40; liver: Lv-3; inner chest area (the space between the heart and the diaphragm): Ren-6 & Ren-15

Treat the Areas, Zones, and Regions

The focus of this book is on areas, zones, and regions, not on points. The reason for this is that we are interested in making a change in the connective tissue structures through manual techniques on the surface of your body. Sometimes, this may be specific in a particular location, but at other times this will be looking at the river and where it is blocked. This does not require pinpoint accuracy in locating a tiny point. Instead, it requires you to feel and explore, sometimes over a wider part, so that you can find the reactive area. You are, therefore, moving away from a prescriptive, off-the-peg solution and into the realm of what the ancient Chinese were intending: Listening to your body.

In order to do this, we can see the body in terms of areas of treatment, and within these areas, as noted above, there can be caverns, roots, and rivers. In order to locate them, you first need to ensure that you are measuring the distances correctly.

Distances

Note that the distances used in finding some of the areas and regions are as follows:

A FINGER-WIDTH: The distance from one side of the middle finger to the other.

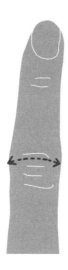

TWO FINGERS-WIDTH: The distance across the index and middle fingers.

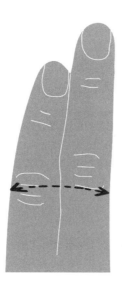

THREE FINGERS-WIDTH: The distance across the middle three fingers together.

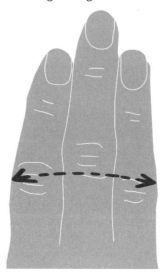

A HAND-WIDTH: The distance across all four fingers together.

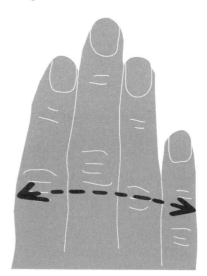

The following are the areas used in this book for self-treatment with manual therapies, and they have been separated into body parts to make them easier to locate. The common Western abbreviated name/number is given first, then the translated name, and then the original Chinese. In China, the abbreviated name/number is not used, and areas are only known by their names.

Find Areas on Your Head

(See also colour insert at back of book.)

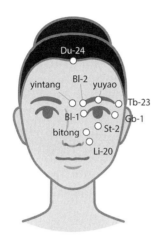

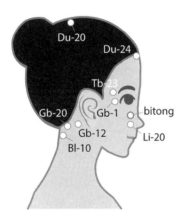

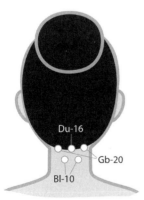

Hairline

DU-24 COURTYARD OF THE SPIRIT (*SHENTING*): On the midline of the head, just behind your hairline at the top of your forehead.

Vertex

DU-20 HUNDRED MEETINGS (*BAIHUI*): On the midline of your head, follow the slanted line of the ear upwards to the top of the head (Heat *shu*).

Occiput

GB-12 MASTOID PROCESS (*WANGU*): While it is placed under and just before the end of the base of the skull, it originally had a wider scope of the whole area beneath the skull bone.

GB-20 WIND POOL (*FENGCHI*): Below the base of the skull, halfway between the centre line and Gb-12.

DU-16 PALACE OF WIND (*FENGFU*): On the midline of the back of your head, below the base of the skull.

BL-10 CELESTIAL PILLAR (*TIANZHU*): One finger-width from the midline of the back of your head, below the occipital protuberance.

Find Areas on Your Face

Eyes

YINTANG: Halfway between your eyebrows.

YUYAO: At the midpoint of your eyebrows.

BL-1 BRIGHT EYES (*JINGMING*): Just above the inside corner of your eye.

BL-2 GATHERED BAMBOO (*ZANZHU*): Directly above Bl-1 on your eyebrow.

ST-2 FOUR WHITES (*SIBAI*): Just below the centre point of the lower eye socket.

GB-1 PUPIL CREVICE (*TONGZILIAO*): Follow the corner of your eye outwards towards the temple, just over the ridge of the eye socket.

Nose

LI-20 WELCOME FRAGRANCE (*YINGXIANG*): Next to and level with the midpoint of the flare of the nostrils.

BITONG: Next to your nose, at the beginning of the flare of the nostrils.

Find Areas on Your Neck and Shoulders

(See also colour insert at back of book.)

QUEPEN: Although in modern TCM this is restricted to the acupoint St-12, it actually refers to the wide area above your clavicle (collar bone) beneath the neck (Heat *shu*).

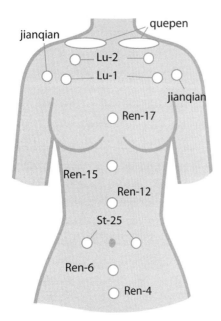

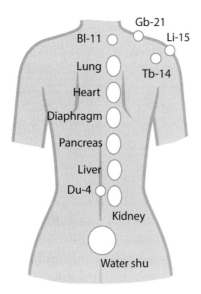

LU-1 MIDDLE PALACE (*ZHONGFU*): Two finger-widths outwards diagonally, below Lu-2, in the muscle ridge (Heat *shu*).

LU-2 CLOUD GATE (*YUNMEN*): In the hollow at the outside end of your collar bone (Heat *shu*).

JIANQIAN: In the shoulder muscle, halfway between the underarm crease and LI-15.

LI-15 SHOULDER BONE (*JIANYU*): Directly under the bone at your shoulder joint on the centre line of your arm (Heat *shu*).

TB-14 SHOULDER CREVICE (*JIANLIAO*): At your shoulder joint, just behind the deltoid arm muscle. At the same level as Li-15 but behind it in the dip.

GB-21 SHOULDER WELL (*JIANJING*): On the top of the shoulder muscle, halfway between the midline of your neck and the end of your shoulder.

BL-11 GREAT SHUTTLE (*DAZHU*): Two finger-widths from the spine, level with the first thoracic vertebra (T1) (Heat *shu*).

Find Areas on Your Chest

REN-17 CHEST CENTRE (*SHANZHONG*): On the midline of the sternum, level with the fourth rib space (the nipples are usually in the space between the fourth and fifth ribs in men).

Find Areas on Your Abdomen

REN-15 TURTLE DOVE TAIL (*JIUWEI*): On the midline of your abdomen, a finger-width below the end of the sternum (breast bone) (Source).

REN-12 MIDDLE CAVITY (*ZHONGWAN*): On the midline of your abdomen, halfway between the end of the sternum and your navel.

ST-25 HEAVEN'S PIVOT (*TIANSHU*): Three finger-widths from the midline of the abdomen or halfway from the farthest line of abdominal muscles (as in those six-pack muscles), level with your navel.

REN-6 SEA OF *QI* (*QIHAI*): On the midline of the lower abdomen, around two finger-widths below your navel (Source).

REN-4 GATE OF ORIGIN (*GUANYUAN*): On the midline of the lower abdomen, a hand-width below your navel or three finger-widths above the top of the pubic bone (the line of bone you hit as you feel down the abdomen).

Find Areas on Your Back

To locate individual vertebrae in the thoracic and lumbar (L1–5) areas of the back, it is a simple case of counting vertebrae. For the thoracic spine, count down 1–12, and for the lumbar spine, 1–5.

LUNG REGION (*BACK SHU AND HEAT SHU*): Halfway between the vertical edge of the scapula (shoulder blade) and the spine, level with the gap between the 3rd and 4th thoracic vertebrae (T3–T4). This is normally found by continuing the diagonal lateral line of the bony spine of the shoulder blade.

HEART REGION (*BACK SHU*): Halfway between the vertical edge of your shoulder blade and the spine, level with the 4th and 5th (T4–T5), and 5th and 6th (T5–T6), thoracic vertebrae. While the heart *shu* is placed at the 5th and 6th, the heart ruler is often placed above it at the 4th and 5th. So this region covers both.

DIAPHRAGM REGION (*BACK SHU*): Following the same vertical line coming down the lung and heart regions, the diaphragm region is rarely used but as it affects a major chest structure through which all river systems pass through, it can be invaluable. It is level with the gap between the 7th and 8th thoracic vertebrae (T7–T8). This is normally found at the same level as the lower edge of your shoulder blades.

LIVER REGION (*BACK SHU*): Extend the same vertical line as above (a hand-width from the spine) and the liver region is level with the

9th and 10th thoracic vertebrae (T9–T10). This region can be extended to cover 10th and 11th thoracic vertebrae (T10–T11), which is the TCM location of the gallbladder *shu*.

PANCREAS REGION (*BACK SHU*): Two vertebrae down from the liver region is the pancreas region. Extend the same vertical line as above, which is around a hand-width from the spine and level with the 11th and 12th thoracic vertebrae (T11–T12). The TCM location of the stomach *shu* is one below, at the area between the 12th thoracic vertebra and 1st lumbar vertebra (T12–L1). So this wide area is the pancreas region.

KIDNEY REGION (*BACK SHU*): It is level with the gap between the second and third lumbar vertebrae (L2–L3). This is normally found by finding the bottom of the ribcage at the sides and bringing your hands together at the spine at the same level. This region can be extended to cover 1st and 2nd lumbar vertebrae (L1–L2), which is the TCM location of the triple burner *shu*. This makes sense as both are heavily involved with the passage of water.

DU-4 GATE OF LIFE (*MINGMEN*): On the midline of the spine, in the space between the second and third lumbar vertebrae (L2–L3). Find the highest points of the hip bone at the sides of the body, and draw an imaginary line across to the spine, and then go up one vertebra.

WATER *SHU* REGION (*SHUI SHU*): This wide area covers the sacrum and the top of your buttocks and incorporates the TCM location of the bladder *shu*.

Find Areas on Your Arms

(See also colour insert at back of book.)

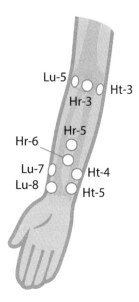

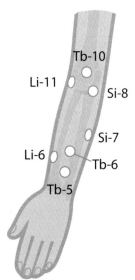

Heart Root Shu/Junction/Source Areas

HT-3 LESSER SEA (*SHAOHAI*): At the end of your elbow crease on the medial side (inside) of your arm (Root *shu*).

HT-4 SPIRIT PATH (*LINGDAO*): Two finger-widths from your wrist, to the inside of the tendon (flexor carpi radialis) (Root *shu*).

HT-5 PENETRATING THE INTERIOR (*TONGLI*): Two finger-widths from Ht-7 on the radial side (outside) of the tendon (Junction).

Heart Ruler Root Shu/Junction/Source Areas

HR-3 MARSH AT THE BEND (*QUZE*): On the ulnar (little finger side) of the tendon (biceps brachii) at the front of your elbow crease (Root *shu*).

HR-5 PASSING BETWEEN (*JIANSHI*): A hand-width up from your wrist between the two tendons (palmaris longus and flexor carpi radialis) (Root *shu*).

HR-6 INNER GATE (*NEIGUAN*): Three finger-widths up from your wrist in between the two tendons as described in Hr-5 (Junction).

Lung Root Shu/Junction/Source Areas

LU-5 FOOT MARSH (*CHIZE*): Just lateral to (on the outside of) the biceps tendon at the front of the elbow crease (Root *shu*).

LU-7 BROKEN SEQUENCE (*LIEQUE*): Two finger-widths proximal (towards your elbow) from Li-5 on the lateral side of your forearm (Junction).

LU-8 CHANNEL GULLY (*JINGQU*): Two finger-widths proximal to (towards your elbow) the wrist on a line from Lu-9 to Lu-5 (Root *shu*).

Small Intestine Root Shu/Junction/Source Areas

SI-8 LITTLE OCEAN (*XIAOHAI*): In the gap between the tip of the elbow (medial epicondyle of the humerous) and the "funny bone" (olecranon process) (Root *shu*).

SI-7 BRANCH OF THE UPRIGHT (*ZHIZHENG*): Just over one-third of the distance between your wrist and Si-8, on the border of the ulna (the inside forearm bone) (Junction).

Triple Burner Root Shu/Junction/Source Areas

TB-10 HEAVENLY WELL (*TIANJING*): Bend the arm at the elbow. The area is a finger-width above the tip of the elbow in the triceps brachii tendon at the back of your arm (Root *shu*).

TB-6 LIMB DITCH (*ZHIGOU*): A hand-width from the posterior wrist crease, along the midline of your arm (between the radius and ulnar bones) (Root *shu*).

TB-5 OUTER PASS (*WAIGUAN*): Three finger-widths up from the posterior wrist crease, along the midline of your arm (between the radius and ulnar bones) (Junction).

Large Intestine Root Shu/Junction/Source Areas

LI-11 POOL AT THE BEND (*QUCHI*): At the lateral end of the elbow crease when the elbow is bent towards you (Root *shu*).

LI-6 VEERING PASSAGE (*PIANLI*): A hand-width from your wrist on a line between Li-5 and Li-11 (Junction).

Finding Areas on Your Hands

(See also colour insert at back of book.)

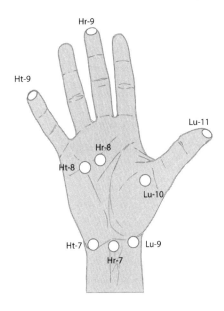

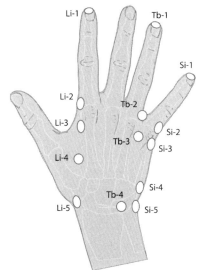

Heart Root Shu/Junction/Source Areas

HT-9 LESSER RUSHING (*SHAOCHONG*): The area around the tip of your little finger (the heart river ends here) (Root *shu*).

HT-8 LESSER PALACE (*SHAOFU*): If you make a loose fist, it is where the tip of your little finger touches the palm, below the MCP joint (Root *shu*).

HT-7 SPIRIT GATE (*SHENMEN*): At the little finger end of the wrist crease, next to the small bone at the base of your hand (Root *shu*).

Heart Ruler Root Shu/Junction/Source Areas

HR-9 MIDDLE RUSHING (*ZHONGCHONG*): The area around the tip of your middle finger (Root *shu*).

HR-8 LABOUR PALACE (*LAOGONG*): If you make a loose fist, it is where the tip of your middle finger touches the palm, below the MCP joint (Root *shu*).

HR-7 GREAT MOUND (*DALING*): At the middle of your wrist between the two tendons as described in Hr-5 (Root *shu*).

Lung Root Shu/Junction/Source Areas

LU-11 LESSER SHANG (*SHAOSHANG*): The area around the tip of your thumb (Root *shu*).

LU-10 FISH BORDER (*YUJILU*): In the fleshy part of the palm (thenar eminence) below the thumb (Root *shu*).

LU-9 GREAT ABYSS (*DAYUAN*): In the wrist joint, below the base of your thumb (Root *shu*, Source).

Small Intestine Root Shu/Junction/Source Areas

SI-1 LESSER MARSH (*SHAOZE*): The area around the tip of your little finger (the small intestine river starts here) (Root *shu*).

SI-2 FRONT VALLEY (*QIANGU*): On the ulnar (inner forearm bone) side of your little finger, just distal (above) the MCP joint (Root *shu*).

SI-3 REAR STREAM (*HOUXI*): Proximal (below) the little finger joint at the lateral side of the hand, between the metacarpal bone and palm muscles (Root *shu*).

SI-4 WRIST BONE (*WANGU*): On the little finger side of the hand, above the wrist, at the other end of the fifth metacarpal bone to Si-3, between the bone and palm muscle (Source).

SI-5 YANG VALLEY (*YANGGU*): At the lateral side of the wrist, between the head of the ulnar and your hand (Root *shu*).

Triple Burner Root Shu/Junction/Source Areas

TB-1 RUSHING PASS (*GUANCHONG*): The area around the tip of your ring finger (Root *shu*).

TB-2 FLUID GATE (*YEMEN*): On the back of your hand, in the web between the ring and little fingers, above the MCP joint (Root *shu*).

TB-3 CENTRAL INLET (*ZHONGZHU*): If you make a loose fist, this point lies on the back of the hand between the metacarpal bones and forms an equal-sided triangle with the MCP joint of the ring and little finger (Root *shu*).

TB-4 YANG POOL (*YANGCHI*): Follow the gap between the metacarpal bones from Tb-3, and it is in the wrist joint before the head of the ulnar (little finger-side forearm bone) (Source).

Large Intestine Root Shu/Junction/Source Areas

LI-1 SHANG NOTE YANG (*SHANGYANG*): The area around the tip of your index finger (Root *shu*).

LI-2 SECOND GAP (*ERJIAN*): Just after the thumb side of the MCP joint (knuckle) of the index finger (Root *shu*).

LI-3 THIRD GAP (*SANJIAN*): Just before (proximal to) the thumb side of the MCP joint (knuckle) of the index finger (Root *shu*).

LI-4 CONVERGING VALLEY (*HEGU*): In the web of flesh between your thumb and index finger (Source).

LI-5 YANG STREAM (*YANXI*): Spread open the fingers of your hand, follow the line of the thumb down to your wrist, and it is in the dip (Root *shu*).

Finding Areas on Your Legs

(See also colour insert at back of book.)

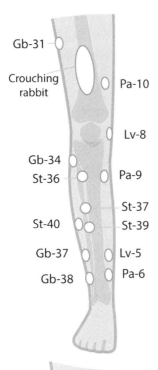

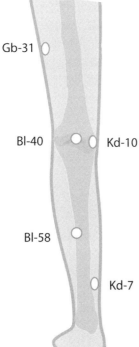

Liver Root Shu/Junction/Source Areas

LV-8 SPRING AT THE BEND (*QUQUAN*): Just after the medial (inside) end of the knee crease when the knee is bent (Root *shu*).

LV-5 WOODWORM CANAL (*LIGOU*): One-third of the distance from the tip of the medial malleolus (inside ankle bone) to the knee crease, between the calf muscle and the tibia (shin bone) (Junction).

Pancreas Root Shu/Junction/Source Areas

PA-9 YIN MOUND SPRING (*YINLINGQUAN*): Found on the same level as the bottom edge of the bony protuberance below your knee. Feel down from the knee, and there is a lump. The area is at the level of the bottom of this lump, and also Gb-34 on the other side of the leg. It is in the muscle just behind the bone on the inside of your leg (Root *shu*).

PA-10 SEA OF BLOOD (*XUEHAI*): In the vastus medialis (thigh) muscle above your knee. Go up the same height as your knee cap (about three finger-widths) and on a line up from Pa-9.

PA-6 THREE YIN INTERSECTION (*SANYINJIAO*): A hand-width up from the tip of the medial malleolus (inside ankle bone), next to the tibia.

Kidney Root Shu/Junction/Source Areas

KD-10 YIN VALLEY (*YINGU*): On the medial side of your knee crease between the tendons (Root *shu*).

KD-7 RETURNING STREAM (*FULIU*): Three finger-widths directly above Kd-3, next to the Achilles tendon (Root *shu*).

Bladder Root Shu/Junction/Source Areas

BL-40 BENDING CENTRE *(WEIZHONG)*: In the middle of the crease at the back of your knee (Root *shu* and Heat *shu*).

BL-58 SOARING UPWARDS *(FEIYANG)*: Just below your calf muscle on a line up from Bl-60 (Junction).

Stomach Root Shu/Junction/Source Areas

CROUCHING RABBIT *(FUTU)*: On the front of your thigh. It has been relegated by TCM to a small acupoint at St-32, but originally was a much larger region along the midline area of your quadricep muscles, so cover the whole area.

ST-36 LEG THREE MILES *(ZUSANLI)*: A hand-width below the bottom of your kneecap, one finger-width outwards from the thicker tibia (shin bone) (Root *shu* and Heat *shu*).

ST-37 UPPER GREAT VOID *(SHANGJUXU)*: A hand-width below St-36, a finger-width from the tibia (Heat *shu*).

ST-39 LOWER GREAT VOID *(XIAJUSHU)*: A hand-width below St-37, a finger-width from the tibia (Heat *shu*).

ST-40 ABUNDANT BRIDGE *(FENGLONG)*: Halfway between the tip of the lateral malleolus (outside ankle bone) and the knee crease, two finger-widths from the tibia (Junction).

Gallbladder Root Shu/Junction/Source Areas

GB-31 WIND MARKET *(FENGSHI)*: On the outside of your thigh, just over halfway between the knee crease and the head of the femur (thigh bone). Stand and put your hands relaxed at your sides. Put your middle finger on an imaginary trouser crease running down the sides of the legs. The area should be here.

GB-34 YANG MOUND SPRING *(YANGLINGQUAN)*: Just below the head of the fibula bone, on the lateral side of your lower leg. A finger-width and a half down from the knobbly head of the bone and in the area towards the centre line of the leg (Root *shu*).

GB-38 YANG ASSISTANCE *(YANGFU)*: Five finger-widths up from the tip of the lateral malleolus (outside ankle bone) at the front edge of the fibula (outside leg bone) (Root *shu*).

GB-37 BRIGHT LIGHT *(GUANGMING)*: One finger-width higher up your leg than Gb-38 (Junction).

Find Areas on Your Feet

(See also colour insert at back of book.)

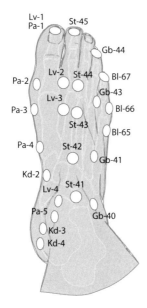

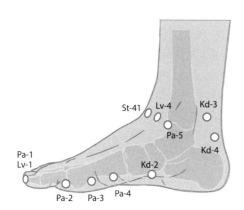

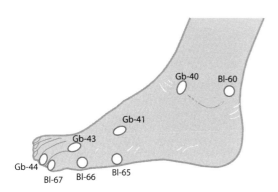

Liver Root Shu/Junction/Source Areas

LV-1 LARGE CONTAINER (*DADUN*): The area around the tip of your big toe (Root *shu*).

LV-2 CIRCULATING BETWEEN (*XINGJIAN*): In the web between the big toe and second toe (Root *shu*).

LV-3 GREAT RUSHING (*TAICHONG*): In the gap between the bones that lead to the big toe and second toe. Follow the gap up from Lv-2, and it is before the two bones meet (Root *shu*).

LV-4 MIDDLE SEAL (*ZHONGFENG*): Located at your ankle, just medial to the medial malleolus (inside ankle bone below the tibia) (Root *shu*).

Pancreas Root Shu/Junction/Source Areas

PA-1 HIDDEN WHITE (*YINBAI*): The area around the tip of your big toe (Root *shu*).

PA-2 GREAT CAPITAL (*DADU*): Just distal to (beyond) the MTP joint on the lateral side (outside) of your big toe, below the bone (Root *shu*).

PA-3 GREAT WHITE (*TAIBAI*): Just proximal (next) to the MTP joint on the lateral side of your foot, below the bone (Root *shu*).

PA-4 GRANDFATHER GRANDSON (*GONGSUN*): At the other end of the first metatarsal bone to Pa-3, in the dip (Junction).

PA-5 SHANG MOUND (*SHANGQIU*): Below the medial malleolus (inside ankle bone), where the horizontal and vertical edges meet medially (Root *shu*).

Kidney Root Shu/Junction/Source Areas

KD-1 GUSHING SPRING (*YONGQUAN*): At the base of the little toe on the sole of your foot. (Root *shu*).

KD-2 BLAZING VALLEY (*RANGU*): Go down from the front edge of the medial malleolus (inside ankle bone) to the side of the arch of your foot, and it is under the navicular tuberosity, the prominent bone you can feel (Root *shu*).

KD-3 GREAT STREAM (*TAIXI*): Halfway between the tip of the medial malleolus and the Achilles tendon (Root *shu*, Source).

KD-4 GREAT BELL (*DAZHONG*): Just below and slightly posterior to (behind) Kd-3 (Junction).

Bladder Root Shu/Junction/Source Areas

BL-60 KUNLUN MOUNTAIN (*KUNLUN*): Midway between the tip of the lateral malleolus (outside ankle bone) and your Achilles tendon (Root *shu*).

BL-64 CAPITAL BONE (*JINGGU*): Feel along the lateral side (outside) of your foot until you come across a bone protruding out. This is the tuberosity of the fifth metatarsal bone. The area is distal (towards your toes) to this protuberance (Source).

BL-66 COMMUNICATING VALLEY (*TONGGU*): On the lateral side of your foot, just proximal (towards your ankle) to the fifth MTP joint (Root *shu*).

BL-65 BUNDLE BONES (*SHUGU*): On the other side of the MTP joint to Bl-66 (Root *shu*).

BL-67 EXTREME YIN (*ZHIYIN*): The area around the tip of your little toe (Root *shu*).

Stomach Root Shu/Junction/Source Areas

ST-41 STREAM DIVIDE (*JIEXI*): In the middle of the front of your ankle, level with the tip of the lateral malleolus (outside ankle bone) (Root *shu* and Heat *shu*).

ST-42 RUSHING YANG (*CHONGYANG*): On the dorsum (top) of your foot, two finger-widths down from St-41, on a line between St-41 and St-43 (Source).

ST-43 SUNKEN VALLEY (*XIANGGU*): On the top of your foot between the second and third metatarsal bone, proximal to (before) the MTP joint (Root *shu*).

ST-44 INNER COURTYARD (*NEITING*): At the web between the second and third toes (Root *shu*).

ST-45 FORMIDABLE PASSAGE (*LIDUI*): The area around the tip of your middle toe (Root *shu*).

Gallbladder Root Shu/Junction/Source Areas

GB-40 MOUND OF RUINS (*QIUXU*): Below the lateral malleolus (outside ankle bone), where the lines of the forward horizontal and vertical edges meet medially (Source).

GB-41 OVERLOOKING TEARS (*LINQI*): On the lateral side of the top of your foot, between the metatarsal bones that lead to the fourth toe and little toe (Root *shu*).

GB-43 RAVINE STREAM (*XIAXI*): In the web between the fourth toe and little toe (Root *shu*).

GB-44 YIN OPENING (*QIAOYIN*): The area around the tip of your fourth toe (Root *shu*).

Treat the Microsystems
Zones on Your Hand

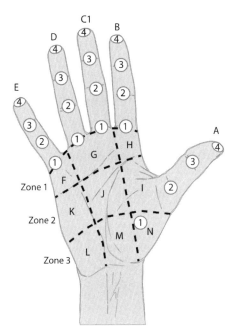

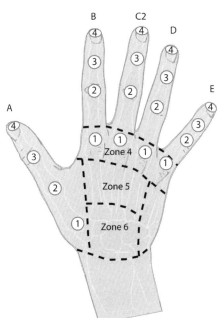

Fingers

An instant way to recognize the organization of the projected body on your fingers is to visualize it as a walking creature. Imagine your middle finger as the head and the other four fingers are the front and back legs. It is the application of an image of the human body using holographic principles, and one that is the core of Korean hand therapy.

The distribution is as follows:

A. THUMB: 1. hip 2. knee 3. ankle 4. toes
B. INDEX FINGER: 1. upper arm 2. elbow 3. wrist 4. fingers
C1. MIDDLE FINGER: 1. throat 2. mouth 3. nose 4. head (*palm*)
C2. MIDDLE FINGER: 1. neck 2. occiput 3. vertex 4. head (*dorsum*)
D. RING FINGER: 1. upper arm 2. elbow 3. wrist 4. fingers
E. LITTLE FINGER: 1. hip 2. knee 3. ankle 4. toes

Hand – Palm Side

ZONE 1 (*UPPER*): F–H: Chest & lung; G: Heart
ZONE 2 (*MID*): K: Liver; J: Pancreas & stomach; K–I: Small & large intestine
ZONE 3 (*LOWER*): M: Kidney, bladder; L–N: Reproductive organs

Hand – Dorsum Side

ZONE 4 (*UPPER*): Neck area: Cervical spine (midline)
ZONE 5 (*MID*): Upper back area: Thoracic spine (midline)
ZONE 6 (*LOWER*): Lower back area: Lumbar spine

Zones on Your Foot

Microsystem treatments on your feet were called "zonal therapy" for a reason, because this is the best way to understand how to use them to treat. Instead of small fixed points, focus your attention on wider zones. The named regions within each zone are so that there is a theoretical connection between the standard foot microsystem maps and this one. However, in general, whenever you see a foot zone mentioned, treat the whole zone. This means looking for any tension within the tissue in that zone, and manipulating it with acupressure or Gua sha treatment, or both. The zones are to guide you.

Some notable changes have been made with my version of the feet. The heart region is usually only found on one foot in a standard microsystem map of the foot. But this does not make any sense. The idea is that if you put your feet together and look at the soles, it should show the body symmetrically, with most of the regions repeated on either side in their respective positions. The heart is a *zang* storage region like the lung, pancreas, liver, and kidney, and by definition, these have to be on both sides. The heart and the pancreas are in the middle of your body, and so straddle both sides; the lung and kidney already have two separate parts; and the spleen is considered part of the liver system so, in effect, the liver is in two parts as well. This is the reason that you will often see the liver and spleen referenced together and the heart on both sides.

The key to understanding the zones is to find the demarcation lines on the soles of your feet. These are the four lines that separate the five zones.

SHOULDER LINE: An imaginary line across the toe joints on the soles of your feet.

DIAPHRAGM LINE: An imaginary line between the ball and the arch of your foot.

WAIST LINE: An imaginary line from the base of the fifth metatarsal (you can find it on the lateral (outside) edge of the sole).

PELVIC LINE: Where the heel starts on the sole on an imaginary line coming down from both ankle bones.

For the purposes of this book, these lines wrap around the whole foot so you can treat on the sole, the lateral or medial sides, or the dorsum (top), and it will still be in the same zone.

Once you have the above four lines clear in your head, then the following distribution should make logical sense.

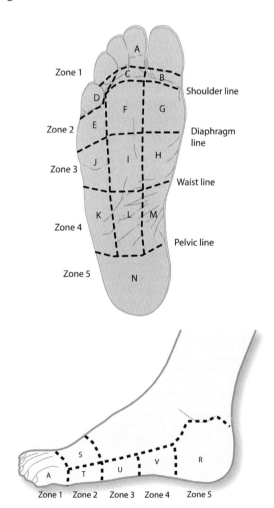

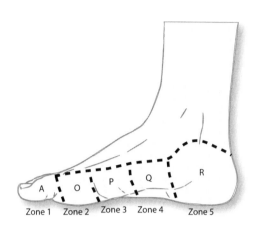

ZONE 1: Above Shoulder Line

Sole

A: Head/face
B: Neck
C: Eye
D: Ear

Medial Side

A-O: Cervical area

ZONE 2: Above Diaphragm Line

Sole

G: Heart
E-F: Lung

Lateral Side

T: Scapula & shoulder

Dorsum side

S: Chest

ZONE 3: Above Waist Line

Sole

J-L: Liver, spleen, & gallbladder
H: Pancreas & stomach
I: Kidney

Medial Side

P: Thoracic area

Lateral Side

U-V: Arm & elbow

ZONE 4: Above Pelvic Line

Sole

L-M: Small intestine
K-M: Large intestine
M: Bladder

Medial Side

Q: Lumbar area

ZONE 5: Below Pelvic Line

Sole

N: Reproductive organs

Lateral/Medial Side

R: Sacrum, coccyx, uterus/prostate

Zones on Your Ear

Maps of the ear microsystem can get very complicated and consist of a great number of areas to treat. For our purposes in this book, with the treatment strategies of acupressure and Gua sha, such detail is neither necessary, nor desirable. For that reason the following eight-zone map of the projected body onto the ear has been simplified and coded. This should make it easier to locate and treat using your ear, without losing the holographic principles of the microsystem.

As with all of the microsystems presented here, the zone is the key. Go to the zone suggested, and look for any reactivity. This means pressing and finding sore areas. The named regions within the zones are as a guide only, and not for you to follow doggedly without reacting to the unique living, breathing person you are treating.

The organization of the ear microsystem should be self-explanatory and make logical sense when you apply the projected body onto your ear.

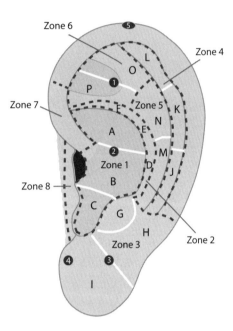

ZONE 1 (Superior & Inferior Concha): Internal Organs

A: Bladder, kidney, pancreas, spleen, large intestine, small intestine, stomach
B: Liver, lung, heart, heart ruler, throat
C: Brain, *sanjiao*

ZONE 2 (Antihelix): Spinal Column

D: Cervical
E: Thoracic
F: Lumbar-sacral

ZONE 3 (Lobule): Head and Face

G: Head area (antitragus)
H: Jaw, ear
I: Teeth, eye

ZONE 4 (Scaphoid Fossa): Upper Limbs

J: Shoulder
K: Arm & elbow
L: Wrist, hand, & fingers

ZONE 5 (Antihelix Body): Front

M: Neck & chest
N: Abdomen

ZONE 6 (Antihelix Crus): Lower Body

O: Hip, knee, ankle, toes
P: Buttocks, uterus

ZONE 7 (Helix Root): Groin Area

Prostate, external genitals, urethra, rectum, ovaries, testes

ZONE 8 (tragus): Sensory Organs

Ear, nose, eye

Support Regions

1: Shenmen
2: Relaxation
3: Sensorial
4: Cerebral

Extra Areas

5: Ear Apex

PART 5

What Are the Main Patterns and How Do You Treat Them?

While everyone has a unique body makeup which is a combination of genetic, environmental, and developed characteristics, we can broadly place what happens within your body into certain universal patterns of balance and imbalance. In this section, we look into these patterns and explore how they materialize in your body and suggest how they can be treated using the various therapies explained earlier in the book.

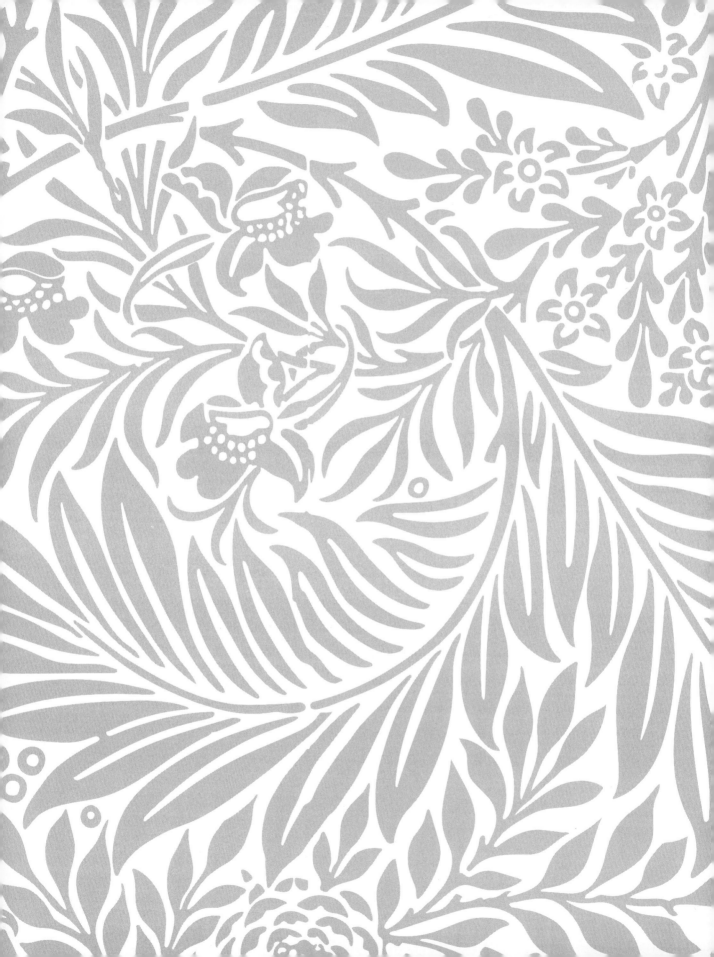

The Main Pattern Groups

Whilst there are intricate relationships and balances within the body on many different levels, they can be grouped together to create a set of generalized patterns common to us all. These patterns of impairment form the basis of health or ill health and often underlie identified health conditions and illnesses.

They can be divided into two groups focussing on conditions of weakness or overflow. Rather than opposites, these patterns can also work hand in hand in the often complex presentations of the body's internal balance.

Patterns of Weakness

These patterns occur when key substances in the body become weakened and impaired.

- General weakness
- *Yang* weakness
- *Yin* weakness
- Blood circulation weakness

Patterns of Overflow

These patterns occur when key substances in the body become too obstructive, abundant or forceful.

- Stagnation
- Heat
- Cold
- Damp/phlegm
- Wind

Patterns of weakness or deficiency are those which need to be restored or built up after having been depleted, and patterns of overflow or excess are those which require release after having been accumulated. Both can feed into each other in a vicious spiral which, if left unchecked, can deepen an impairment and can lead to more worrying symptoms. For patterns of weakness the situation is one of the banks of the river crumbling, or the water being dried up, or the flow being slow and without force; and for patterns of overflow, the river has burst its banks, or has been blocked by debris or is flowing too fast.

How this might manifest in terms of signs and symptoms within your body is that when the affected river system goes offline, whether through deficiency or excess, it triggers a set of markers along its river course to show you what is happening inside. When the situation is one of weakness, there is a general trend for these markers to show your body lacking something; perhaps it is colour, energy, moisture, or strength. And when the situation is one of overflow, the markers show a tendency for an excess of fluids, tension, temperature, and motion. In this way, many signs and symptoms can be very revealing about the possible nature and location of the impaired systems affected.

The patterns are not exclusive, and there can be several present at the same time in the same person. If this is the case, as regards treatment, you start with the dominant one.

Patterns of Weakness

General Weakness

Signs and Symptoms
Pale skin that has lost its vitality; tiredness; low energy; weakness in your arms and legs; pale, loose stools; no appetite; feeling bloated after eating; occasional shortness of breath; catch a cold easily.

Can Include or Lead To
Underlies a host of medical conditions, both acute and chronic—anything from nasal allergies and chronic fatigue syndrome to depression and persistent back pain.

Common Causes
Worrying, overstudying, being inactive, stooping over a desk for long periods, too much cold or raw food, eating in a hurry and at irregular times, emotional stress, chronic diseases, overuse of antibiotics for a cold or flu, smoking, or childbirth.

An Explanation
This pattern is an extremely common one, as most people exhaust their capacity at some point in their lives. Some of us do it all the time! The basic idea is that there is not enough water in the rivers, and so not enough power to circulate around the body properly.

And we have to restore, replenish, and coax the body back to moving smoothly with the *yin/yang* breath motion. Any intervention we do should be *yin*-type; we should avoid *yang* interventions, which can be too draining for the body.

Our strength comes from the food we eat, from the air we breathe, and from the reserves we were born with. If our diet is not appropriate or the quantity of air too low (through bad posture, for example) or if we lead a stressful lifestyle, sometimes there is not enough to keep pace with demand.

This condition often develops gradually over time and is not unlike a car running on empty. It will become slow, sluggish, parts will seize up, and the engine will smoke and rumble, even over short distances.

If there is not enough energy to power the body, it often means that the pancreas, lung, or kidney systems have become weakened, either directly, through an improper diet, smoking, or doing too much, or indirectly, through the effect of emotional stress, which tends to affect the liver system and create stagnation patterns.

Whatever the cause, the most effective ways to strengthen the body are those that most people have some degree of control over – diet, exercise, and lifestyle. And a few simple changes can make all the difference.

Food Therapy

Dietary Factors That Can Worsen General Weakness
- Irregular eating patterns, especially eating late at night and overeating, and drinking

too much during meal times can all weaken the digestive process.

- Cold-natured foods, such as salads, raw fruit, fruit juice, wheat, raw vegetables, tomatoes, tofu, sweet food, beer, brown rice, cold drinks from the refrigerator, and iced water, are weakening if consumed in excess.

- Too many damp-forming, congesting foods, such as dairy products, ice cream, concentrated orange juice, bread, and peanuts, also add to the weakness. In particular, processed products containing sugar or corn syrup, flaked or puffed grains (breakfast cereals, for example), wraps, cookies, chocolate, white flour, and white pasta.

Dietary Factors That Can Improve General Weakness

- Follow a diet similar to the ideal diet as detailed in the Food Therapy section. Complex carbohydrates, such as whole grains and legumes, are important as they support your body over an extended period of time. They should be combined with large quantities of vegetables and with a small amount of good-quality protein.

- Food should be enjoyed and chewed slowly in a calm atmosphere, and you should follow many of the guidelines in the Food Therapy section.

- Soups and stews are preferable, as they often help strengthen and aid digestion.

- Your digestive process can be strengthened with lightly cooked, simple food, such as the following:

  ▸ FRUIT: Cooked or stewed fruits, such as cherries, peaches, figs, grapes, coconut, and dates.

  ▸ VEGETABLES: Cooked vegetables, such as pumpkins, carrots, peas, potatoes, squashes, yams, sweet potatoes, leeks, olives, mushrooms, garlic, onions, and fennel, preferably fresh and not frozen.

  ▸ GRAINS: Cooked white rice, oats, porridge (oatmeal), millet, corn, barley, and malt (but not cereal bars and most boxed breakfast cereals).

  ▸ HERBS AND SPICES: Warming herbs and spices, such as fresh ginger, sage, thyme, and nutmeg.

  ▸ LEGUMES, SEEDS, AND NUTS: Lentils, chickpeas (garbanzos), black beans, walnuts, and chestnuts.

  ▸ MEAT AND SEAFOOD: Small amounts of beef, lamb, chicken, ham, liver and kidney; also eel, herring, mackerel, salmon, trout, tuna, and anchovies.

  ▸ DRINKS: Jasmine tea (especially with meals) and drinks at room temperature or above.

  ▸ OTHERS: Bee pollen and royal jelly.

Manual Therapy

For weakness, a *yin*-based treatment, not one that is *yang*-based, is most appropriate. This means gentle, flowing movements that allow your body to adjust at its own pace rather than harsh interventions that force it to act.

In terms of Gua sha, light scraping is appropriate, especially if weak or frail. This can improve the circulation of blood, which is often sluggish when there is a weakness. Scraping should, therefore, be gentle and more connected with increasing microcirculation in the tissue beneath the skin than trying to extract the red marks of *sha* on the skin surface.

There is a technique in Japan called *kanpu masatsu* (dry towel friction) whereby, as the name suggests, a small towel is held at both ends and rubbed on the skin to create friction and a sense of warmth (see following page). This is the style of Gua sha needed here. The goal is to increase circulation in the connective tissue streams and tributaries that will feed into the river system.

The main focus of the Gua sha treatment should be on the digestive centre so that the stomach and pancreas systems as well as the kidney system are strengthened. A general strengthening treatment is required that includes all the systems.

On Your Head

Scrape over your head as if the Gua sha tool were a comb. Start at the midline at Du-24, and go backwards over your head towards your neck at Du-16, and then repeat in parallel lines moving towards your ears, first going back on one side of your head and then on the other.

On Your Back

Note that this should be done on you by someone else due to the difficulty of reaching your back. Gently scrape down the back area with enough force to move circulation but not enough to cause large amounts of *sha* to appear on the skin. Cover all of the back *shu* regions in the wide muscle area either side of the spine. You can also thumb-press down the back muscles either side of the spine and gently hard-press any tight areas, whether or not they are back *shu* regions.

On Your Arms

Gently thumb-press or scrape down the *yin* river systems (lung, heart, and heart ruler) on the inside of your arm. You do not need to be too specific. Just knead or push any sore areas you find along the way. Do each of these river systems separately in a downwards motion. In particular, check the root *shu* areas for reactivity in your lower arm (lung: Lu-5 and Lu-8; heart: Ht-3 and Ht-4; heart ruler: Hr-3 and Hr-5).

On Your Legs

Thumb-press or use a tool to scrape up the pancreas and down the stomach river systems in your lower leg. Check for any areas of soreness or tightness, and gently knead those areas. Especially check the root *shu* areas in these river systems on your lower leg at St-36 and St-41, and Pa-9 and Pa-5.

On Your Hands

Gently massage the whole hand. Use the Hand Circulation sequence in Chapter 13. Gua sha is particularly useful for gentle, circulatory treatment on your hand, especially if you are treating yourself. Use the same principles as with the hand massage above, but scrape with the side of the tool using short scrapes towards your fingers. Follow the line of each of your fingers and especially around the joints.

On Your Feet

As with the hands, cover the whole foot using the Foot Circulation sequence in Chapter 13. Use Gua sha to scrape along the soles of your feet, following the lines of your toes as instructed.

On Your Ears

As with the hands and feet, cover the whole ear by doing the Ear Circulation in chapter 13, either using Gua sha or your fingers.

KANPU MASATSU (Dry Towel Friction)

For this sequence you will need a soft towel or cloth around 1m (3ft) in length. The size most used is 1m x 35cm (14in). A thicker towel is recommended for areas where you want to give stronger stimulation, such as the back.

While kanpu masatsu was traditionally done on bare skin, this can be irritating and provide too strong a treatment, so rubbing over light clothing is recommended.

Neck

STEP 1: Fold the towel, put it on your neck, and stroke downwards from the nape to the base of your neck.

STEP 2: Extend the towel, and holding both ends, pull it tight on the back of your neck, and move it gently from side to side to create light friction on your neck.

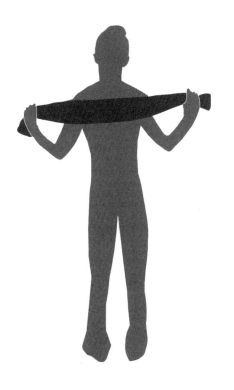

Back

STEP 3: Keeping the towel extended, and holding both ends, rub left and right at the back of your shoulder down to your shoulder blade.

STEP 4: Cross the towel on your back, and hold both ends, so that one arm is above your shoulder and the other is at your waist, and rub the entire back evenly. Repeat on the other side.

STEP 5: Fold the towel about the width of your back and, using both arms simultaneously, rub both sides of your back downwards towards your buttocks and side of your hip.

STEP 6: Repeat step 3 in the lower part of your back from side to side.

Abdomen

STEP 7: Fold the towel to a size that can be held with both hands, and rub your stomach/ abdomen area in a circle.

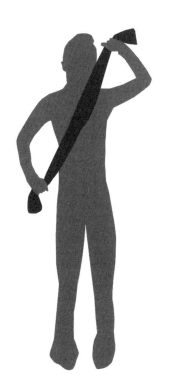

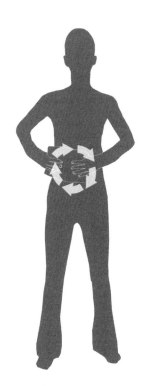

STEP 8: Press the towel near your navel, and rub downwards. Continue this downwards motion over the whole stomach/abdomen area.

STEP 9: Hold both ends of the towel (as in Step 3), and rub the entire stomach/abdomen area from side to side.

Arms

STEP 10: Follow the *yin* rivers to your fingers. Fold the towel into a size that is easy to hold, and rub from the inside of your arm down towards your palm, and then rub the entire palm of your hand. Wrap each finger in the towel, and rub the sides of your fingers using your other hand to rub the towel along them.

STEP 11: Follow the *yang* rivers to your shoulder. Start by rubbing the sides of your fingers as in Step 10, and then rub the back of your hand with the folded towel. Continue up the lateral side of your arm to your shoulder.

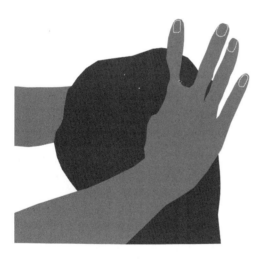

Legs

STEP 12: Follow the *yin* rivers to your inner thigh. Put the towel around each toe, and move it left and right, while holding both ends of the towel to rub the sides (twisting the towel can make it easier). Drape the towel under the sole of your foot, and rub the entire sole evenly,

moving the towel with both hands. Then rub up the medial side of your ankle, lower leg, and finish at your inner thigh.

STEP 13: Follow the *yang* rivers to your toes. Rub down from your lateral side and back of your thigh to your outer ankle. Rub down the top and sides of your foot to your toes, and repeat the towel rubbing of each toe as above.

Each of the steps in the above sequence can be repeated 10 times (1 set), and you can do up to three sets in a session of dry towel rubbing. The stiffer you make the towel, the stronger the treatment, so use enough force to feel comfortable by gently and slowly breathing deeply. A good time to do the sequence is either after you wake up in the morning or/and before going to bed. If you rub directly on your skin, ensure that the skin is dry to avoid irritation.

Exercise Therapy

Follow exercises 1–5 of the Five Qualities of Nature stretches, ideally on a daily basis, but do them slowly and gently (see p. 101 ff.). These stretches can help to strengthen the river systems that are weak.

The following sotai *exercises can also be very beneficial to strengthening weakness:*

❶ *Swing Your Bottom*
Kneel on the floor and rest your bottom on your heels. Move your bottom to one side, and then slowly swing it across to the other side. Continue this movement for up to a few minutes.

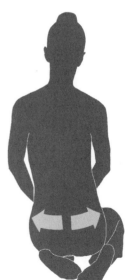

❷ Crouch Twist

Crouch on the floor, with your arms straight and palms and both knees touching the floor. Move your bottom to the right side, and at the same time twist your left shoulder down. Then slowly swing your bottom across to the left, and twist your right shoulder downwards. Repeat this swinging motion for up to a few minutes.

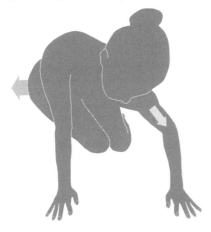

❸ Swing Your Waist

Stand facing a wall, and press gently with both palms. Your arms should be slightly bent and your body upright. Swing your bottom slowly from side to side, while keeping your hands and feet stationary.

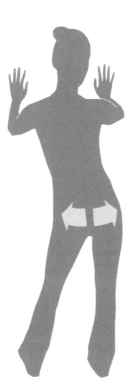

❹ Bend Your Hip

Stand with your arms at your sides and your feet shoulders'-width apart. Put your right hand on your right hip, and bend your body from the hip to the right. Return to the original position, and then repeat the same sequence on the other side. Repeat several times on both sides.

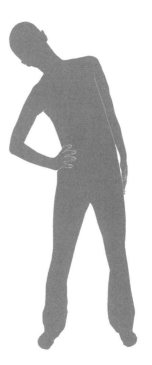

❺ Arm Swing

Stand with your arms at your sides and your feet shoulders'-width apart. Breathe in and, as you breathe out, put your right hand on your right hip, and lift your left arm as you bend to the right. Swing your arm so that it reaches above your head to the left, and continue to breathe out. Return to the original position, and then repeat the same sequence on the other side. Repeat several times on both sides.

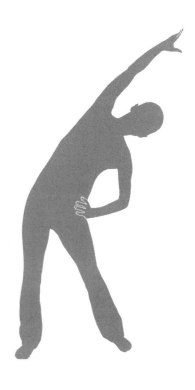

Lifestyle Therapy

1. It is essential to take regular moderate exercise outside in the fresh air rather than indoors. A British review concluded that exercising in the natural environment gives greater feelings of revitalization, increased energy, and less tension, anger, and depression than indoors.[53]

2. Breathing deeply, especially when in the fresh air, can strengthen your lungs but is so rarely practised. Most of us, most of the time, take shallow breaths and need to be reminded to fill our lungs.

3. If seated for extended periods—at work or school, for example—take frequent breaks and actively move around. There is more information on this in the Lifestyle Therapy section.

4. Living with the seasons and with the motion of breath is very important in cases of weakness. This means matching what nature does. When winter comes, it is a time of stillness, contemplation, and preparation.

   New plans can take hold in spring, when the upwards motion leads you into summer, when you should be more active, and when autumn arrives, you bring things to a gentle close for winter. There is more on this in the Qualities of Nature section and also in chapter 10.

Yang Weakness

Signs and Symptoms
Lower backache, weak and cold knees, feeling cold in your back or abdomen, weak legs, apathy, tiredness, impotence, a desire to lie down, chronic digestive problems, diarrhoea, frequent visits to the toilet, being indecisive, and lacking motivation.

Can Include or Lead to
Cystitis, nephritis, prostatitis, urethritis, sexual problems such as frigidity, impotence and premature ejaculation, depression, anxiety, recurrent lumbago, sciatica, rheumatoid arthritis, impaired hearing, and tinnitus.

Common Causes
A chronic illness, old age, too much cold or raw food, exposure to a cold or damp environment, overexercise at a young age, worry, overthinking, stress, lack of exercise, or being constitutionally weak.

An Explanation
Breath motion must be balanced within your body in order to maintain good health. Sometimes, an impairment develops that tips the scales to one side or the other. This could result from a host of factors, from an improper diet that weakens digestion to a sedentary lifestyle that affects circulation patterns.

When the *yang* motion becomes hindered, it can no longer balance *yin*, and so signs and symptoms of characteristics associated with *yin* become much more evident. Hence when *yang* is weakened, your body shows more tiredness, cold feelings, lack of drive, and essentially much of what appears in the General Weakness section, but with the addition of a real sense of coldness.

In order to help your body get more in sync with its *yin/yang* breath, it is essential to strengthen *yang* by making dietary changes. Diet is often one of the main contributing factors to this type of weakness.

Food Therapy

Dietary Factors That Can Worsen Yang Weakness

- Eating cold-natured foods such as salad is often considered an essential part of a healthy diet, but if you have a yang weakness it is not unlike using freezing water to melt ice. For this reason, avoid cool or cold-natured foods, especially raw fruit and raw vegetables, as they can weaken the digestive yang motion when overconsumed.

Also avoid or reduce these foods:

- ▸ **FRUIT:** Citrus fruits, such as grapefruit, lemons, limes and tropical fruits, such as mangos, kiwis, and bananas.
- ▸ **VEGETABLES:** Raw vegetables, salads, tomatoes, summer squash, cucumbers, spinach, and Brussels sprouts.
- ▸ **HERBS AND SPICES:** Peppermint and excessive amounts of salt.
- ▸ **DRINKS:** Fruit juice, carrot juice, green or black tea, strong alcohol, and iced drinks, including iced water.
- ▸ **OTHER:** Dairy products, including ice cream; chocolate; tofu; vinegar; and refined sugars.

Dietary Factors That Can Improve Yang Weakness

- As with General Weakness, in order to strengthen the *yang* motion, a diet of mostly vegetables and grains and only a small amount of meat or high-quality protein is needed. To strengthen *yang* motion, eat warming, pungent foods to help digestion; salty foods to strengthen the kidney system; and sweet foods to strengthen the pancreas, including the following:

  FRUIT: Stewed fruits, in particular apricots, cherries, peaches, plums, raisins, and dates.

  VEGETABLES: Lightly cooked onions, leeks, garlic, parsnips, sweet potatoes, onions, pumpkins, squash, carrots, peas, fennel, turnip, and garlic, preferably fresh and not frozen.

  GRAINS: Cooked grains, such as rice, oats, roasted barley, and millet (but not cereal bars and most packaged breakfast cereals).

  LEGUMES, SEEDS, AND NUTS: Black beans, chickpeas (garbanzos), hazelnuts, walnuts, pistachios, and chestnuts.

  HERBS AND SPICES: Warm spices, such as cloves, black peppercorn, ginger (fresh and dry), cardamom, rosemary, turmeric, nutmeg, black pepper, cloves, and cinnamon.

MEAT AND SEAFOOD: Chicken, lamb, beef, mackerel, tuna, anchovies, salmon, prawns, and shellfish.

DRINKS: Fennel tea and red grape juice. All drinks should be at room temperature or above.

OTHERS: Soups and honey.

Manual Therapy

One of the most useful therapeutic tools when there is *Yang* Weakness is to use gentle heat, particularly on the lower back. Any combination of gentle massage and heat is usually well received.

Do the Dry Towel Friction sequence detailed in General Weakness.

ON YOUR BACK: Using light force, scrape or thumb-press down the back muscles either side of the spine. Cover all of the back *shu* regions and hard-press any areas of tension afterwards. You will need help to do this on your back.

ON YOUR FRONT: With slight pressure, palm-circle in a clockwise direction around Ren-12. Hard-press and circle Ren-6, Ren-12 and Ren-17 on the centre line of the body.

ON YOUR ARMS: Gua sha or thumb-press down the lung, heart ruler, and heart rivers on the inside of the arm. Knead any areas of tightness or tension you find, especially around the root regions.

ON YOUR LEGS: Thumb-press or use a Gua sha tool to scrape up the pancreas and down the stomach river systems in your lower leg. Check for any areas of soreness or tightness, and gently knead those areas. Especially check the root *shu* areas in these river systems on your lower leg, at St-36 and St-41, and Pa-9 and Pa-5. Press and knead the area around Kd-3 and Kd-4 at your ankle.

ON YOUR HANDS: Do the Hand Circulation sequence in chapter 13. Press and knead the following areas if sore: Zone 1- lung (F–H), heart (G); zone 2 – liver (K), stomach, pancreas (J), large intestine (K–I); zone 3 – kidney (M).

ON YOUR FEET: Do the Foot Circulation sequence in chapter 13. Use your fingers or a Gua sha tool. Press and knead Kd-1 at the base of the little toe. Also hard-press zone 2 – lung and heart (E–G); zone 3 – kidney (I); and stomach and pancreas (H).

GINGER FOOT SOAK: Use a foot soak to improve circulation and add warming agents to the water. Boil water with 50g (1.7oz) of sliced ginger (about the size of your thumb), and take it off the heat when you smell the ginger aroma. Let it cool to a lower temperature, then it is ready to use in the soak.

HEAT YOUR FEET

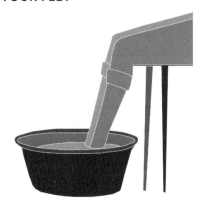

Using a hot foot bath to regularly soak your feet is something that is part of Chinese culture, and this is one of the techniques I used in my clinic in North Africa for many years. We had one of the rooms devoted to hot foot baths, where patients would soak their feet in buckets with soothing Chinese herbs. The root *shu* regions on your feet, ankles, and lower legs mean that this is less about making you warm (and not at all about detoxifying) and more about increasing blood circulation all over your body.

You can buy electric foot bath devices, but here are instructions if you wish to do it the more natural way:

- Your equipment consists of a big bottle or flask of very hot water, another of cold water (unless you are next to a source of running water), a blanket, a towel, any herb/spice/oils to add, a thermometer (preferably infrared), a plastic sheet or tray, and a tub large enough to comfortably lie your feet in.

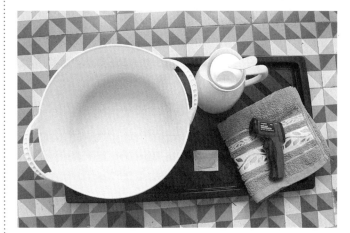

- Put the plastic sheet or tray under the bucket and then fill the bucket only enough to submerge your toes with hot water. Combine hot with cold water so that the temperature is tolerably hot. If you wish, herbs, spices, oils can be added. Place your feet in the bucket, and adjust the water temperature until comfortable.
- Put one foot on the other, and move your feet to one side of the tub. Now pour in more hot (and some cold) water on the other side of the tub so that it covers your ankles (or higher if your tub is tall). The water temperature should be 38–45°C (100–113°F), and it should feel hot but not too hot that you cannot submerge your feet. This is where an infrared thermometer is useful, as you can use it from a distance.

- Once the desired heat has been reached, either cover the bottom part of your body with the blanket or have the blanket on your lap. As the water temperature gradually drops, use the bottle of hot water to top up the bucket (but remember to move your feet to the side as before). Then repeat this sequence for 15–30 minutes, or until you feel that you are sweating.
- Once you have finished, lift your feet out and onto the towel and then dry them. Once you are dressed, lie down and rest for 20–30 minutes.
- Foot soaks can be done daily and at any time. Many people benefit from taking a foot bath in the evenings before bed.

Herbal bags specially made for soaking are available, or make your own by adding ingredients like apple cider vinegar, rice vinegar, Epsom salts, mugwort, ginger, safflower, cinnamon, orange peel, peppermint, lavender oil or rosemary oil, to name but a few.

CAUTION: Do not soak if you suffer from circulatory or blood vessel disorders, impaired sensation (neuropathy), have a pacemaker or electrical implants, have swelling in your feet or legs, varicose veins, any open injuries, or rashes or sores on your feet or legs.

Caution, too, for children, pregnant women, and anyone with diabetes, who may need to either avoid foot baths, or seek medical advice before starting them (see the Diabetes section for more information).

Do not take a food bath straight after meals, allow an hour for digestion.

A sudden increase in blood circulation can cause dizziness during your foot bath. If that happens, remove your feet immediately and lie down. To avoid any incidents, remember to move your feet to the side when pouring

in hot water into the other side. Check the temperature carefully before submerging your feet.

ON YOUR EARS: Cover your whole ear by doing the Ear Circulation sequence in chapter 13, either with a Gua sha tool or your fingers. Pay particular attention to zone 1 (A–C), and press and circle the support region, *shenmen* (1).

Exercise Therapy

Follow exercises 1–5 of the Five Qualities of Nature stretches (see p. 101 ff.). Ideally, do the sequence daily and without exertion. Do any of the supplementary exercises in the General Weakness section.

Lifestyle Therapy

1. It is very important to dress appropriately for the season and weather, keeping warm, especially around the lower back and abdomen. If it feels comfortable, use a heat source, such as a hot water bottle or heat pad, to maintain warmth.
2. It is essential to take gentle regular exercise to regulate your circulation but nothing more until you regain your energy reserves. Do not push yourself unless really necessary. When you feel tired, stop.
3. Try to minimize *yang*-type physical activity, such as jogging, running, aerobic exercise, martial arts, boxing, team or ball sports, or weight training. And instead choose more *yin*-type physical activity, such as yoga, walking, Pilates, stretching, tai chi or qigong, or gardening.
4. Rest is important. The force that drives your body to be active is not strong enough, so if you try to behave as if there is nothing wrong and try to do many things, the problem will be exacerbated, and you will be creating a negative spiral.

Yin Weakness

Signs and Symptoms

Lower backache; sweating at night; dizziness; dry mouth at night; dull headache at the back of your head; vertigo; tinnitus; poor memory; deafness; thirsty; sore back; aching in your bones; dark, scanty urine; constipation; strong dreams; dry cough; and feeling worse in the evenings.

Can Include or Lead to

Insomnia, migraines, high blood pressure, glaucoma, diabetes, tremors, hypochondriac pain, chronic gastritis, gastric neurosis, recurrent lumbago, anxiety, deafness, and impaired hearing.

Common Causes

Emotional stress; overwork; too much sexual activity; long-term worrying; a stressful, busy life; a chronic illness; lack of routine; going to bed late; playing computer games, or using a computer for extended periods.

An Explanation

With a busy lifestyle, it can be relatively easy for the breath pattern to show an impairment, and what often happens is that the *yin* motion is unable to provide an effective counterweight to the motion of *yang*.

Yin can be impaired because of the presence of long-standing internal heat, and whether akin to a gentle simmer or a full-blasting furnace, it will over time burn up and hinder the motion of *yin*. This heat commonly develops from an obstruction pattern resulting from overwork, stress, or unresolved emotional issues.

When *yin* is exhausted, the *yang* motion cannot be contained, as it would be in a balanced system. This means that hot, agitated signs of *yang* can appear in your body, especially when the breath motion of the day moves into its *yin* phase in the evening and at night. This is when *yin* is supposed

to be the dominant motion and signs and symptoms of *yang* become clearly evident.

In order to restore the balance of *yin*, changes in eating habits and lifestyle often have to be made to reduce any overstimulation and direct sources of heat.

Food Therapy

Dietary Factors That Can Worsen Yin Weakness

- Hot or warm-natured foods, especially those that are pungent, bitter, and sour, including foods such as citrus fruits, cinnamon, cloves, and ginger, lamb, coffee, red wine, and spirits.

  Avoid roasting and deep-frying, as these encourage more heat.

Dietary Factors That Can Improve Yin Weakness

- A wide and varied nourishing diet will help the digestive process and the body's ability to transform food into the five flavours. After being transformed, the nutrition from the salty flavour gets sent down to the kidney system, where it is stored and forms the basis of both the *yin* and *yang* of the body. To help *yin*, it is therefore important to strengthen the stomach and pancreas.

- The diet for General Weakness would form a good basis for this, with its stress on complex carbohydrates and vegetables and only a small amount of high-quality protein. The difference here is the addition of more fruit and high-quality, very nutritious, fatty foods such as dairy products (from a cow, goat, or sheep), which strongly benefit the motion of *yin*.

- The predominance of sweet and sour cooling foods needed to strengthen *yin* can have negative effects; too many cool-natured foods can damage the stomach and pancreas. Ideally, foods should involve more stews and steaming. In addition to food to strengthen, more of an emphasis on high-quality protein and the following foods will help strengthen *yin* motion:

▸ **FRUIT:** Apples, pears, grapes, pineapples, tomatoes, blackberries, strawberries, wolf or goji berries, bananas, and watermelon.

▸ **VEGETABLES:** Peas, spinach, seaweed salad, and asparagus (in moderation—too much asparagus can affect the kidney system).

▸ **GRAINS:** Corn, rice, and wheat, including pasta and noodles.

▸ **LEGUMES, SEEDS, AND NUTS:** High-quality protein and omega 3-rich foods like flax, pumpkin, sunflower and black sesame seeds, walnuts, chestnuts, and kidney-shaped foods, such as black beans and kidney beans.

▸ **MEAT AND SEAFOOD:** Good-quality pork, duck, fish, and shrimps strengthen *yin,* but only when eaten in small amounts (about 10 percent of your diet).

▸ **DRINKS:** Red fruit juice, citrus juice, milk (goat's or sheep's milk is less damp-forming), and homemade fruit smoothies.

▸ **OTHER:** Olive oil, cheese, eggs, omelettes, and a small amount of salty foods, such as miso, sea salt, sauerkraut, or Korean kimchi.

CAUTION: Many people have *yin* weakness inside, but outside have lots of damp (otherwise known as fat). If so, avoid some of the more damp-forming foods and drinks from the above lists. See the section on Damp/Phlegm for more details.

Manual Therapy

ON YOUR HEAD : Scrape over your head as if the Gua sha tool were a comb. Start at the midline at Du-24, and go backwards over your head towards the neck at Du-16, then repeat in parallel lines, moving towards your ears—first go back on one side of your head and then on the other.

ON YOUR BACK: Thumb-press or scrape down the back muscles either side of the spine. Cover the whole area of the back *shu* regions. You will need the help of another person with this.

ON YOUR ABDOMEN: Palm-circle clockwise with both hands on top of each other around your navel for 10 cycles. Repeat several times.

ON YOUR ARMS: Gua sha or thumb-press down the heart and heart ruler rivers on the inside of your arms. Knead and hard-press any areas of tension or tightness that you come across.

ON YOUR LEGS: Thumb-press up to Kd-10 along the kidney river on the inside of your lower leg. Thumb-press or scrape down the stomach river on the outside of your lower leg from St-36 to St-41. Knead and hard-press any areas of tension or tightness that you come across.

ON YOUR HANDS: Do the Hand Circulation sequence in chapter 13. Press and knead the following areas if sore: Zone 1 – lung, heart (F–H); zone 2 – stomach, pancreas, liver (K–J); zone 3 – kidney (M).

ON YOUR FEET: Do the Foot Circulation sequence in chapter 13. Use either Gua sha or your fingers. Press and knead the following if sore: Zone 3 – kidney, liver/spleen, stomach, and pancreas (J–H).

ON YOUR EARS: Do the Ear Circulation sequence in chapter 13. Use either Gua sha or your fingers. Press and knead the following if sore: Zone 1 – especially A and B; support region – *shenmen.*

Exercise Therapy

Follow exercises 1–5 of the Five Qualities of Nature stretches (see p. 101 ff.). Ideally, repeat the stretches on a daily basis, especially exercise 4, which strengthens the kidney system and can help rebalance the yin motion.

Lifestyle Therapy

1. Listen to your body. If it is telling you that it has had enough, do not ignore it. It is very easy to push yourself for all sorts of reasons, whether at work, home, or study, but if you are tired, then to preserve your *yin*, you have to rest.
2. When *yin* is weak, it often helps to reduce all sources of stimulation. This means getting serious (at least temporarily) about shutting down the computer, switching off your mobile phone, and avoiding media of any kind. You may gasp with horror at being disconnected from the 21st century, but these activities have a very strong draining effect on *yin*, especially when they are part of your daily habits.
3. Note also that some medical drugs, such as nonsteroidal anti-inflammatories, can damage the *yin* motion of the stomach system when taken regularly.

Blood Circulation Weakness

Signs and Symptoms

Pale lips, dizziness, numb arms or legs, blurred vision, "floaters" in your vision, insomnia and difficulty falling asleep, poor memory, muscular weakness, muscle cramp, headaches, weak nails, painful or light periods, and dry eyes, hair, and skin.

Can Include or Lead to

A whole range of conditions, most notably anaemia, neuroses, dysmenorrhea, amenorrhea, sleepwalking, and mental instability.

Common Causes

A diet lacking in nourishment for blood; overexercise; heavy bleeding, especially during childbirth; anxiety; worrying over things you cannot change; going to bed late; too much watching television, looking at a computer screen, or playing video games.

An Explanation

For clarity, the pattern "blood circulation weakness" is not referring to an actual physical lack of blood in your blood vessels. The same quantity of blood is present as normal in your body, but it is the quality that is different; it is this quality that has been weakened. Basically, the water that is flowing in the river is not adequate to provide nutrients to the farmlands around it.

One of the systems implicated in circulation weakness of this kind is the lung system, which through its expansion and contraction motion of breathing brings force to the movement of blood. Another is the heart system, which through its rhythmic beat gives it its timing. The stomach, pancreas, and digestive process, in combination with the lung system, allow your body to extract what it needs to nourish blood from the food you consume and the air you breathe. The liver system is where the stores of blood are replenished. Weakness in any one of these can have a ripple effect on how strong the force of blood is.

If there is not much force to your blood circulation, it can nourish only the areas of your body close to where it is created and stored. Any parts that are farther away, such as your head, hands, and feet, can become prone to malnourishment and, hence, sometimes show symptoms like dizziness, numbness, and cramp.

Not all circulation signs and symptoms are due to weakness, however. Cold hands and feet, for example, are more likely to be an obstruction pattern blocking the smooth flow of circulation to the extremities than they are to be a weakness.

In order to strengthen blood circulation, changes usually have to be made to dietary habits to include simpler, more nutritious meals, and also changes to lifestyle habits so that your body has time to rest and rejuvenate.

Food Therapy

Dietary Factors That Can Worsen Blood Circulation Weakness

- Warm or hot foods that are also bitter or pungent, such as cinnamon and coffee, have a drying effect on body fluids and can weaken blood circulation.
- Sugary foods, foods with chemical additives, and foods containing high amounts of saturated fats can adversely affect the liver and pancreas systems, and thus, by definition, blood circulation.
- Spices like dry ginger, pepper, and cinnamon, and drinks like black tea, coffee (decaffeinated included), hot chocolate, energy drinks, soft drinks, and strong alcohol can all have a heating effect on your body and weaken circulation.

Dietary Factors That Can Improve Blood Circulation Weakness

- Ideally, a lightly cooked diet consisting of neutral foods that are sweet to build up the pancreas system and sour for the liver system should be followed. Vegetables should form the main part of your diet, especially those high in folic acid, such as dark leafy greens and broccoli. Support this with complex carbohydrates, such as rice and lentils or other strengthening grains or legumes. There is a stronger focus here on high-quality protein, such as meat, seafood, eggs, nuts, and seeds.
- The natural colour of foods sometimes plays an important role in how they react in the body. This is particularly true of blood-enriching foods. Dark red and dark green are the key colours of fruit and vegetables for strengthening blood.
- Many of the following foods strengthen blood:
  - **FRUIT:** Many naturally red fruits, such as red apples, grapes, cherries, wolfberries, and plums, and also dried apricots, dried figs, prunes, lychees, and coconut. Seasonal fruit is preferable.
  - **VEGETABLES:** All green leafy vegetables, such as spinach, cabbage, and broccoli; naturally red (ish) vegetables, such as carrots and beetroot; and seaweed and fennel. Preferably fresh and not frozen.
  - **GRAINS:** Rice, porridge (oatmeal), oats, and millet.
  - **HERBS AND SPICES:** Parsley and watercress.
  - **LEGUMES, SEEDS, AND NUTS:** Lentils, mung beans, black sesame seeds, pumpkin seeds, and sunflower seeds.
  - **MEAT AND SEAFOOD:** High-quality (organic or chemical-free) animal protein, such as chicken; beef; liver; shellfish, such as mussels, oysters, and clams; sardines; crab; eel; and octopus.
  - **DRINKS:** Small amounts of some alcohol, such as stout and red wine; rosehip tea; hibiscus tea; red grape juice; and water at room temperature or above.
  - **OTHERS:** Bee pollen and royal jelly; soups, stocks or broths; eggs; and fermented foods, such as sauerkraut, kimchi, yogurt, and miso.

Manual Therapy

As for any weakness pattern, the intervention should be *yin*-based (more gentle), and any *yang*-based (stronger) treatments should be avoided unless the pattern is one of a combination of overflow and weakness.

First, do the Dry Towel Friction sequence detailed in General Weakness.

ON YOUR HEAD : Scrape over your head as if the Gua sha tool were a comb. Start at the midline at Du-24, and go backwards over your head towards the neck at Du-16, then repeat in parallel lines, moving towards your ears; go back on one side of your head and then on the other.

ON YOUR BACK: Gua sha or thumb-press down the muscles of the back on either side of the spine, and knead any areas of tension afterwards. Cover all of the back *shu* regions.

ON YOUR ARMS: Encourage circulation by following the river systems in your arms. Thumb-press or use a Gua sha tool (gently) down the three *yin* rivers to your wrist, one at a time, and also up the three *yang* rivers to your shoulder.

ON YOUR LEGS: As above with the arm, encourage circulation by following the river systems. Thumb-press or use a Gua sha tool (gently) up the three *yin* rivers to your groin, and down the three *yang* rivers to your ankle, one at a time.

ON YOUR HANDS: Do the Hand Circulation sequence in chapter 13. Knead any sore areas, including zone 1 – heart (G); zone 2 – liver, pancreas, stomach, and large intestine (K–I).

ON YOUR FEET: Do the Foot Circulation sequence in chapter 13. Also knead zone 2 – heart (G); zone 3 – liver/spleen and pancreas (J-H), if sore.

Use a regular foot soak to improve circulation and add soothing oils like lavender (see *Yang Weakness* for more information).

ON YOUR EARS: Do the Ear Circulation sequence in chapter 13. Use either a Gua sha tool or your fingers. Press and knead the following if sore: All of the main systems involved are sections A and B in zone 1.

Exercise Therapy

Follow exercises 1–5 of the Five Qualities of Nature stretches (see p. 101 ff.). Do the sequence daily, slowly and methodically. It is also very important not to overdo the exercises as this can be counter-productive.

Lifestyle Therapy

1. Relaxation and rest are as good as any treatment for this pattern, and should not be underestimated. Time should be found in even the busiest of schedules to relax and rest.
2. Try to stabilize your day-to-day activities and follow the natural breath pattern of the day. For example, make sure you eat and sleep at the same time every day. See chapter 10 for more information on following the daily breath pattern.

19

Patterns of Overflow

Stagnation

Signs and Symptoms
Feeling bloated, tight chest, depressed, irritable, easy to upset, burping, wind, nausea, a lump in the throat, tense and stressed, irregular periods, swollen and painful breasts, premenstrual tension, muscle tension in the neck and back, and pain that comes and goes.

Can Include or Lead to
A whole host of conditions, but especially those of pain, depression, high blood pressure, migraines, menstrual disorders such as premenstrual syndrome, endometriosis, amenorrhea and dysmenorrhea, indigestion, gastritis, hepatitis, neurosis, and chronic fatigue syndrome.

Common Causes
Emotional stress, especially when emotions are repressed; frustration that has been building up; resentment; overwork; work stress; lack of regular exercise; and bad posture.

An Explanation
The motion of breath should move smoothly and harmoniously with the circulation patterns around the body, so that all the cogs that make up the various systems are turning in the right directions.

Invariably something turns up somewhere in the complicated interactions among the systems of your body to interrupt the process and form a stagnation pattern. When stagnation happens, it can be due to an obstruction in the flow of blood caused by an injury. Any kind of accident, injury, twist, sprain, strain, or muscle-pull can block the flow of blood and lead to the build-up of pressure from behind. This usually manifests as bruising, blood clotting, and pain.

Often, injuries "heal" without this obstruction pattern within them being resolved. When this happens, despite a normal appearance, pain can continue, or the area can gradually become weaker due to the inability of the circulation to properly reach the affected tissue.

This is a very common pattern in continuing chronic pain at the site of an old injury. It is also often complicated by the addition of the climates, and especially wind, cold, or damp, which can lodge in the area because it has become a backwater, disconnected from the main circulation. This was looked at in detail in chapter 8.

Stagnation also appears in the absence of any injury and can be caused by emotional stress, which may build up over time and fester in the body, manifesting in tissue and blocking the smooth flow. This is often the origin of features like cysts, fibroids, and masses in the abdomen, as repressed emotions find a place to express themselves within the body.

When stagnation appears, it can often be accompanied by agitation, heat, and pain. The situation is not unlike the road system of a major

149

city. Outside of rush hour, the cars move freely, but when commuters all leave work at the same time and head home, the traffic builds up. A traffic accident can then create major hold-ups, whereby the cars in the midst of the jam have their engines running and honk their horns and drivers become thoroughly frustrated.

Stagnation can be very much about getting stuck and agitated. Physically tight muscles can cause pain and discomfort but, mentally, emotions can also get stuck, and it can be difficult to "snap out of it" when irritable, stressed, or depressed.

In order to lessen stagnation of an emotional nature, an awareness of the importance of letting out emotions is essential. Unexpressed emotions tend to fester and deepen any stagnation. Changes in dietary habits also often have to be made, especially when the digestive systems are involved, and also a commitment to regular exercise, which will boost circulation patterns.

Food Therapy

Dietary Factors That Can Worsen Stagnation

- Overeating and an irregular diet involving comfort eating or skipping meals will weaken the stomach system and worsen any stagnation.
- Some foods are harder to digest than others, and with a stagnation pattern, they are best reduced or avoided altogether. The following foods are common examples:
  - ▸ Oversalted, processed, or sweetened foods and foods high in saturated fats and oils, such as tinned meat, vegetables, or ready-to-eat meals, cream, cheese, sandwich spreads, red meat, pizza, French fries, nuts, and margarine, and rich, greasy food such as lamb, beef, and creamy or cheesy sauces.
  - ▸ Some people with this pattern crave spicy, hot food because eating it will temporarily move circulation and make them feel better. This is not a good idea, however, as obstructions tend to generate heat. If hot

food is then added to this heat, the pattern may worsen. For this reason, it is best to avoid any hot spices like chilli, cayenne, Tabasco sauce, and pepper.
  - ▸ Also for this reason, it is preferable to avoid coffee and other sources of caffeine, fizzy soft drinks, fruit-flavoured soft drinks, and alcohol.

Dietary Factors That Can Improve Stagnation

Certain eating routines can make a difference in reducing stagnation when connected to the stomach and pancreas systems:

- Eating less is one of the most important strategies. Ideally, your stomach should be only two-thirds full after meals.
- Eating calmly, without distractions, and chewing food well will ease its passage through the body and reduce the likelihood of a stagnation pattern.
- A very important point for people with a tendency towards stagnation is to avoid being too fixated on diet. Part of the imbalance of this pattern is the tendency to stick unwaveringly to a set of instructions. It is, however, important to be relaxed about any change in diet and not be rigid about what you can or cannot eat. The resulting stress of worrying about your diet may mean you end up with more of the same pattern you are trying to relieve!
- A strong digestive process can help stabilize the liver system, so food that nourishes the stomach and pancreas systems as detailed in General Weakness will also help this pattern. The focus of your diet should be on grains and vegetables, supported by small amounts of protein. Pungent spices can be added to encourage the movement of circulation.
- The following foods can be of great benefit in removing Stagnation:
  - ▸ **FRUIT:** Grapefruit, citrus peel, peaches, cherries, plums, and hawthorn berries.

- **VEGETABLES:** Watercress, leeks, onions, beetroot, carrots, garlic, radishes, cabbage, turnips, aubergines (eggplants), cauliflower, broccoli, Brussels sprouts, and celery.
- **HERBS AND SPICES:** Turmeric, basil, cardamom, marjoram, cumin, horseradish, rosemary, cloves, caraway, coriander, and chives.
- **LEGUMES, SEEDS, AND NUTS:** Chestnuts, pine nuts, and black sesame seeds.
- **MEAT AND SEAFOOD:** Prawns, crab, and shrimps.
- **DRINKS:** Red wine, fennel tea, jasmine tea, aniseed tea, dill tea, and chamomile tea.
- **OTHER:** Apple cider vinegar.

Manual Therapy

Unlike patterns of weakness, patterns of overflow require more of a *yang* intervention. This means that the treatment is stronger, more pressured, and designed to break blockages and get the circulation moving again.

The location of the treatment is related to the river system involved, and the obvious place to start in establishing this is to identify which of the rivers are located close to any places of obstruction. The nearest rivers have to be involved in some way, whether directly or indirectly.

These are the rivers to identify if there is any tightness or soreness along them and to press or knead these areas.

ON YOUR HEAD: Hard-press or scrape with the Gua sha tool with short up and down strokes, along the occiput area, including Gb-12, Gb-20, Du-16, and Bl-10.

ON YOUR BACK: Wherever the obstruction pattern is, the back is involved in some way, so it is a useful place to explore. Look for areas that feel different with touch. Perhaps they feel tighter or sore, or look different. In general, scrape or thumb- or finger-press down the

muscle areas on either side of the spine, and knead any sore areas. Look at all of the back *shu* regions, and feel for any reactivity.

ON YOUR FRONT: Gua sha down the sternum, especially around Ren-17, and expect *sha* to appear.

ON YOUR LEGS: Thumb-press along the *yang* rivers (stomach, gallbladder and bladder) down the whole leg. Knead any tight areas you find, especially at Bl-40, St-36, and Gb-34.

ON YOUR ARMS: Thumb-press up the *yang* rivers (large intestine, triple burner and small intestine) to your shoulder and knead any sore areas.

ON YOUR HANDS: Do the Hand Circulation sequence in chapter 13. Use your fingers or a Gua sha tool. Also knead zone 1 – chest, lung, and heart (F–H); zone 2 – liver, pancreas, and stomach (K–J); and any sore areas.

ON YOUR FEET: Do the Foot Circulation sequence in chapter 13. Use your fingers or a Gua sha tool. Also press and knead the following, if sore: Zone 2 – lung and heart (E–G); zone 3 – liver/spleen, gallbladder, stomach, and pancreas (J–H).

VINEGAR FOOT SOAK: Use a foot bath regularly to help improve circulation, and add ingredients like apple cider vinegar or rice vinegar. You can use one tablespoon for every litre of water. See Heat Your Feet in *Yang* Weakness for more information on how to do foot soaks.

ON YOUR EARS: Do the Ear Circulation sequence in chapter 13, either with Gua sha or use your fingers to knead. Look for any sore, reactive areas but, in particular, check the whole of zone 1; zone 2 – cervical, thoracic, and lumbar-sacral areas (D–F); zone 3 – head area (G); support region – *shenmen* (1).

Exercise Therapy

Do exercises 1–5 of the Five Qualities of Nature on a daily basis, preferably after waking. Especially useful are exercises 2, 3, and 5 (see p. 101 ff.).

Lifestyle Therapy

1. Emotions play a major part in this condition, and the ability to release or express repressed emotions or remove the cause of these emotions can often have a dramatic effect. This could be anything from confiding in someone to formal therapy.

2. Lack of exercise is a major contributing factor to stagnation, so it is essential to do regular exercise. This may mean leaving the car at home and walking, swimming, cycling, dancing, running—whatever is practicable and enjoyable.

3. Some very tense people prefer to play equally tense sports such as squash—and end up no less tense afterwards than before. It is important, therefore, that there is a sense of relaxation in the exercise or the effects will not be beneficial.

4. In general, movement and warmth help move circulation. So gentle exercise and stretching and avoiding the cold are usually important in maintaining the natural flow in the body.

5. Stress and overwork can often be unavoidable but, in order to improve this pattern, it is necessary to adapt your life or working life to lessen them. This can often appear impossible in the busy life most of us lead, but there are always things that can be changed if you have the desire and will to change them.

Damp/Phlegm

Signs and Symptoms

Heavy limbs, heavy head, tiredness, reduced appetite and weak digestion, frequently blocked nose, persistent cough, a stuffy feeling in the chest, feeling bloated, being overweight, inability to concentrate, dull aches in joints, swellings and lumps, muzzy or dull headaches, dizziness, ringing in your ear(s), a yellow colour around the mouth, and urine might be cloudy.

Can Include or Lead to

Obesity, arthritis, gastroenteritis, chronic gastritis, chronic colitis, irritable bowel syndrome, Crohn's disease, chronic bronchitis, rhinitis, sinusitis, asthma, bronchiectasis, oedema in your legs and ankles, urinary tract infection, cystitis, urinary tract or kidney or gallbladder stones, prostate disorders, numbness, bone deformities and nodules.

Common Causes

A diet high in processed, fatty foods, exposure to the weather, living in a damp environment, repeated lung infections, emotional stress, over-thinking, overstudying, or a long chronic illness.

An Explanation

Body fluids are essential to ensure our bodies are properly lubricated. Sometimes, however, your body overproduces and accumulates excess body fluids in the form of endogenous damp. This is like a moist field rich in nutrients becoming flooded with water from a nearby river, and as it is unable to drain the excess water away, remaining muddy and boggy.

An excess of damp is often caused by an impairment in the digestive process. The stomach and pancreas systems are unable to process and digest food efficiently, usually as a result of a rich diet of fried, processed, damp-forming foods. The greater the strain on these two digestive systems to sort through the food material, the greater the likelihood that they will generate damp and store it in the form of fat.

As we have seen before, damp is a climate pattern and can also come in from outside the body via the mouth and nose, along with wind. This could manifest as a cold, flu, headache, or even a lung infection. It can also come from being in a damp environment, staying in wet clothes, or not drying wet hair.

Damp is a sticky, thick substance, more like glue than water, and it can be very difficult to get rid of. Phlegm often develops from dampness, and has a tendency to thicken and harden with heat. Both can linger in your body, sometimes slowing down or blocking essential functions, and can collect in your joints, causing pain. This is often in the background of medical conditions like high cholesterol, heart disease, and obesity.

The most effective way to help remove damp and phlegm is to remove the source. For most people, this can be addressed through their dietary habits, but it could also be simple solutions in lifestyle, such as not sleeping with wet hair.

Dietary Factors That Can Worsen Damp/Phlegm

- Overeating and eating late at night can weaken the stomach system and lead to stagnation in the digestive process.
- Excess drinking during meal times can often literally flood the stomach system and slow it down. It is then less likely to process food efficiently and more likely to accumulate damp.
- Most of the foods that help generate damp in your body are nutrition-dense, so much so that the body can become overwhelmed with too much nutrition at once. Fruit juice is one example of this. Many fruits combine sweet and sour flavours, and this alone can have a dampening effect on the body, and a glass of fruit juice, which usually contains the juice of several pieces of fruit, concentrates this still further. Normally, the stomach and pancreas systems cannot process this level of concentration efficiently and, as a result, it is often stored as damp.
- The following foods are considered highly nutritious and, therefore, damp/phlegm-forming when overconsumed:
  - ▸ **FRUIT:** Bananas, oranges, avocados, and too many dried fruits like dates and figs
  - ▸ **VEGETABLES:** Raw vegetables
  - ▸ **GRAINS:** Wheat, bread, many kinds of cereal bars, and oats, especially when served with milk and sugar

  - ▸ **MEAT:** Naturally fatty meat, such as pork, lamb, duck, and beef
  - ▸ **LEGUMES, SEEDS, AND NUTS:** Roasted peanuts
  - ▸ **DRINKS:** Beer; concentrated fruit juice, especially orange and tomato; milkshakes; yogurt drinks; fruit-flavoured soft drinks; and cow's milk.
  - ▸ **OTHER:** Foods high in saturated and hydrogenated fats, deep-fried food, and any greasy foods; all dairy produce (from a cow), including cream, butter and spreads, cheese, and ice cream; also mayonnaise, tofu, white sugar, yeast, concentrated sweeteners, processed foods with artificial flavours (often packaged food targeted at children and usually claiming to be "vitamin-enriched"); milk chocolate; eggs; and virtually all junk food.

Dietary Factors That Can Reduce Damp/Phlegm

- All food should be cooked and served warm.
- The diet essentially needs to strengthen digestion as in General Weakness, as fully functioning stomach and pancreas systems will help prevent damp from collecting in the first place. As many of the grains tend to be sweet-natured, overconsumption can aggravate damp, so be cautious not to consume them in excess. Most of the diet should be composed of vegetables, with a reduced amount of grains and small amounts of animal protein.
- In addition to the foods that strengthen, some warming and drying foods are beneficial, especially if also sweet, bitter, or pungent. These have the welcome effects of drying up or expelling the damp/phlegm and consist of many of the following foods:
  - ▸ **FRUITS:** Damp – lemons, pears, cherries, grapes, cranberries, and papayas. Phlegm – persimmons, grapefruit, orange peel, apple peel, and tangerine peel.

▸ **VEGETABLES:** Cooked vegetables, such as celery, lettuce, pumpkins, artichokes, turnips, button mushrooms, garlic, onions, broad beans, radishes, and seaweed

▸ **GRAINS:** Dry grains, such as barley, corn, rye, rye crispbread; also rice, which encourages the production of urine and helps rid the body of excess damp

▸ **HERBS AND SPICES:** Watercress and drying and warming spices, such as black pepper, parsley, horseradish (wasabi), cloves, nutmeg, and mustard

▸ **LEGUMES, SEEDS, AND NUTS:** Almonds, walnuts, kidney beans, and aduki beans

▸ **MEAT AND SEAFOOD:** Small amounts of mackerel, anchovies, clams, chicken, turkey, and white fish

▸ **DRINKS:** Barley water, chamomile tea, jasmine tea, and green tea

Manual Therapy

While damp and phlegm, like all climates, can attach anywhere and be treated like an obstruction pattern, they are also closely connected with the stomach and pancreas systems. This is the focus of the treatment in this section.

ON YOUR BACK: Scrape down the lung, pancreas, and liver back *shu* regions on the upper and mid back. These are not areas you can reach yourself, so you will need the help of another person to do it.

ON YOUR FRONT: Finger- or thumb-press down the midline of the abdomen. Knead any sore areas, especially around Ren-4, Ren-6 and Ren-12.

ON YOUR ARMS: Thumb-press down the lung river along the upper and lower arms. Press and knead any sore or tense areas around and below Lu-5.

ON YOUR LEGS: Use a Gua sha tool to scrape down the front of your thigh. This is the area of Crouching Rabbit and is part of the stomach river system. Thumb-press down the stomach and up the pancreas rivers on your lower leg. Press and knead any sore areas, including the root shu regions Pa-9 and St-36, and the junction region, St-40.

ON YOUR HANDS: Do the Hand Circulation sequence in chapter 13. Use your fingers or a Gua sha tool. Knead any sore areas, especially in zone 2 – stomach, pancreas, and intestine areas (K-I). Also check the thenar eminence area at Lu-10 (N-I), and knead if sore.

ON YOUR FEET: Do the Foot Circulation Sequence in chapter 13. Use your fingers or a Gua sha tool. Check the following areas and knead if sore: Zone 1 – lung (E-G); zone 2 – stomach, pancreas, liver/spleen (J-H); zone 4 – small intestine and large intestine (K-M). Also press and knead, or scrape with a Gua sha tool, around the root *shu* and source regions of the pancreas and stomach in your foot. These include St-41, St-42, St-43, St-44, and St-45, and Pa-1, Pa-2, Pa-3, and Pa-4.

ORANGE PEEL FOOT SOAK: Add 15–30g of orange or tangerine peel to hot water and boil it for about 10 minutes. Pour the boiled water and tangerine peel into the footbath. Add an appropriate amount of cold water to comfortably start soaking your feet. See Heat Your Feet in *Yang* Weakness for more information on how to do foot soaks.

ON YOUR EARS: Do the Ear Circulation sequence in chapter 13. Use either your fingers or a Gua sha tool. Check the following areas and knead if sore: B & C in zone 1.

Exercise Therapy

Do exercises 1–5 of the Five Qualities of Nature stretches daily (see p. 101 ff.). Exercises 1, 2, and 5 strengthen the lung, pancreas, and liver systems, all of which are strongly implicated with damp and can thus be supported.

Lifestyle Therapy

1. Regular gentle exercise improves circulation and helps your body process dampness.
2. Avoid any bad habits, such as not drying your hair after washing it and going to bed with wet or damp hair. The damp can easily enter your body via the head and neck.
3. Watch where you sit outside. Grass is a great place to picnic on a sunny day, but it retains moisture, and can happily pass that moisture on to your clothes and into your body.
4. In general, warmth and dryness are important factors to combat damp, so stay warm and dry as much as you can.
5. Smoking is a direct cause of phlegm and heat in the lung system, and the only way to prevent this from building up is to stop completely. So if you suffer from phlegm-type symptoms and smoke, better stop.
6. The bitterness and coldness of antibiotics can damage the pancreas and stomach systems when these medications are taken regularly. Much of the bacteria being targeted by antibiotics is beneficial to the digestive process and enhances your body's immunity. When damaged, your digestion is much more likely to accumulate damp/phlegm and digestive issues.

Heat

Signs and Symptoms

MILD: Headache at the temples, behind the eyes, on one side of the head, or only at weekends; migraine; dizziness; ringing in the ears; insomnia; irritability; and a tendency to get angry easily; eyes and face may appear red, and urine may be dark.

SEVERE: Feeling hot, thirsty, skin conditions with red eruptions, skin hot to touch, a bitter taste, a sore throat, dark and scanty urine, dizziness, headache, a flushed face, agitation, a tendency to get angry easily, tinnitus, bloating, wind, constant hunger, bleeding gums, and sour regurgitation.

Can Include or Lead to

Vertigo, ear and hearing problems, Ménière's disease, menopausal problems, chronic hepatitis, gastritis, ventricular and duodenal ulcers, stomatitis, chronic cholecystitis, high blood pressure, hyperthyroidism, halitosis, gingivitis, diabetes, eczema, dermatitis, acne, insomnia, asthma, bronchiectasis, cystitis, and conjunctivitis.

Common Causes

Long-term repressed emotions, in particular anger or frustration over a long period of time; stress; overwork; a diet with too much greasy, fried food; smoking; drinking too much alcohol; being overexposed to a hot environment; and catching a cold that never went away.

An Explanation

Heat can appear from a variety of sources. It can develop over time, often as a consequence of a strong imbalance in breath motion, whereby, without an effective counterbalance from *yin*, there is a tendency for the *yang* motion to dominate. The relationship here is not unlike that of a car engine and its coolant system. When you drive the engine heats up, but the amount of heat is regulated by the water in the radiator. If the car is not well maintained, however, the water levels might drop, and the next time you go for a drive there is nothing to stop the engine temperature from rising. The car might then sputter to a halt in a cloud of steam.

Yin is often impaired, due to heat, which can be generated from stagnation or from an inappropriate diet of heating, fatty foods. There is then a counterflow motion as *yang* rises, like hot steam, all the way through the body up to your head, and as a result often causes symptoms in the top part of the body, such as headaches and dizziness.

Heat can also come from obstruction —in fact, this is the most common cause—and with it, the irony that a major cause of heat obstruction in your body is from a transformed cold pattern; hence, heat can come from cold. In general, though, obstruction can also be the result of factors such as stress, improper eating habits, and overwork, which interrupt particular river systems and lead to muscle tightness and discomfort. The longer the blockage has been going on, the more sustained and widespread the heat, which can rise upwards causing conditions such as insomnia, headaches, and a bitter taste.

Heat can also be generated from diet. Too many hot-natured, oily, processed foods can damage the *yin* motion of the stomach system. *Yin* Weakness can generate warmth, which, over time, becomes heat, and can cause symptoms such as constant hunger, nausea, thirst, and bleeding gums.

Colds, flu, and other lung-related conditions can also generate heat. This heat can be confined to the lung system, as in a barking cough or asthma, or it can spread and go deeper into the layers of the body and cause conditions such as dry constipation and abdominal pain. This is the pattern of external climates attaching to areas that lack proper circulation and remaining there.

The obvious solution for too much heat is to use a counterbalance, and dietary changes can be made to add more cold- or cool-natured foods and reduce those that are hot or warm. Any imbalance between the motions of *yin* and *yang* has to be addressed, or the same process will happen again. This usually involves dietary changes and self-treatment, as detailed here and in the *Yin* Weakness section.

Food Therapy

Dietary Factors That Can Worsen Heat

- Overeating creates stagnation and adds to the heat.
- Frying, roasting, or barbecuing foods will increase their heat-producing properties.
- All hot- or warm-natured foods, no matter their individual flavours, will generate heat. The obvious ones to avoid are:
  - **HERBS AND SPICES:** Chillies, cinnamon, ginger, black pepper, salt, garlic, mustard, and horseradish.
  - **LEGUMES, SEEDS, AND NUTS:** Peanuts.
  - **MEAT AND SEAFOOD:** Red meat, especially lamb, veal, shrimps, and prawns.
  - **DRINKS:** Bitter drinks like coffee and tea, especially green tea, and also beer, red wine, and strong alcohol.
  - **OTHER:** Chocolate, heated vegetable oils, cheese, curries, eggs, and creamy food.

Dietary Factors That Can Improve Heat

- An ideal diet to reduce heat should be high in cooling fruits and vegetables. Be very cautious, however, about eating too many cold, raw foods, as they can impair the digestive process and end up causing more heat!
- Cool- or cold-natured foods that are also sweet, bitter, or sour will help reduce heat, such as the following:
  - **FRUIT:** Cool-natured fruits, such as grapefruit, lemons, kiwis, watermelons, pears, bananas, and any tropical fruits.
  - **VEGETABLES:** Cool-natured vegetables, such as asparagus, lettuce, aubergines (eggplants), spinach, cabbage, potatoes, peas, watercress and tomatoes; celery, cucumber and beetroot also encourage urination, which can help reduce heat.
  - **GRAINS:** Millet, rice, barley, and wheat.
  - **LEGUMES, SEEDS, AND NUTS:** Mung beans.
  - **SEAFOOD:** Clams.
  - **DRINKS:** Water with lemon juice, pear juice, elderflower tea, chamomile tea, and peppermint tea.
  - **OTHER:** Tofu and yogurt.

Manual Therapy

ON YOUR HEAD: Using Du-20 as the anchor point, use a Gua sha tool to scrape downwards, using short strokes. Go in several different directions, but always start at Du-20. This covers the Heat *shu* regions on the top of your head.

ON YOUR FRONT: For heat in the chest and arm areas, scrape outwards, above and below your clavicle, and the sides of your neck into your shoulder (the area of Open Basin), downwards from Lu-2 to Lu-1, and the area around *Jianqian*. In the arm, scrape or press and knead the Heat *shu* area around Li-15.

ON YOUR BACK: For heat in the chest area, scrape down Bl-11 and the lung back *shu* region, both of which have strong heat clearing properties.

For general heat, scrape down all of the back *shu* regions on your back, as they are primarily used to treat heat and cold patterns. It is very common for *sha* to appear on your skin and for you to feel the heat emanating from the areas of *sha*. The position of these regions means that another person would need to treat you.

ON YOUR LEGS: For heat in your stomach, scrape down the stomach river in the lower leg, and press and knead the Heat *shu* regions, if tense or sore: St-36, St-37, St-39, and St-41. For heat in your legs, scrape another Heat *shu* region, Bl-40, at the back of your knee. Another technique is to slap the area with the tool to create redness and *sha*.

ON YOUR HANDS: Thumb-press or use a Gua sha tool to scrape downwards on each of your five fingers and thumb. Scrape from the root *shu* regions at the tips (Lu-11, Hr-9, Ht-9, Li-1, Tb-1, and Si-1) to the palm on the front and to the knuckles on the back. Repeat several times. Knead any sore areas especially zone 1 – heart and chest (F-H).

ON YOUR FEET: Thumb-press or use a Gua sha tool to scrape downwards from the root *shu* regions at the tips of the toes in zone 1 (Pa-1, Lv-1, St-45, Gb-44, and Bl-67) to the MTP joints in zone 2 and on the sole of the foot, towards the heel, until you reach zone 5.

ON YOUR EARS: Gua sha down zones 5, 4, and 3 to the end of your ear lobe. Press and knead ear apex (5) at the top of your ear.

Exercise Therapy

Follow exercises 1–5 of the Five Qualities of Nature stretches daily (see p. 101 ff.). Generally strengthening all of the river systems can help reduce heat.

Lifestyle Therapy

1. Heat often does not just appear out of the blue one day; it builds gradually, like a pressure cooker, until one day the lid pops off. Quite often, actions in your life need to change to reduce the likelihood of this. If you suffer from a pattern of heat, it is time to think about making some changes in your life. Smoking and drinking alcohol, stress at work, a simpler, less rich diet—recognize and try to remove some of the reasons behind the heat.

2. There is a strong emotional component to heat, especially when that emotion is being in some way repressed. Smoldering resentment and frustration at being passed over for a job promotion, for example, can quite easily be the pressure increase that pops the lid. It is very important not to let strong emotions like this take hold inside. Usually this means sharing how you feel with family, friends, or people you trust.

Cold

Signs and Symptoms

Severe pain or stiffness, better with warmth and worse with pressure, an aversion to the cold, desire for warm drinks, contraction of tendons, cold arms and legs, thin watery discharges, diarrhoea, and vomiting.

Can Include or Lead to

Joint pain, arthritis, back pain, irritable bowel syndrome, uterus disorders, and prostate problems.

Common Causes

Exposure to the cold; sitting on cold, wet surfaces; a diet of excess cold-natured foods; or long-term illness.

An Explanation

Cold conditions in your body tend to be associated with pain because of the contracting action of cold on muscles, tendons, and body tissues. It can affect any of the river systems, blocking them and lingering in joints and tense muscles.

Cold is one of the climates, and depending on where you are in the world and what environment you live in, can be a major cause of obstruction patterns in your body. Many people have pathogenic cold somewhere in their bodies, which is often stuck in an area of tissue lacking effective circulation (see the discussion of "backwater" in chapter 8), so that your body cannot easily remove it.

Sometimes cold can have a recent origin, such as feeling a chill after being out on a cold winter's day, but other times it relates to an event that happened a long time ago. It could be something as simple as sitting on a cold step or wearing inappropriate clothing, but once cold has entered and your body is not able to remove it, it can stay for life.

I have climbed Mount Fuji in Japan three times—once with my wife, once with my brother-in-law, and once with my sons. Despite scheduling the climb during the stifling heat of summer, each time the temperature at the summit before sunrise dropped to subzero. The first trip with inadequate clothing and equipment was perhaps the coldest experience of my life. It was so cold you had the feeling that it was 50:50 as to which was coming first—freeze to death or sunrise. The body is, however, resilient, and the first rays of light from the east made the cold instantly go away. I was lucky in that this cold experience had no long-term effect on my body, but many people can trace a pain, feeling, disorder, or just some kind of imbalance to an extreme cold event of this kind.

You often know whether cold is part of a pattern of obstruction because of the sharp, contracting pain that can be experienced.

It is easy to dismiss cold as something that will just go away once you heat yourself up, but the ancient Chinese were clear in their appraisal that this cold is not the same as the "temperature" cold. It is not the cold that goes away when you sit in front of an open fire or a warm radiator; this cold is a motion, not just a temperature. It contracts and constricts wherever it is, and once it is attached, the application of heat might not be enough to dislodge it.

Having said that, the most common way to treat cold is by adding warmth—not through "temperature" warmth but strong *yang* treatment on the outside of the body and specific types of food on the inside. Of course, regular warmth can also help in the process.

Food Therapy

Dietary Factors That Can Worsen Cold

- Raw foods, such as salads and fruit, can easily lead to digestive impairment. Fruits should be stewed and all vegetables cooked.
- Cooling foods, such as bananas, grapefruit, persimmons, melons, soya products, tomatoes, watermelons, cucumbers, lettuce, ice cream, and yogurt, will increase cold.

Dietary Factors That Can Improve Cold

- Warming cooking styles, such as roasting, grilling, and cooking with alcohol, will help dispel cold. As *Yang* Weakness is a pattern that is related to cold, much of the dietary advice discussed earlier regarding *Yang* Weakness also applies here. Add more warm and sweet foods, such as:

▸ **FRUIT:** Cherries and lychees.
▸ **VEGETABLES:** Onions, turnips, sweet potatoes, and leeks.
▸ **HERBS AND SPICES:** Ginger, nutmeg, basil, and black pepper.
▸ **MEAT AND SEAFOOD:** Lamb, chicken, anchovies, shrimps, and mussels.
▸ **NUTS:** Chestnuts and walnuts.
▸ **DRINKS:** Wine and strong alcohol (in small quantities).
▸ **OTHER:** Vinegar.

Manual Treatments

To remove the climatic cold that has entered your body, you might think that an obvious part of treatment would be to apply heat, but this is not necessarily the case. Heat will help, but the cold that gets into your body is not temperature-related, as explained above. It is not cold as in zero degrees Centigrade or 32 degrees Fahrenheit but is instead, a motion that holds tissue together tightly. This is the important point about cold, and this is why it can be challenging for your body to remove it.

ON YOUR BACK: The back shu areas on your back are primarily used to remove heat and cold from the core storage systems of your body. This is not only because of the direct connection between these regions and the systems themselves but also because it is the closest and safest exit pathway to the main core of your body.

Let us suppose that cold is stuck in tissue. It is contracted and painful, but you manage to treat it and that cold is removed. It does not disappear in a puff of smoke—Chinese medicine is not about magic; it is about natural processes mirrored in the world around us.

Instead, what happens is that the natural intelligence in your circulation system (*zheng qi*) will try to push it out, as it would with any pathogenic climate, pollutant, or foreign entity. If your treatment were on the front of the body, then you would be encouraging the movement in that direction, and if it were on the back, then in the reverse direction. The path of least resistance is out the back, away from all the storage regions.

While you can thumb-press down the back muscles either side of your spine, and knead any sore areas, including around the *shu* regions, the most efficient and most effective treatment is to scrape down the back with Gua sha. Gua sha was developed as a treatment specifically for situations of this type, so it is always best to start with the most appropriate treatment.

Scrape downwards along the muscles of the back. For obvious reasons, this has to be done on another person or another person on you. The red marks of *sha* may appear. It is best to avoid scraping over the scapula area and directly on the spine as they can be painful areas. Cover all the back *shu* regions.

ON YOUR LEGS: The movement of the *yang* river systems (stomach, gallbladder, and bladder) in your legs is down, towards your feet. With cold patterns, it is important to ensure that the leg rivers are moving freely and there are no impairments that will block them or cause them to be sluggish. This is because it is this downwards motion that the body can use to expel cold, which from its very nature has a descending quality.

Use Gua sha or thumb-press down the stomach, gallbladder, and bladder rivers on your legs. Do each river system separately, and go all the way down to your feet. The Crouching Rabbit region on your quadricep muscles, on the front of your thigh, is a large area that can invariably feel tense and sore due to the frequent use of these powerful muscles. Check there first, and also check the following areas: St-36 and St-40 on the stomach river; Gb-34, Gb-37, and Gb-38 on the gallbladder river; and Bl-58 on the bladder river.

ON YOUR HANDS: Do the Hand Circulation sequence in chapter 13. Use a Gua sha tool, and repeat until you feel the warmth of circulation in your fingers and hand. Knead any sore areas.

ON YOUR FEET: Do the Foot Circulation sequence in chapter 13. Use your fingers or a Gua sha tool, and repeat until you feel warmth in your feet.

Cold is contracting but also descending, so the obvious motion for your body to use to expel cold is one that moves downwards. This is why regular foot treatment is a useful technique for this pattern as it enhances the local circulation of your feet and allows your body to process cold out.

Foot soak therapy can help with this, especially with the addition of warming and moving agents such as ginger. You can follow the instructions for a Ginger Foot Soak in *Yang Weakness*.

ON YOUR EARS: Do the Ear Circulation sequence in chapter 13. Use your fingers or a Gua sha tool. Repeat until you feel warmth in your ears.

Exercise Therapy

Do exercises 1–5 of the Five Qualities of Nature stretches on a regular basis, as these can encourage circulation in the river systems (see p. 101 ff.).

Lifestyle Therapy

1. Wear appropriate clothing, especially during the change in seasons, when wind and cold can easily enter the body.

2. It is important to note that some medical drugs have a cooling effect on the body. Antibiotics, tranquilizers, diuretics, and anaesthetics can often be a source of climatic cold.

Wind

Signs and Symptoms

Sudden onset of dizziness; tiredness; sneezing; nasal discharge or nasal congestion; shivering; colds; itchy eyes, nose, and throat; fever; joint pain; headache; aversion to wind and cold; sudden change of symptoms; skin eruptions; tics, muscle spasms, convulsions, and tremors.

Can Include or Lead to

Common cold, influenza, laryngitis, allergic rhinitis, asthma, sinusitis, upper respiratory tract infection, eczema, urticaria, stroke, trigeminal neuralgia, shingles, Parkinson's disease, arthritis, and epilepsy.

Common Causes

Exposure to the weather; sitting in drafts; a diet high in processed, fatty foods; or long-term illness.

An Explanation

Wind has the same effect inside your body as it does on the outside: You may be sailing on the calm waters of a lake or strolling through rocky trails in the still mountains, but in a moment, a gust of wind can change everything. As the breeze picks up, the lake becomes choppy, and the trees sway to and fro, and before you know it, a gale is blowing, and everything is moving and shaking.

When wind is active inside your body, this is the type of instability it describes. Indeed, many of the terms for sudden catastrophic changes, such as stroke or epileptic seizures, were considered diseases of wind by the ancient Chinese.

The type of wind was categorized by its direction, and through careful observation of seasonal change, eight winds were specified that affect individual storage systems (see chapter 6 for more information about this). For example, the Cold Wind from the north affects the kidney system and bones, shoulder, and back muscles, while the Dry Wind from the west affects the lung system and skin. Implied in these descriptions is a great deal more than just being out in that type of wind, though, and when seen within the context of the qualities of nature, the wind directions are actually telling us the origin of a problem and can help to treat it.

In essence, wind carries things. In winter, you can feel the cold carried within the North Wind in your bones, and in summer, the humid heat in the South Wind on your face. It is the bus that transports its passengers to their destination, and these passengers are climate patterns: Cold, heat, damp, and dryness.

The most common pattern for wind to enter your body is via the nose and mouth, and it follows the general pattern of when you catch a cold or flu. Wind is the vehicle that carries other climates into your body, so it is often accompanied by cold, heat, and damp.

If the defence system of your body (*wei qi*) is strong and efficient, then your symptoms will reflect the conflict between *wei qi* and the climate pattern, as your body attempts to eject wind. If there are any vulnerable areas of tissue that are not served properly by the river circulation system, wind can attach itself to the tissue and begin to disrupt circulation. If wind enters with cold, you might have shivers and feel cold; if wind enters with heat, you might have a fever and a dry mouth and throat.

If you have pain or discomfort in a particular place, such as your knee, you may have the feeling that the pain jumps or comes and goes. Perhaps one day it is on the left knee and the next it is on the right. Or maybe it is a tingling sensation in your hand that becomes a tingling sensation in your foot.

The progression of an illness pattern is not a gradual process; it is quite sudden, and involves the movement of wind within the circulation of your body as it transports the factors of the obstruction pattern. This is not some fancy way to dress up changes in the nervous or immune systems, both of which can be involved in aspects of the physiology that change easily; instead, it is about applying the natural unpredictable and rapidly changing motions that affect the ecology of our bodies in a real way.

Movements of this type and those that may lead to spasms and involuntary movements are often attributed to the liver system, which is connected to wind within wood, its natural quality. It is thought that this close relationship to wind allows your body to generate its own motion of wind. This is something that happens in nature frequently, such as wildfires. As a wildfire spreads, hot air rises so quickly that it creates a vacuum below it, and this vacuum is rapidly filled with fire, creating an updraft and its own dramatic wind system, or "firestorm".

This is the essential process in the liver system, too. When the *yin* motion of the liver is impaired, blood circulation becomes weak, and as the *yang* motion cannot be contained, it has a tendency to become hyperactive, agitated, and create updraft heat. Within this motion of weakness, a wind "firestorm" appears and can lead to wind-like symptoms in your body, such as contractions, tremors, and tics.

Underlying this *yin* weakness in the liver system is a weakness in the kidney system, which can develop over time and is part of the general decline in kidney *yin* and *yang* motions as you move through life. This can often explain a slight tremor in old age.

Food Therapy

Dietary Factors That Can Worsen Wind

- Foods that can stagnate and weaken the liver system and encourage wind include highly processed foods containing hydrogenated fats, nuts, and dairy products. See Stagnation for more details.

- Prawns, shrimps, shellfish, eggs, crab, and buckwheat can easily agitate wind and should be avoided.

Dietary Factors That Can Improve Wind

- Foods that can improve circulation within the liver system include watercress, onions, turmeric, horseradish, and black pepper. See Stagnation for more details.
- Cool-natured, sweet foods, such as apples, pears, tomatoes, peas and asparagus, strengthen *yin*. See *Yin* Weakness for more details.
- Also, many of the following individual foods can help reduce wind:
  - ▸ **FRUIT:** Coconut, strawberries.
  - ▸ **VEGETABLES:** Celery and aubergine (eggplant).
  - ▸ **GRAINS:** Oats.
  - ▸ **HERBS AND SPICES:** Basil, fennel, ginger, sage, and anise.
  - ▸ **LEGUMES, SEEDS, AND NUTS:** Pine nuts, sunflower seeds, black sesame seeds, water chestnuts, and black soybeans.
  - ▸ **MEAT AND SEAFOOD:** Bass (perch) and rabbit.
  - ▸ **DRINKS:** Chamomile tea.

Manual Therapy

ON YOUR NECK: Scrape up and down along the horizontal area below the occiput. Scrape over Gb-12, Gb-20, Bl-10, and Du-16; the movement of the tool should be like a toothbrush when brushing your teeth. Also scrape from these areas down your neck. Cover the back and sides of your neck, and scrape into your shoulder (do not scrape the front of your neck).

ON YOUR FRONT: Scrape downwards from Lu-2 to Lu-1, and down the sternum to Ren-17. Press and knead any areas of tension.

ON YOUR BACK: Scrape down from Bl-11, through the lung, heart, and diaphragm back *shu* regions and into the mid-back. If wind is present, it is very common for *sha* to appear on your skin. The position of these regions means that another person would need to treat you.

ON YOUR ARMS: Thumb-press up the triple burner and large intestine rivers from the source region at Tb-4 and root *shu* at Li-5 at your wrist, to Tb-14 and Li-15 at your shoulder. Press and knead any areas of tension.

ON YOUR LEGS: Scrape down or thumb-press the gallbladder river along your leg, in particular Gb-31 in your upper leg and Gb-34 in your lower leg. Press and knead any areas of tension. Thumb-press or scrape down the stomach river from St-36 to St-41. Press and knead any areas of tension.

ON YOUR HANDS: Do the Hand Circulation sequence in chapter 13. Use either Gua sha or your fingers. Also press Li-4 and zone 1 (F-H) and knead any areas of tension.

ON YOUR FEET: Do the Foot Circulation sequence in chapter 13. Use either Gua sha or your fingers. Wind often affects the upper body first, so press and knead any areas of tension in zones 1 and 2.

ON YOUR EARS: Do the Ear Circulation sequence in chapter 13. Use either Gua sha or your fingers.

Exercise Therapy

Follow exercises 1–5 of the Five Qualities of Nature stretches daily (see p. 101 ff.). Generally strengthening all of the river systems can help prevent wind.

Lifestyle Therapy

It may seem obvious but stay out of the wind. If it is a windy day, ensure that you wear appropriate clothing so that vulnerable areas such as your neck are protected. If you have any symptoms of a cold or flu (wind and cold or heat), follow the advice in the Colds and Flu section.

PART 6

How Do You Treat Common Medical Conditions?

Chinese medicine focuses on facilitating the smooth motion of breath throughout the body, as covered in the previous section. It is equally useful for treating weakness or overflow patterns that have already taken hold, often with a familiar Western medical name. In this section, I have included those conditions that, in my experience, are the most common and show how the same principles can be applied in treating them.

20

Head, Neck, and Shoulder Area

Headaches

Symptoms

Pain, ache, or discomfort in the head; dizziness; eye pain; earache; tender face or head; sensitivity to light.

Can Include or Lead to

Migraine, otitis, trigeminal neuralgia, sinusitis, tumour, and spondylitis.

When to See Your Doctor

If the pains are severe, get worse, and are accompanied by vomiting, a stiff neck, light sensitivity, limb weakness, or tingling.

Common Causes

Stress, dehydration, lack of exercise, anxiety, medication, allergies, tight muscles, and emotional stress, especially anger.

An Explanation

Headaches manifest in different ways. There is no catch-all treatment for them. This is because headaches are usually caused by an impairment in breath motion within the body, not necessarily the head, and that impairment will vary from person to person.

The exact symptoms of a headache can usually give us useful information about what has happened in the body and what may be causing it.

If the headache is accompanied by cold-like or flu-like symptoms, it is often the case that wind has entered the lung system. Wind can affect your head by causing pain and dizziness. A clear sign of wind being present is the strong desire to stay away from wind, whether it be a gentle breeze or an air conditioner fan.

An acute headache, in which the pain is intense, piercing, or throbbing, suggests heat rising. This is especially so if the headache is mainly felt at the temples on both or either side, and also behind the eyes. Sometimes, there is also an accompanying sensation of heat in the head. This kind of headache can be triggered by emotional stress or the end of the working week.

Stagnation in the circulation system of your body occurs in exactly the same way as when a river gets blocked: Something tangible is within the tissue that is obstructing the smooth movement of your circulation along a particular river system (often within the liver and gallbladder rivers). This can be brought on by a whole range of factors, from emotional stress and overwork to bad posture and lack of exercise. This kind of headache can feel tight and penetrating, possibly at the forehead or temples, and can be worse before a period, in stormy weather, and with emotional stress but relieved with physical activity and as the day draws on.

Damp and phlegm can also cause headaches. The sticky nature of these substances can arise from an impaired stomach and pancreas system as a result of an inappropriate diet, or it can stem from a build-up within the lung system and cause a distinctive heavy feeling in the head. This is often described as a muzzy sensation, like cotton wool surrounding your head, and can be accompanied by difficulty in concentrating and thinking clearly. This kind of headache is often felt at your forehead and can feel worse lying down or in wet weather.

Weakness patterns often underlie pain in your head. An impairment of blood circulation, especially within the liver system, can cause a headache. When this happens, blood does not have the power to nourish your whole body properly, and often a dull headache at the top of your head results. This may feel worse after menstruation, studying, or physical activity. There could also be a weakness in the kidney system. This often happens in old age, as your kidneys start to wane. This kind of headache may feel dull or empty, come on later in the day, or be relieved by lying down and resting.

Food Therapy

Dietary Factors That Can Affect Headaches

Follow the relevant diets for the general patterns, according to the type of headache. For example, for damp patterns, see the Damp/Phlegm section; for hot patterns, see Heat; and so on.

Manual Treatment

The location of the headache can be very helpful in establishing which of the river systems may be involved. Although not always applicable, the following is a general guide:

- **ON THE SIDES OF YOUR HEAD**: Gallbladder system
- **ON YOUR FOREHEAD**: Stomach system
- **AT THE BACK OF YOUR HEAD**: Bladder system
- **AT THE TOP OF YOUR HEAD**: Liver or kidney system

The nature of the pain can also give valuable clues:

- **DULL ACHE:** Kidney system
- **TIGHT, CONTRACTING PAIN:** Cold pattern
- **MOVING DISCOMFORT:** Wind pattern
- **MUZZY FEELING:** Damp/Phlegm pattern

ON YOUR HEAD: While a general treatment on your head can be counterproductive, it can be soothing to press, knead, and hard-press certain key areas; for example, the eye areas (*yintang, yuyao,* Bl-1, Bl-2, St-2, and Gb-1) and the occiput areas (Gb-12, Gb-20, Bl-10, and Du-16). Look for any areas that are relieved by pressing.

ON YOUR NECK AND SHOULDERS: Often treating your neck and shoulders can help relieve a headache. Almost all river systems come through the neck area, and it can be an area of great tension. If you can release that tension and allow the breath motion to move freely and circulation to flow within the space created, then it can be very helpful. Scrape down the back and sides of your neck and into your shoulder area with a Gua sha tool. Avoid scraping at the front of your neck.

ON YOUR ARMS: If possible, use the knowledge of how rivers connect. Look at the parents of the rivers you think might be most associated with the symptoms; for example, if your headache is on one side, it may be connected to the gallbladder river. The parent river of the gallbladder is *shaoyang,* and the other part of *shaoyang* is the triple burner on your arm. In this way, you can respond to the body by finding tense areas and treating them with kneading or with scraping with a Gua sha tool.

ON YOUR LEGS: As above with the arm, use river connections. For example, if you think your headache is connected to the gallbladder river, the paired river in the wood natural quality is liver; therefore, look for any tension in both the gallbladder and liver river systems in your legs, and knead the area.

ON YOUR HANDS: Press and knead the following hand areas, if sore: Li-4 area; all of zone 4, which covers the neck area; zone 1 – chest (F-H); C1 & C2 at the joints of the middle finger (1-4).

ON YOUR FEET: Do the Foot Circulation sequence in chapter 13. Knead any sore areas, including zone 1 – neck, head, and face (A); zone 2 – heart (G) and shoulder (T); zone 3 – liver/spleen, gallbladder, and kidney (J-H). Zone 1 above treats the root *shu* areas (Pa-1/2, Lv-1/2, Kd-1, Gb-44/43, St-45/44, and Bl-67/66).

ON YOUR EARS: Press and knead the following areas, if sore: Zone 3 – head area (G); zone 5 – neck (M); support region – *shenmen* (1).

Exercise Therapy

Headaches can often be related to the state of several systems at the same time, so it is useful to do exercises 1–5 of the Five Qualities of Nature stretches daily (see p. 101 ff.).

Lifestyle Therapy

Causes of a headache are numerous, so there is no one cure-all remedy for them—the key is to know the trigger, if there is one. The following can help prevent headaches:

1. Posture should be correct for the activity being done. Long-term hunching over a desk, for example, may cause backache, a sore neck, and headaches.
2. Your work environment should be adjusted, if necessary. Migraines can sometimes be caused by some types of computer screens.
3. Dehydration is a common cause of headaches. This can often be avoided by drinking enough, so that you never actually feel thirsty. If you feel thirsty, you are often already dehydrated.
4. Keep a food diary to record what you eat and drink over a set period of time; for example, a month. If, over that time, a food triggers a headache, you can then narrow down the potential cause, as the headache will likely begin 12–24 hours after you consumed the food.
5. Regular doses of painkillers, such as codeine, paracetamol, ibuprofen, and aspirin, can actually cause headaches. They can be effective at reducing the pain of a headache, but like all strong drugs, have their own withdrawal symptoms—one of which is something called a "rebound headache". This means that as the drug works its way out of the body, the body then reacts with a headache. This can then result in the need to take strong painkillers again to relieve this rebound headache, sometimes leading to a vicious cycle of taking strong painkillers to relieve the effects of taking strong painkillers.
6. Finding time for rest and relaxation is often helpful. If you find that you do not have time for relaxation, lifestyle adjustments may have to be made.

Dizziness

Symptoms
Feeling lightheaded or giddy, blurred vision, floaters or spots in your vision, and loss of balance.

Can Include or Lead to
Viral ear infections, vertigo, Ménière's disease, hypertension, arteriosclerosis, and neurosis.

When to See Your Doctor
If the symptoms are severe and persistent.

Common Causes
Overwork, stress, exhaustion, emotional stress, a diet with too many damp/phlegm-forming foods, depression, anxiety, severe blood loss, a long chronic illness, or drug side effects.

An Explanation

Dizziness is usually due to an impairment in the breath motion. When *yin* motion becomes weak, the rising and agitating action of *yang* becomes much more active, and can move up quickly to disturb the equilibrium in your head. Strong emotions, such as anger or aggression, can also create a similar pattern. Dizziness is worse when stressed and is often due to a stagnation pattern that has forced *yang* upwards.

When blood circulation is impaired, it is slow and cannot bring enough fresh, nutrient-rich blood up to your head in time. This is the reason for the feeling of temporary dizziness some people get when standing up quickly. It also is the source of the mild dizziness that may come from doing too much or staying up too late and will often improve with rest.

When there is a lot of damp/phlegm in your body, it can slow blood circulation and prevent *shenming, qi,* and the other substances, nutrients, and minerals that travel within your blood from effectively reaching your head. This can sometimes be accompanied by a lack of clarity and an inability to concentrate. It can also result in very strong dizziness with nausea.

Food Therapy

Dietary Factors That Can Worsen Dizziness

To prevent *yang* from rising, avoid hot, pungent spices, such as cinnamon, ginger, and black pepper. See Heat for more details.

When circulation is weakened, avoid too many bitter, sour, salty, and hot foods. Avoid salads, raw fruit and vegetables, and dairy produce. See General Weakness and Blood Circulation Weakness for more details.

For damp/phlegm patterns, avoid damp- or phlegm-forming foods, such as wheat, dairy, bananas, peanuts, processed foods, orange or tomato juice, and fatty meat, such as pork. See Damp/Phlegm for more details.

Dietary Factors That Can Improve Dizziness

To prevent the upward movement of *yang*, eat more sour and bitter cooling foods, such as kidney beans, black sesame seeds, watercress, mushrooms, eggs, and rhubarb. See Heat and the Sour and Bitter food lists for more details.

Your general circulation can be strengthened with neutral and warming foods, such as rice, pumpkin, chickpeas (garbanzos), parsnips, and cooked fruit. See General Weakness for more details.

To remove damp/phlegm, add more of the following to your diet: barley, rye, pumpkin, broad beans, celery, aduki beans, and radishes.

Manual Therapy

ON YOUR HEAD: Press *yintang,* and knead upwards to the hairline. Press the midpoint at the top of your forehead (Du-24) and knead outwards along the hairline.

Press and knead with four fingers together from the temples, around the back of the ear to the occiput (the base of the skull). At the occiput area, either thumb- and hard-press or use a Gua sha tool to scrape up and down along the area below the bone (Gb-12, Gb-20, Bl-10, and Du-16). Press Du-16, just under the occiput, and knead in a downwards motion to where your neck meets your shoulders.

ON YOUR BACK: Use Gua sha to scrape down the back and sides of your neck and the back *shu* regions, in particular the upper regions (lung, heart, and diaphragm). Also thumb-press, knead, and hard-press any areas of tension.

ON YOUR LEGS: Generally feel along the river systems in your legs, and check for any areas of tightness or tension. Pay particular attention to the *yang* rivers (stomach, gallbladder, and bladder) in your lower leg.

ON YOUR HANDS: It is no coincidence that the areas around the metacarpal-phalangeal joints have actions connected to your neck and head. This is the common position of the neck in the projection of the body onto the hand. Knead or press with a Gua sha tool: Zone 1 and zone 4 (cover the whole knuckle area); C1 & C2 on the middle finger (1–4).

ON YOUR FEET: The metatarsal-phalangeal joints and the toes above them on your feet represent the neck and head area. This is the potent area of the start and finish of all the leg rivers, and they are the root *shu* areas (Pa-1/2, Lv-1/2, Kd-1, Gb-44/43, St-45/44, and Bl-67/66).

- Knead any sore areas in zone 1, around the joints on the soles of your feet and also on the toes. Press around the toes but not on the nail itself.
- Use a downwards scraping motion over this area with your Gua sha tool. Also use the tool to press into any tight areas, especially in the soles of your feet.
- Also do the complete Foot Circulation sequence in chapter 13.

ON YOUR EARS: Press and knead any reactive areas in zone 2 – spinal column region (D-F); zone 5 – neck (M); zone 3 – head and face region on the ear lobe (H-I).

Exercise Therapy

Do exercises 4 and 5 of the Five Qualities of Nature stretches (see p. 102 ff.). These help to strengthen the water (kidney and bladder) and wood (liver and gallbladder) systems.

Lifestyle Therapy

1. Keep in mind that widely used drugs such as tranquilizers, antidepressants, and diuretics can cause dizziness. If this is the case, you should discuss with your doctor about changing or reducing their use.
2. Reduce your workload and level of stress, if possible. Knowing when to stop or when

the body has had enough is a key point in reducing some kinds of dizziness.
3. For dizziness due to Blood Circulation Weakness, standing quickly can make you feel light-headed, so get into the routine of holding something solid and changing positions slowly.

Sleeping Disorders

Symptoms

Inability to sleep, difficulty falling asleep, waking up at night, waking up early, strong dreams or nightmares, not feeling rested after sleeping, fatigue, poor appetite, and dizziness.

Can Include or Lead to

Insomnia, anxiety, and depression.

When to See Your Doctor

If accompanied by severe mental or emotional symptoms.

Common Causes

Emotional stress, overwork, late nights, overexercise, overthinking, excessive study, and pressure from work.

An Explanation

Insomnia is very much connected to the day–night breath pattern inside your body. In the daytime, the *yang* motion of breath gives you the force needed for your body to function in its everyday tasks. In particular, it needs *yang* to think, see, smell, hear, and touch effectively.

When night falls and *yang* motion of breath gives way to *yin*, *yang* retreats from the areas it reinforced throughout the day and disconnects from the senses enough for your body to fall asleep.

If, however, the *yang* motion is unable to become dormant for the night, your senses are still awake and your body cannot easily switch off.

The problem here is not so much with *yang* but that the *yin* motion is not strong enough to hold *yang* in place. There is an imbalance in the *yin/yang* breath motion. And as *yang* is the motion that takes you through the daytime hours and provides you with the active force to work, study, exercise, and do all the movement-based tasks you need to do, it is not the motion to take you into the night. This is a common cause of waking up during the night, or early in the morning, as the heat from this agitated *yang* moves upwards and outwards.

There is a similar cyclical movement in blood that, if not working properly, causes insomnia. As in the case of *yang*, the force of blood is sent around your body during the day to allow you to do your everyday activities. At night this force of blood, which by its nature has a *yin* motion, settles in the liver system and adds to the sense of calm that allows your body to drift to sleep. If the blood circulation is too weak, however, it cannot gather in the liver and will "wander" around your body, keeping it awake.

Food Therapy

Dietary Factors That Can Worsen Sleeping Difficulties

- Stimulants like coffee, black tea, tobacco, fizzy soft drinks, energy drinks, alcohol, and recreational drugs can agitate the *yang* motion and worsen insomnia.

Dietary Factors That Can Improve Sleeping Difficulties

- Blood-strengthening foods include beetroot, seaweed, black sesame seeds, Guinness stout, and green leafy vegetables. See Blood Circulation Weakness for more details.
- *Yin*-strengthening foods include sardines, chicken, sweet potato, black beans, wolfberries (goji berries), and apples. See *Yin* Weakness for more details.

Manual Therapy

ON YOUR HEAD: Rub your palms together until warm, then cover both eyes until the warmth dissipates. Repeat several times. The heat is generated from the two root *shu* regions (Ht-8 and Hr-8) on your palm and is emanating from the heart river. By doing this, you can help to regulate any heat in the heart system.

Then press, knead, and hard-press the eye areas (*yintang*, *yuyao*, Bl-1, Bl-2, St-2, and Gb-1).

From *yintang*, knead upwards to your natural hairline along the *du* reservoir. Press Du-24 at the midpoint of your forehead, and knead or scrape outwards along the hairline towards the sides of your head.

Gua sha over the top of your head. Start at the hairline above your forehead, at Du-24, and scrape backwards, past Du-20, towards the nape of your neck, at Du-16. Use short scraping motions, and follow parallel lines, from areas along your hairline, so that you cover most of the head above your ears.

Press and knead with four fingers together, from the temples, around the back of the ear to the occiput.

At the occiput, press, knead, and hard-press the occipital areas (Gb-12, Gb-20, Bl-10, and Du-16), or use a Gua sha tool to scrape in short, up-and-down motions across them.

ON YOUR ARMS: Thumb-press or scrape along the heart and heart ruler river systems, from your upper arm to the root *shu* areas at your wrist (Ht-7 and Hr-7).

ON YOUR FRONT/BACK: While seated, rub your navel area on the front, and Gate of life (Du-4) on your back, with the palm of your hand until it feels warm.

Scrape down and across your shoulders (covering Gb-21 area) and down the back *shu* regions on the back. Press and knead any areas of tension afterwards.

ON YOUR LEGS: Generally feel along the river systems in your legs, and check for any areas of tightness or tension. Pay particular attention to the *yang* rivers (stomach, gallbladder, and bladder) and in your lower leg.

ON YOUR HANDS: Press and knead each of your fingers, moving down to your knuckles. Then use a Gua sha tool to scrape downwards in the same way, covering all sides of your fingers. This covers the root *shu* regions (Li-1/2, Si-1/2, Tb-1/2, Ht-9/8, Hr-9/8, and Lu-11/10).

Press and knead the following areas: Zone 1 – chest and heart (F-H); zone 2 – liver (K); zone 3 – kidney (M).

ON YOUR FEET: Rub the kidney area in zone 3 (I) on the soles of your feet with the palm of your hand. Then press with a slowly increased pressure and release. Repeat this several times.

Do the Foot Circulation sequence in chapter 13. Use your fingers or a Gua sha tool. Cover the root *shu* regions on the foot (Pa-1/2/3, Lv-1/2/3, Kd-1/2/3, Gb-44/43, St-45/44/43, and Bl-67/66/65).

Recent research from Asia looked at soaking feet to help insomnia. They studied the use of home-based footbaths with a water temperature of 40°C (104°F) for 30 minutes, 1–2 hours before bedtime, to promote sleep in people with traumatic brain injuries. The results showed that it had a positive effect on sleep onset and waking after sleeping, and that it was recommended as an alternative intervention for insomnia.[54] For more information about using foot soaks, see Heat Your Feet in chapter 17 and refer to *Yang* Weakness.

ON YOUR EARS: Do the Ear Circulation sequence in chapter 13. Use your fingers or a Gua sha tool. Press and knead any reactive areas in zone 1; zone 3 – head and face region on the ear lobe (G-I); support region – cerebral (4), relaxation (2), and *shenmen* (1).

Exercise Therapy

A useful technique to help sleeping disorders is to relax your muscles with the following gentle exercises:

❶ Relax Your Arms, Shoulders, and Upper Body
Stand naturally, with your arms hanging at your sides. Raise your arms forward to shoulder level, clench your hands, and tense the muscles of your upper arms while breathing in at the same time.

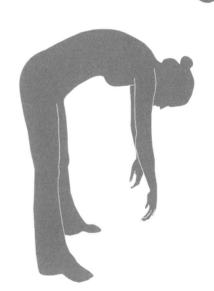

Bend over, allow your arms to hang, then swing them to and fro in order to make the muscles of the upper arms and shoulder joints relax fully, exhaling at the same time. Repeat this several times until you feel relaxed.

❷ Relax Your Head, Neck, and Shoulders

From a seated position, interlock your hands, place them on the back of your head, and push your head backwards as you simultaneously pull your hands forward in the opposite direction. Tense the muscles of your head and neck as you inhale, then relax the head, neck, and shoulders, and breathe out. Repeat this several times.

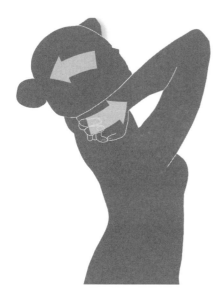

❸ Relax Your Back and Sides

Lie face up with your arms at your sides, palms down. Tense your back and side muscles, while breathing in, then relax and breathe out. Repeat several times.

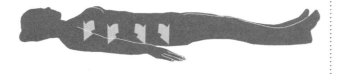

❹ Relax Your Front

Lie face up, link your fingers, and put both hands on the back of your head. Raise your head slightly, and contract your abdomen muscles. Then lower your head and relax, while breathing out. Repeat several times.

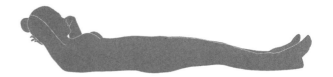

❺ Relax Your Legs

From a seated position, put your hands on your knees, then push down on each thigh, stamp the floor, and tense your leg muscles, while breathing in. Then relax, and breathe out. Repeat several times.

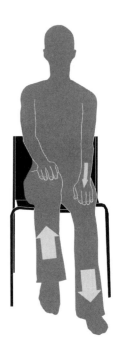

❻ Relax Your Fingers and Toes

Lie on your side, with your legs and arms bent slightly and your head resting on the arm closest to the ground. Then contract your fingers and toes, and breathe in. Relax, and breathe out.

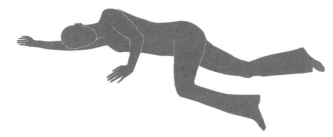

❼ Relax Your Whole Body
Stand with the feet close together and your arms hanging in front of your body, with the fingers of both hands interlocked. Then lift your heels, raise your arms upwards, and contract the muscles all over your body, breathing in at the same time.

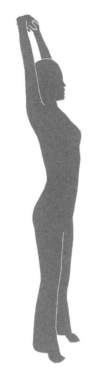

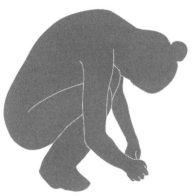

Lower your arms, move the hands apart, squat, and drop your head forward, allowing the muscles all over your body to fully relax, while breathing out. Repeat several times.

Lifestyle Therapy

1. Playing video games, watching TV, and staring at a computer screen late at night or for long periods during the day impedes *yin* motion and should be avoided when there are sleep problems.

2. Avoid taking naps during the day to make up for lost sleep, as this may worsen the pattern. Remember that the problem is often one of an imbalance between the motions of *yin* and *yang*, so doing *yin* activities not habitually done in *yang* time, and vice versa, can mess with your body's balance. This is something that nightshift workers and long-haul travellers know only too well.

3. Try to stop what you are doing and just rest at least half an hour before you go to bed. No reading, watching television, talking, or fiddling with electronic devices. Just sit, and let your body and mind calm down. Of course, this may not be possible all the time, but the intention should be there.

Anxiety

Symptoms
Constant worry and nervousness, an inability to concentrate, an inability to sleep, dizziness, palpitations, restlessness, phobias, panic attacks, and irritability.

Can Include or Lead to
Depression, hyperthyroidism, hypoglycaemia, PMT, menopausal symptoms, and post-traumatic stress disorder.

When to See Your Doctor
If the symptoms are severe.

Common Causes
Strong emotions, such as sadness or grief, depression, stress, overwork, pressure to work hard, too much caffeine, eating too many damp/phlegm-producing foods, a side effect of medication or withdrawal symptoms, menopause, hyperthyroidism, heavy bleeding, or sudden shock or trauma.

An Explanation

There is no one body expression for anxiety. The exact nature of the anxiety differs according to which of the body systems are causing the anxiety symptoms.

The most common condition underlying feelings of anxiety is an impairment of the heart system. Typical indicators of this are if the anxiety gets worse when tired and if there are accompanying palpitations or cardiac symptoms. This is also often the background to many panic attacks and phobias.

Sometimes the fire–water balance between the heart and kidney systems leads to both being impaired, especially the *yin* motion. When this happens, *yin* cannot act as a balanced counter-weight to the motion of *yang*, leading to agitation and lack of peace. An element of shock is usually present, which can bring on palpitations with this pattern.

In addition to patterns of weakness, there can be heat or damp/phlegm in other parts of the body, which can both rise and affect the heart system. This is often referred to as a "mist" and is like the steam rising out of the spout of a boiling kettle. It can easily be caused by any of the other patterns, or it may have a separate cause, such as a dietary one. This mist clouds the heart system and affects your mind, causing a lack of clarity, nervousness, and waking up before dawn.

Anxious feelings can also come from body-wide stagnation, which affects the general circulation and can encourage blockages and obstructions wherever the body will allow it. This is usually related to an impairment of the liver system and affects the ability of your body to follow the emotional breath cycle, causing it to get stuck or move sluggishly.

Food Therapy

Dietary Factors That Can Worsen Anxiety

- Food or drink containing caffeine, such as chocolate, caffeinated soft drinks, energy drinks, coffee, and black tea, agitate the *yang* motion and can potentially worsen anxiety. Coffee, in particular, has a bitter flavour that can disperse and weaken the heart system.
- Dairy products, tofu, and alcohol can worsen anxiety, particularly if there is a phlegm or heat pattern. It is also important to strictly limit meat consumption for the same reason. See Damp/Phlegm and Heat for more details.
- Warm, pungent foods, such as chillies, black pepper, cayenne pepper, basil, cloves, cinnamon, cumin, rosemary, marjoram, and nutmeg, can exacerbate a *yin* weakness pattern. See *Yin* Weakness for more details.
- Salads, raw fruit and vegetables, dairy products, ice-cold drinks, and foods that can weaken *yang* must be avoided, particularly when there is weakness in the heart system. See General Weakness for more details.

IMPORTANT NOTE Do not get overly anxious about the food you eat. You want to get rid of anxiety, not add to it. A little of the above is fine once in a while.

Dietary Factors That Can Improve Anxiety

- To reduce damp/phlegm and heat, follow a diet of easy-to-digest fresh foods, including leafy greens, radishes, persimmons, watercress, turnip, and seaweed. See Damp/Phlegm and Heat for more details.
- Kidney *yin*-strengthening foods include pork, kidney beans, black beans, and seaweed. See *Yin* Weakness for more details.
- Heart-strengthening foods are those that generally strengthen your body, such as rice, cooked fruit, carrots, and chickpeas (garbanzos). See General Weakness for more details.

Manual Therapy

ON YOUR HEAD: Using Du-20 as an anchor point, use a Gua sha tool to scrape downwards, using short strokes. Go in several different directions but always start back at Du-20 each time. This covers the heat *shu* regions on the top of your head, which can help with calming agitation.

From *yintang*, knead upwards to your natural hairline along the *ren* reservoir. Press Du-24 at the midpoint of your forehead, and knead or scrape outwards along the hairline, towards the sides of the head.

Press and knead with four fingers together, from the temples around the back of the ear to the occiput.

At the occiput, press, knead, and hard-press the occipital areas (Gb-12, Gb-20, Bl-10, and Du-16), or use a Gua sha tool to scrape in short up-and-down motions across them.

ON YOUR BACK: Gua sha down the heart, diaphragm, liver, and kidney back *shu* regions. Press, knead, and hard-press any areas of *sha*, or tension.

ON YOUR ARMS: Thumb-press along the heart and heart ruler rivers down to the root *shu* regions at your wrist (Ht-7 and Hr-7). Knead any areas of tension.

ON YOUR HANDS: Do the Hand Circulation sequence in chapter 13. Also knead zone 1 – chest, lungs, and heart (F-H).

ON YOUR FEET: Do the Foot Circulation sequence in chapter 13. Also knead zone 1 – head/face (A-D); zone 2 – heart (G); zone 3 – liver/spleen (J) and pancreas (H) areas, if sore.

ON YOUR EARS: Do the Ear Circulation sequence in chapter 13. Use your fingers or a Gua sha tool. Press the following areas, knead if sore: Zone 3 – head area (G); zone 5 – neck (M); zone 1 – heart (B); and support region – *shenmen* (1). Also use the ear treatment advice in Heat in chapter 19.

Exercise Therapy

1. *Follow the same relaxation pattern to the exercises in the previous section on insomnia.*
2. *Do the exercise Bend Backwards from the section on Chest Pain (see p. 205). This exercise is good for releasing tension and Stagnation in your upper back.*
3. *Do exercises 3 and 4 of the Five Qualities of Nature stretches (see p. 102 f.).*

Lifestyle Therapy

It is vital to reduce external stressors and find ways to relax. But relaxation is more than just the absence of stress; it must be proactive. Be sure to get regular exercise, such as walking, and introduce enjoyable activities, such as painting, which calm the mind and offer a distraction from worrying.

Depression

Symptoms

In general, feeling pessimistic about life, tired, unmotivated, miserable, sad or weepy, unable to think clearly, and lacking in energy.

A more useful distinction here may be to list the possible depression symptoms by their natural quality correspondence. This often gives a clearer indication of where the imbalances may lie:

WOOD: Changeable moods, frustrated, feeling stuck or trapped, feeling aggressive, unable to relax, sighing, or timid.

EARTH: Feeling insecure, worrying, a lack of support, repetitive thinking, or unable to find a solution.

METAL: Grief, sadness, a lack of self-worth, inability to let go, or a sense of pointlessness.

FIRE: A lack of joy, feeling rejected, feeling hurt, an inability to communicate well, feeling agitated, or being on the defensive.

WATER: Fear, dread, an inability to cope, a sense of being overwhelmed, or feeling helpless.

Can Include or Lead to

Clinical depression, mood disorders, dysthymia, seasonal depression, and bipolar disorder.

When to See Your Doctor

If the symptoms are severe, or if there are any suicidal thoughts or urges.

Common Causes

Exhaustion, emotional strain, stress, overwork, an improper diet, shock, bereavement, a long-standing illness, pain, and sometimes a constitutional tendency.

An Explanation

Sometimes, when your body is confronted by strong emotions, you keep them inside rather than allowing them to be released. When this happens, a physiological reaction can occur. Over time, unexpressed emotions fester in your body in the form of a Stagnation pattern.

Stagnation slows down your body's internal functions, creating obstruction patterns and preventing blood from circulating freely. Emotions have their own circulation pattern, and they too begin to stagnate. It gradually becomes more and more difficult to move from one emotion to another. Instead, like a wheel following a rut in the road, you get stuck in one emotion and are unable to move out of it. This condition is likely to result in many of the Wood-type symptoms above.

Stagnation of emotions can also be cavused by a climate pattern, whereby wind, cold, heat, or damp remain attached within tissue. The subsequent restricted circulation through the affected area can, in turn, affect a river system and start a ripple effect. If there is also too much damp/phlegm in your body due to an improper diet, this too can add to the stagnation. Damp and phlegm are heavy and sticky and can slow down the body's processes.

If your body has run out of any of the essential substances it needs to function, it will begin to feel weaker, both physically and mentally. This is also true on a deeper level, as our vitality depends on having the correct balance of substances in the body. When the balance is weak, the result can be a lack of drive or will on a very profound almost spiritual level.

Dietary Factors That Can Worsen Depression

- Processed, tinned, fatty foods cannot be digested efficiently by a weakened stomach system and can easily lead to stagnation or the accumulation of damp and phlegm. Both of these can lead to the obstruction pattern that can cause depression.
- A five-year British study found a link between the consumption of processed foods, such as desserts, fried foods, processed meats, and high-fat dairy products and the development of depression. According to the study, participants who followed a processed foods diet were 58 percent more likely to be suffering from depression.[55]
- It is, therefore, important to avoid damp-forming foods, such as processed, junk foods, deep-fried food, wheat, fatty meat such as pork, and beer in your diet. See Damp/Phlegm for more details.

Dietary Factors That Can Improve Depression

- Rice, carrots, onions, cooked fruit, lentils, chickpeas (garbanzos), and other foods that strengthen the stomach and pancreas systems can be beneficial in removing one of the underlying causes of depression. See General Weakness for more details.
- The following foods can also help improve circulation: Grapefruit; citrus peel; watercress; onions; beetroot; spices like turmeric, cardamom and coriander; black sesame seeds; and chamomile tea.

Manual Therapy

The Dry Towel Friction sequence detailed in General Weakness can help with circulation.

ON YOUR HEAD: At the occiput, press, knead, and hard-press the occipital areas (Gb-12, Gb-20, Bl-10, and Du-16) or use a Gua sha tool to scrape, using short up-and-down motions across these areas, then scrape or thumb-press down the back and sides of your neck.

ON YOUR BACK: Gua sha down the heart, diaphragm, and liver back *shu* regions. Press, knead, and hard-press any areas of *sha,* or tension.

ON YOUR LEGS: Thumb-press or scrape down the gallbladder river, from your hip to your ankle. In particular, check the Gb-31 area in your upper leg and Gb-34 area in your lower leg, but press and knead any areas that feel tight. Also thumb-press up the liver river, from your ankle to your knee, and knead any sore areas, including Lv-8.

ON YOUR HANDS: Do the Hand Circulation sequence in chapter 13. Also knead and press zones 1 and 2.

ON YOUR FEET: Do the Foot Circulation sequence in chapter 13. Press and knead zone 2 – heart and chest (E-G); zone 3 – liver/ spleen, pancreas, and kidney (J-H) if sore.

MUGWORT FOOT SOAK: Foot soaks can help improve circulation in the body, especially if there is a stagnation pattern. Use 50g (1.7oz) of fresh mugwort leaves (or 30g (1oz) of dried mugwort leaves), and place them in 1500 ml (50fl oz) of water to boil. Turn down the heat and simmer for about 15 minutes, then remove mugwort leaves and pour the water into the tub. See Heat Your Feet in *Yang* Weakness.

ON YOUR EARS: Do the Ear Circulation sequence in chapter 13. Press the following areas and knead if sore: Support regions – shenmen (1), relaxation (2), sensorial (3) and cerebral (4); zone 1 – superior and inferior areas (A-B); zone 2 – spinal column (D-F).

Exercise Therapy

1. *Do the exercise Bend Backwards from the Chest Pain section (see p. 205). This exercise is useful for releasing tension in the upper back.*
2. *Do exercises 1–5 of the Five Qualities of Nature stretches on a daily basis (see p. 101 ff.). This can help improve the circulation of the river systems and strengthen weakness.*

Lifestyle Therapy

1. The motion of grief and sadness is downwards. To counteract this, it is important to enhance the rising, uplifting motion of the east and the liver system. Exercise can help with this. Regular gentle exercise can help increase circulation and reduce any blockage resulting from damp/ phlegm. The better your circulation, the better the chances of movement in your emotions. The recommended minimum exercise levels for adults is 30 minutes a day, five times a week; for under 18s, at least an hour a day.
2. Overwork can be bad for your mental health. A UK study found that people who work for 11 or more hours a day are twice as likely to suffer from major depression as those working a standard eight-hour day.[56]

Facial Pain

Symptoms

Pain on one side of the temple, jaw, forehead, or face; a burning feeling; a red face; tiredness or burning in the eyes; toothache; muscle spasms; dizziness; and bad breath.

Can Include or Lead to

Trigeminal neuralgia, supraorbital neuralgia, mumps, and rhinitis.

When to See Your Doctor

If the symptoms are severe.

Common Causes

Exposure to the weather; an injury or accident; stress; overwork; emotional stress, especially anger; overworrying; an improper diet of greasy foods; too much alcohol; or a long chronic illness.

An Explanation

Pain in the face is normally caused by an obstruction pattern and counterflow in the facial river systems. There are a variety of common causes for this blockage, both internal and external, which are related to the location and intensity of the pain.

Your face is a part of your body that is rarely covered up and, therefore, exposed to the world around you most of the time. Sometimes, an impairment in the protective action of *wei qi*, which defends your body from the environment, allows a climate (wind, cold, or heat) to penetrate the pores of your skin. This is, however, perfectly normal and should not cause undue pain. But if any of those climates, floating around within the circulation of the connective tissue, find an area of tissue that is not properly connected to the rivers that run within it, they can attach themselves there. It can be difficult for your body to remove them, as no river can reach them, and it will then create an obstruction pattern in your face.

If cold has entered your facial tissue, it can cause extreme pain by contracting the muscles and tendons of your face; heat can cause redness and a burning sensation; and wind may move the pain around or cause tics or muscle spasms.

A common situation in facial pain is that there is also a pattern of heat rising from below. It can be from an impairment in a system, such as the liver system after sustained emotional stress. Unexpressed emotions can fester within the liver system, and over time build heat to such an extent that there is a counterflow, which rises to your face, causing intense burning pain. This type of facial pain is usually very sharp and gets worse with strong emotions.

A similar heat pattern can rise from the stomach and pancreas systems if there is a history of following a diet of greasy, hot, damp-forming foods. The stomach system is often implicated in facial pain as the stomach river runs across your face and jawline and influences the areas of your face commonly involved. It can sometimes get worse after eating certain types of hot foods and can be accompanied by bad breath.

Dietary Factors That Can Worsen Facial Pain

- Grilling, roasting, and deep-frying encourage heat in the body.
- Hot-natured, spicy foods, such as ginger, coriander, turmeric, and other spices, lamb, chillies, coffee, chocolate and spirits, can also cause heat. See Heat for more details.
- Dairy products, bananas, peanut butter, processed junk foods, and some fruit juice are damp-forming foods. See Damp/Phlegm for more details.
- Oily food can strongly affect the liver system and provoke heat.

Dietary Factors That Can Improve Facial Pain

- Food should be lightly cooked or boiled in water.
- Cold or cool-natured foods can help soothe heat. These include foods like cranberries, grapefruit, melons, bean sprouts, celery, cucumbers and lettuce, peppermint, marjoram, green tea, chamomile tea, and oolong tea. See Cold for more details.
- Salty foods, such as barley, miso, and soy sauce, and bitter foods, such as grapefruit rind, asparagus, watercress, rye, and vinegar, can be generally cooling. See Salty and Bitter food lists for more details on diet.

Manual Therapy

ON YOUR FACE: If pressing areas on your face feels comfortable, finger-press along the stomach river and circle the masseter muscle at the angle of your jaw and at the joint area in front of your ear. Follow the cheek bone around from *bitong* to your temple area and from *yintang*, across your eyebrows to the temple.

If it feels comfortable, press, circle, and knead the eye areas (*yintang*, *yuyao*, Bl-1, Bl-2, St-2, and Gb-1) and nose areas (*bitong* and Li-20).

CAUTION: Treating your face directly can sometimes worsen the pattern. If in any doubt, use the alternative areas to treat.

ON YOUR HEAD: If there is heat present in your face, use the heat *shu* on the top of your head to help cool it. Using Du-20 as the anchor point, use a Gua sha tool to scrape downwards, using short strokes. Go in several different directions but always starting at Du-20.

ON YOUR ARMS: Thumb-press the large intestine, small intestine, and triple burner rivers up to the root *shu* areas (Li-11, Si-8, and Tb-10) at your elbow. This covers the root *shu* and junction regions in the lower arm. Press and knead any areas of tension.

ON YOUR LEGS: Thumb-press or scrape with a Gua sha tool down the stomach river from Crouching Rabbit to St-41 at your ankles. Press and knead any areas of tension.

ON YOUR HANDS: Press the following areas and knead if sore: All of zones 1 and 4; C1 & C2 on your middle finger (1-4).

ON YOUR FEET: Press and knead each toe on the top of the foot, from the joint up to and around the toenail. These are the root *shu* regions (Pa-1/2/3, Lv-1/2, Kd-1, Gb-44/43, St-45/44, and Bl-67/66) and the frontal sinus area. Also press and knead zone 1 – head/face, eye, ear, nose and neck (A-D).

ON YOUR EARS: Press the following areas, and knead if sore: Zone 3 – face and head area (G-I); zone 8 – sensory organs; support regions – relaxation (2) and *shenmen* (1).

Exercise Therapy

Do exercise 2 of the Five Qualities of Nature as this can strengthen the stomach river system, which runs across the throat and face (see p. 101 f.).

Lifestyle Therapy

Stress and emotional factors often feature heavily in facial pain. Wherever possible, these should be worked through to try and stop them being the cause of internal heat. Look at ways of managing stress and of unburdening yourself of emotions that you have kept in for a long time. This may mean anything from talking to those close to you to seeking professional psychological help.

Nasal Allergies

Symptoms
Sneezing, a stuffy nose, an itchy nose and throat, eye irritation and weeping, a headache and runny nose, irritability, and insomnia.

Can Include or Lead to
Allergic or non-allergic rhinitis, hay fever, rhinorrhea, nasal congestion, conjunctivitis, and pharyngitis.

When to See Your Doctor
If there are severe symptoms.

Common Causes
Lack of exercise; smoking; overwork; an inherited condition; too many cold-natured, phlegm-forming foods; repressed emotions, in particular grief; repeated use of antibiotics in childhood; overthinking; and worry.

An Explanation

Nasal allergies are widespread. More than one-third of the populations of Europe and Australasia are thought to suffer from nasal allergies.[57] In the United States, that number is 60 million people, an estimated 40 percent of them being children.[58]

To start with, it is important to distinguish what is causing the allergy. The standard conventional medical approach is to see the symptoms as due to external agents, such as pollen, dust, animal fur, smoke, chemicals, or other irritating environmental conditions, and if you could remove these triggers, then the allergic problem is resolved. Medications are used to suppress the body's reaction to these, when this is not possible.

A much better approach is to see not the external agents as the cause but the body's reaction to the external agent, and in particular the lung system, which stretches all the way up to your nose. In this way, rather than the priority being the allergen, which you may have less control over, the priority is the lung imbalance, which can be changed.

Indeed, an impairment in the lung system is the typical cause of the symptoms of an allergy. In someone with a normally functioning system, the external agents that cause the allergic reaction have little impact, as the natural function of defending your body (*wei qi*) is activated. But when impaired, your lung system cannot maintain *wei qi,* and it is easily compromised by climate patterns.

Typically this means wind, which manages to find its way into your nose, and due to a faulty area of tissue circulation, embeds within the lung system. A clear indicator is tiredness, lethargy and a tendency to catch colds. If wind enters with cold, it can cause sneezing and a runny nose; if it enters with heat, it can cause an itchy throat and eyes and thirst.

A climate pattern can remain in the lung system indefinitely, free to disrupt your nose at will and this is the situation for many people suffering with rhinitis. As wind is already in residence, when any subsequent wind arrives, it simply attaches at the same place. Over time, the obstruction caused by this climate pattern causes heat and easily accumulates damp/phlegm, which can harden.

This pattern can quite literally be fed from below as the result of an inappropriate diet. Cold-natured, damp-producing foods, accompanied by bad eating habits, will impair the pancreas system and lead to an accumulation of mucus in the lung system, and by default, the nose. A key indicator of this is when symptoms are triggered by smoke, perfume, or fumes, as strong smells disperse the lung system and agitate the damp/phlegm.

Food Therapy

Dietary Habits That Can Worsen Nasal Allergies

- Overeating cold-natured, damp-forming foods, such as dairy products, bananas, tofu, soya milk, and fatty foods can impair the stomach and pancreas systems and increase phlegm in the lung system. See Damp/Phlegm for more details.

Dietary Habits That Can Improve Nasal Allergies

- Lightly cooked, simple foods strengthen the stomach, pancreas, and lung systems. See General Weakness for more details.
- Add foods that remove phlegm and help clear your sinuses, such as radishes, turnips, onions, watercress, garlic, ginger, and horseradish. See Damp/Phlegm for more details.

Manual Therapy

ON YOUR FACE AND HEAD: Circle your face with a Gua sha tool or your fingers to relax the facial muscles. Press on Du-24 on the midline of the forehead, then finger-press outwards on both sides to the temples, and circle the temple area. Repeat at equally spaced areas on the midline up to the middle of the eyebrows.

Hard-press *yintang*, Bl-1 and Bl-2, *bitong*, and Li-20. From the eyebrows to the midpoint of your nose, gently finger-press outwards along the eye socket to the temples, then circle the temple area. From the midpoint of your nose to the bottom of the chin, finger-press outwards to the corner of your jaw bone and then circle.

ON YOUR NECK AND SHOULDERS: Finger-circle outwards at the base of the skull towards the ear and back again. Now use a tool or thumb-press along and focus on the occiput areas (Gb-12, Gb-20, Bl-10, and Du-16). Hard-press and knead any tense areas.

Finger-circle or scrape down your neck in the muscles on either side of the spine, and go into the shoulder area.

ON YOUR BACK: Gua sha down the lung back *shu* region. Press and knead any areas of tension, or *sha,* afterwards. You need help to do this on yourself.

ON YOUR ARMS: Thumb-press down the lung river from Lu-5 at your elbow to Lu-9 at your wrist, and as the large intestine is the paired river, thumb-press up the large intestine river from Li-5 at your wrist to Li-11 at your elbow. Press and knead any areas of tension.

ON YOUR LEGS: The parent river of the lung is *taiyin,* so treat the other part, the pancreas river in the lower leg. Thumb-press up the pancreas river to Pa-10, and knead any areas of tension.

ON YOUR HANDS: Press and knead the following areas if sore: Zone 1- lungs and chest (F-H); C1 – throat, mouth, nose, and head (1-4).

ON YOUR FEET: Do the Foot Circulation sequence in chapter 13. Press and knead the following areas: Zone 1 – head/face, nose, ear, eye (A-D); zone 2 – lungs and chest (E-G).

Thumb-press up the pancreas river from Pa-1 to Pa-5, which covers most of the root *shu* regions and the junction region.

ON YOUR EARS: Press and knead the following areas if sore: Zone 8 – nose and eye areas; zone 3 – head area (G); zone 1 – A & B; support regions – relaxation (2) and *shenmen* (1).

Exercise Therapy

Do exercises 1 and 2 of the Five Qualities of Nature stretches daily (see p. 101 f.). These help strengthen the lung, large intestine, stomach, and pancreas systems.

Lifestyle Therapy

One of the keys to nasal allergy prevention is not to let your body become weakened in the first place. That is easier said than done, of course, as it involves taking regular exercise, eating sensibly (according to the guidelines above), managing stress so that you can remain relatively calm and relaxed, and expressing your emotions in a positive way—basically following your path, or the Way.

Sinus Problems

Symptoms
Blocked nose, nasal discharge (often yellow or green), no sense of smell, strong headaches, sinuses painful to touch, and a lack of clarity in thinking.

Can Include or Lead to
Sinusitis and nasal polyps.

When to See Your Doctor
If there is a nasal discharge after a head injury.

Common Causes
Stress; repressed emotions; worry; overthinking; an improper diet with too many greasy, hot-natured foods or too many sweet foods; or repeated infections.

An Explanation

If you have sinus problems, you are not alone. Sinusitis is one of the leading forms of chronic disease, with an estimated 18 million cases and at least 30 million courses of antibiotics per year in the US alone.[59]

Wind is the main external cause of sinusitis. It enters the lung system via your mouth or neck, reducing the drainage of fluid from your sinuses and nose. Heat often accompanies any climate pattern and cooks up these fluids into a thick, sticky mucus soup. Unless this mucus is thoroughly cleared, either naturally or with the help of treatment, the pattern will keep repeating itself.

Apart from the climate pattern generating it, heat can come from a variety of sources. Repressed emotions over time will cause a stagnation pattern in the liver system that will generate heat, as will continual stress at home and work. Eating too many heating foods, such as deep-fried foods, lamb, and alcohol, can also be a cause.

The mucus that often accompanies this pattern is a physical manifestation of damp/phlegm. The degree of additional damp/phlegm produced depends on your diet and the efficiency of the stomach and pancreas systems. If your diet consists of too many damp- or phlegm-forming foods, it is highly likely that this excess will be sent up to the lung system.

Taking certain medications long term can also be problematic. People suffering from sinusitis, for example, often take antibiotics to address the condition. Antibiotics clear heat and can improve the symptoms for a while by cooling the sinuses, but they do not clear damp/phlegm. As a result, sinusitis is highly likely to return because the climate pattern, of which the mucus is a symptom, remains unaffected by the antibiotics and ripe for more disruption.

Repeated use of antibiotics can also impair the stomach and pancreas systems directly, and this has a very important implication for sinusitis. When impaired, the stomach and pancreas systems are less efficient in helping the digestive process to sort through fluids and get clogged up with dampness themselves.

This can have a direct ripple effect on the lung system, which is where all this extra sticky substance has to be stored. It quickly becomes impaired and unable to send excess fluid down to the kidney system to be processed. Instead, much of it finds its way up into the sinuses.

Food Therapy

Dietary Factors That Can Worsen Sinus Problems

- Hot-natured and damp-forming foods, such as saturated fats, pizzas, deep-fried foods, and beer, can become sources of phlegm. See Damp/Phlegm and Heat for more details.

Dietary Factors That Can Improve Sinus Problems

- Follow a strengthening diet to build up the weakness in the lung and pancreas systems. See General Weakness for more details.
- Eat foods that expel phlegm, such as citrus peel, persimmons, radishes, grapefruit, and pears. See Damp/Phlegm for more details.

Manual Therapy

ON YOUR FACE AND HEAD: Circle your face with a Gua sha tool or your fingers to relax the facial muscles.

Press on Du-24 on the midline of the forehead, then finger-press outwards on both sides to the temples, and circle the temple area. Repeat at equally spaced areas on the midline up to the middle of the eyebrows. Hard-press *yintang*, Bl-1 and Bl-2, *bitong*, and Li-20.

From the eyebrows to the midpoint of your nose, gently finger-press outwards along the eye socket to the temples, then circle the temple area. From the midpoint of your nose to the bottom of the chin, finger-press outwards to the corner of your jaw bone and then circle.

On your neck and shoulders, finger-circle outwards at the base of the skull towards your ear, and back again. Now use a tool or thumb-press along and focus on the occipital areas (Gb-12, Gb-20, Bl-10, and Du-16). Hard-press and knead any tense areas. Finger-circle or scrape down your neck in the muscles on either side of the spine, and go into the shoulder area.

ON YOUR BACK: Gua sha down the lung and pancreas back *shu* regions. Press and knead any areas of tension or *sha* afterwards. You will need help to do this on yourself.

ON YOUR ARMS: Thumb-press or scrape down the lung river, from Lu-5 at your elbow to Lu-9 at your wrist, and as the large intestine is the paired river, up the large intestine river, from Li-5 at your wrist to Li-11 at your elbow. Press and knead any areas of tension.

ON YOUR LEGS: Thumb-press up the pancreas river from Pa-5 to Pa-10, and knead any areas of tension.

ON YOUR HANDS: Press and knead the following areas if sore: Zone 1 – lungs and chest (F-H); C1 – throat, mouth, nose, head (1-4).

ON YOUR FEET: Press and knead zone 1 – head/face, eye, ear on the toes (A-D); zone 2 – lung and chest (E-G).

Thumb-press up the pancreas river from Pa-1 to Pa-5, which covers most of the root *shu* regions and the junction region.

ON YOUR EARS: Press the following areas if sore: Zone 8 – nose; zone 3 – face and head (G-I).

Exercise Therapy

Do exercises 1 and 2 of the Five Qualities of Nature stretches daily to help strengthen the metal and earth system (see p. 101 f.).

Lifestyle Therapy

1. Some people benefit from regularly washing out their sinuses with warm, salty water—the idea being that water should go in and come out the other nostril or the mouth and clean out lingering mucus.
2. Add 1–2 level teaspoons of pure sea salt to one-half litre of lukewarm (previously boiled or sterile) water.

NOTE A quarter- to a half-teaspoon of baking soda can also be added to prevent any burning sensation that can occur. Pour the saline solution into a syringe, dropper, plastic squeeze bottle, or neti pot, lean over a sink, tilt your head, place the tip of the implement gently in the tip of your nostril, and allow gravity or pressure from the bottle, dropper, or syringe to wash out the sinuses.

Eye Disorders

Symptoms
Vary according to condition.

Can Include or Lead to
Orbital neuralgia, glaucoma, uveitis, cataracts, trachoma, conjunctivitis, iritis, keratitis, scleritis, endophthalmitis, and herpes zoster on the eyelid.

When to See a Doctor
If the symptoms are severe.

Common Causes
Stress, overwork, too long in front of a computer monitor, emotional stress, playing video games, exposure to the weather, late nights, lack of sleep,

doing too much, an inappropriate diet of either too many greasy, hot-natured foods or cold-natured raw foods, or a chronic illness.

An Explanation

A glance at the trajectories of the river systems to and from your eyes should be enough to tell you how they influence, and can be influenced, by a range of different rivers. The river systems most related to your eyes are the heart and liver systems, which come up internally into the eye, but also the small intestine, gallbladder, triple burner, bladder, and stomach rivers, which all start or finish in close proximity to your eye.

Underlying most eye patterns is a weakness of the *yin* motion of the liver and/or the kidney systems. This impairment has usually been there a long time, often with mild symptoms, including dry, bloodshot eyes, which can be blurred, sore, and sometimes with spots in your vision, known as floaters, which are like marks on the lens of a camera. Like most *yin* patterns, it may also feel worse in the afternoon or at night.

Over time, the slow burning heat generated by this *yin* weakness can develop into a raging fire, and symptoms like red, painful, watering eyes with a sensation of heat and pressure from within the eyes, often means that the heat has transformed within the liver system and is burning upwards. This pattern frequently gets worse when under emotional stress.

An inappropriate diet can also indirectly create problems in your eyes. A diet consisting of too many hot, greasy foods or too many cold, raw foods can create an impairment in the stomach and pancreas systems and lead to an accumulation of damp/phlegm which, over time, can combine with a heat or cold pattern to affect your eyes.

Food Therapy

Dietary Factors That Can Worsen Eye Problems

- Deep-fried foods, spices, lamb, coffee, and alcohol increase heat and worsen some eye conditions. See Heat for more details.
- Foods that are highly nutritious and sweet, such as dairy products, orange and tomato juice, and pork, worsen phlegm and mucous. See Damp/Phlegm for more details.

Dietary Factors That Can Improve Eye Problems

- Cooling foods, such as tomatoes, watermelon, cucumber, lettuce, radishes, and mangos, soothe heat. See Heat for more details.
- Barley, celery, pumpkin, turnips, lemons and onions, reduce phlegm and mucous. See Damp/Phlegm for more details.
- Cool-natured, sweet foods, such as apples, pears, tomatoes, peas, and asparagus, strengthen *yin*. See *Yin* Weakness for more details.

Manual Therapy

ON YOUR HEAD AND FACE: Rub your hands together vigorously until they feel warm and then place the palms over your eyes for 10 seconds. Repeat this several times.

Press *yintang* in the middle of your eyebrows, and finger-press outwards along the eyebrow to the temples, then circle your temples. Repeat this several times, and then hard-press Bl-2 and *yuyao*.

Repeat this movement from Bl-1, and finger-press outwards around the eye socket to your temples, and circle again. Repeat this several times, and then hard-press Bl-1, St-2, and Gb-1. Repeat from Bl-1, but go below the eye socket around your cheekbone to the temples. Circle the temples again. Repeat this several times.

Finger-circle outwards at the base of the skull towards the ear and back again. Now use a tool or thumb-press along and focus on the occiput areas (Gb-12, Gb-20, Bl-10, and Du-16). Hard-press and knead any tense areas.

ON YOUR ARMS: Thumb-press or scrape down the heart and heart ruler rivers to the wrist root *shu* areas (Ht-7 and Hr-7). Press and knead any areas of tension.

ON YOUR LEGS: Thumb-press up the liver and kidney rivers to Lv-8 and Kd-10, respectively, and scrape down the gallbladder and bladder rivers from your upper leg down to your ankle at Gb-40 and Bl-60. Knead any areas of tension, especially around your knees.

ON YOUR HANDS: Press and knead the following areas, if sore: Zone 1- heart (G); zone 2 – liver (K).

ON YOUR FEET: Press and knead the following areas if sore: Zone 1 – eye, head/face (A-D); zone 2 – heart (G); zone 3 – liver/spleen, stomach and pancreas (J-H).

ON YOUR EARS: Press and knead the following areas if sore: Zone 3 – eye area (I); zone 8; zone 1 – A; support region – relaxation (2) and *shenmen* (1).

Exercise Therapy

Do exercise 5 of the Five Qualities of Nature stretches daily (see p. 103). This is to help strengthen the wood systems: The liver and gallbladder. The balance of the liver system is closely associated with the delicate balance of your eyes.

Lifestyle Therapy

Many people are putting great demands on their eyes on a daily basis without even realizing it, particularly those who sit in front of screens for hours at a time. Studies in the United States have shown that regular computer users have a severely diminished blinking frequency. Normally, we tend to blink about 18 times per minute, but when using a computer or playing a video game, this reduces to only four times per minute.[60]

As blinking is an action designed to protect your eyes, it is essential to take frequent breaks to rest them and return to blinking properly.

For swollen eyelids, soak thin slices of cucumber in salty water (two tablespoons of sea salt dissolved in a cup of water). Put these over your closed eyes for 10 minutes. Repeat daily. Warmth also soothes your eyes, and a rolled-up hot towel placed over your eyes for several minutes can help.

Ear Disorders

Symptoms

Fullness or pain inside or outside the ear, redness, swelling, discharge, a ringing or buzzing sound, partial hearing loss, deafness, dizziness, and headache.

Can Include or Lead to

Otitis media, inflammation, wax build-up, glue ear, abscess, infection of the auditory canal, and mastoiditis.

When to See a Doctor

If the symptoms are severe, the earache continues for more than a few days, or is accompanied by a high fever.

Common Causes

Exposure to the weather; an improper diet of greasy foods; emotional stress, especially anger or frustration; injury; or accident.

An Explanation

Owing to the exposed position of your ears on the sides of your head, wind entering the ear and bringing with it heat, damp, and cold patterns is often the source of ear problems. Any combination of these factors will cause an obstruction in circulation in or around the ear, often with associated pain or discomfort. The most common pattern is for wind and heat to attach within the ear, with accompanying sore throat symptoms.

Common internal causes of earache involve the liver and gallbladder systems, which can become sluggish and blocked when emotionally stressed. The stagnation in these two systems can lead to a build-up in heat, which races upwards via the gallbladder and triple burner rivers (the parent *shaoyang* river) running around your ears. This then hits an obstruction pattern in the river, impairs circulation around your ears, and causes severe pain. It often feels like the problem is deep within the ear. It can also be accompanied by swelling, redness, and fever.

A diet that contains too many sweet, greasy foods can impair the stomach and pancreas systems and lead to an accumulation of damp/phlegm. This damp/phlegm can easily find its way upwards into the ear and quite literally block it, causing mild pain. There is often an ear discharge with this pattern. It is a very common pattern in children.

For cases of earache that are gradual, mild in nature, and involve symptoms of deafness, low ringing noise in the ear, and feelings of tiredness, it is quite possible that the pain is coming from a weakness in the kidney system. Each of the *zang* storage systems is connected to parts of the body, and a weakness in a particular system (for example, the kidney) can adversely affect the corresponding body part (in this case, the ear). The efficiency of the kidney system, therefore, can directly affect the ear and quality of hearing.

Food Therapy

Dietary Factors That Can Worsen Earache
- Overeating and irregular eating habits lead to stagnation in the digestive process, which can develop into a body-wide stagnation pattern. See Stagnation for more details.
- Cow's milk dairy products, concentrated orange juice, and fatty meat such as lamb can create phlegm and mucous build-up in your body. See Damp/Phlegm for more details.

Dietary Factors That Can Improve Earache
- A balanced diet that strengthens the digestive system should be followed, including many of the foods in General Weakness within the structure of a balanced general diet.
- Radishes, celery, rye, pumpkin, garlic, and aduki beans reduce dampness and phlegm. See Damp/Phlegm for more details on diet.

Manual Therapy

ON YOUR HEAD: Finger-press up the side of your neck to the base of your ear, then come behind it on the skull and finger-press around your ear to the front. This is following the triple burner river system. Press and knead any areas of tension, especially above the ear in the temporalis muscle.

Finger-circle outwards from Du-16 at the base of the skull towards the ear and then hard-press and knead or scrape up and down along the occipital areas (Du-16, Gb-12, Gb-20, and Bl-11).

ON YOUR ARMS: The parent river of the gallbladder is *shaoyang,* which means that you need to thumb-press or scrape the triple burner river up your arm to Tb-14. The parent river of the kidney is *shaoyin,* which means that you need to thumb-press or scrape down the heart river to Ht-7.

ON YOUR LEGS: Thumb-press or scrape down the gallbladder and bladder rivers to Gb-40 and Bl-60 at your ankle and up the kidney and liver rivers to Kd-10 and Lv-8 at your knee. Press and knead any areas of tension.

ON YOUR HANDS: Press the following areas, and knead if sore: C1 & C2 on your middle finger (1-4).

Scrape or thumb-press from Tb-1 to Tb-3 (root *shu* regions) and onto Tb-4 (source region). Press and knead any areas of soreness and tension around them.

Scrape or thumb-press from Ht-9 to Ht-7 (root *shu* regions). Press and knead any areas of soreness and tension around them.

ON YOUR FEET: Press the following areas, and knead if sore: Zone 1 – ear, head/Face (A-D); zone 2 – cervical area (O); zone 3 – kidney, gallbladder and liver/spleen (J-I).

Scrape or thumb-press from Gb-44 to Gb-41 (root *shu* regions) and onto Gb-40 (source region). Press and knead any areas of soreness and tension around them.

Scrape or thumb-press from Kd-1 to Kd-3 (root *shu* regions). Press and knead any areas of soreness and tension around them.

ON YOUR EARS: Press the following areas, and knead if sore: Zone 8 – ear; zone 1 – upper (A); support region – *shenmen* (1).

Exercise Therapy

Do exercises 4 and 5 of the Five Qualities of Nature stretches daily (see p. 102 f.). This is to strengthen the wood and water systems. The gallbladder and kidney systems, in particular, are associated with the state of your ears and hearing.

Lifestyle Therapy

1. Whenever possible, your ears and neck should be protected from exposure to the natural elements, especially from the wind.
2. Avoid repeated use of antibiotics, as they can damage the pancreas system and can lead to the accumulation of dampness and phlegm. These sticky substances can easily find their way to the ear and prolong the problem.

3. If there is a possible stress or emotional component to the ear disorder, try to find ways to limit its extent. Think about where stress might be coming from, if not obvious.

Toothache

Symptoms
Pain or increased sensitivity of the teeth, headache, swelling, bleeding gums, insomnia, and agitation.

Can Include or Lead to
Dental cavities, acute or chronic pulpitis, periodontal abscess, and pericoronitis.

When to See a Doctor
If the symptoms are prolonged and severe.

Common Causes
An improper diet of greasy, fatty foods; too much alcohol; stress; too many dairy products; old age; or a lack of oral hygiene.

An Explanation
Often the cause of toothache is obvious, and you only need a simple method of pain reduction before or after a dental visit. Sometimes, however, the pain in the teeth has no clear dental cause and can be a symptom of something else happening in the body. For example, treatment to relieve stiff shoulders often also relieves toothache.

The two river systems most connected to the teeth are the large intestine and stomach. The former is associated with the upper teeth, and the latter is associated with the lower teeth, and you just have to check the trajectories of these rivers to see why. This is the reason treatment to the neck and shoulder area can sometimes relieve toothache as you are potentially removing the obstructions that might be affecting the teeth.

The obstruction can be climatic if wind enters your body and attaches itself within these rivers in your face. This can happen on a windy day, when your body's defences are low, or when blood circulation becomes so weak that it actually generates its own wind pattern. Like all wind-type patterns, there is a tendency for the pain to come and go or move from one place to another.

Sometimes, severe toothache can be due to heat rising via the stomach system. The heat is usually from an accumulation of heat in the stomach and intestine area over some time, normally caused by an inappropriate diet. If this is the case there will probably be other signs of digestive heat, such as constipation.

The kidney system ensures that your bones and teeth are properly nourished to make them strong and durable. When the *yin* motion in the kidney system weakens, your teeth can also become weak, loose, wobbly, or even fall out. This pattern can also lead to a dull toothache that comes and goes.

Food Therapy

Dietary Factors That Can Worsen Toothache

Hot-natured, spicy foods, such as black pepper, chilli, ginger and paprika, worsen heat in the body, as do fried or roasted foods. See Heat for more details.

Dietary Factors That Can Improve Toothache

- Cold-natured foods, such as bananas, tomatoes, grapefruit, cucumbers, lettuce, and radishes, lessen heat in the body. See Heat for more details.
- Foods such as beetroot, dark leafy greens, peas, apricots, dates, pears, and honey strengthen *yin* and blood circulation. See Blood Circulation Weakness and *Yin* Weakness for more details.

Manual Therapy

ON YOUR NECK: As almost all the rivers pass through the neck, it makes sense to start there. Use a Gua sha tool, and scrape down the muscles at the back and sides of your neck. Press and knead any areas of tension afterwards.

ON YOUR ARMS: Thumb-press or scrape up the large intestine river from Li-5, and knead any areas of tension, especially around the root *shu* at the elbow (Li-11).

ON YOUR LEGS: Thumb-press or scrape down the stomach river to St-41 at your ankle. Press and knead any areas of tension, especially in the area of Crouching Rabbit.

ON YOUR HANDS: Press the following areas, and knead if sore: Zone 2 – stomach, pancreas, and large intestine (K-I). Hard-press Li-4, the source region of the large intestine river.

ON YOUR FEET: Press the following areas, and knead if sore: Zone 1 – head/face (particularly, the tops of the fourth and fifth toes), cervical area (A-D); zone 3 – stomach and pancreas (H); zone 4 – large intestine (K-M). Hard-press St-42, the source region of the stomach river.

ON YOUR EARS: Press the following areas, and knead if sore: zone 3 – teeth (I), jaw (H); zone 1 – B; support regions – relaxation (2) and *shenmen* (1).

Exercise Therapy

Do exercise 2 of the Five Qualities of Nature stretches daily (see p. 101 f.). This can help strengthen the stomach and large intestine systems, which are often indicated in toothache.

Lifestyle Therapy

1. If the source of the pain is tooth decay, or another obvious dental-related reason, the pain will probably not go away completely until this is treated by your dentist. If not, the advice on stress and emotions in Facial Pain may be relevant here.
2. The strength of your teeth is associated with the kidney system, so your lifestyle should be one that does not compromise the storage

area of your *yin/yang* resource. This means listening to your body and following the rhythms of the day—basically, avoiding staying up late, overworking, spending too much time looking at screens, and doing *yang* activities during the *yin* part of the day.

Sore Throat

Symptoms
Swollen, sore throat and/or tonsils, redness, feeling hoarse, pain when swallowing, dry throat, dry cough, and difficulty in speaking.

Can Include or Lead to
A cold; flu; acute infections, such as laryngitis, pharyngitis, and tonsillitis; vocal cord polyps; fibroma; or cancer of the larynx/throat.

When to See a Doctor
If the symptoms of pain and/or soreness last more than a couple of weeks or become severe.

Common Causes
Exposure to the weather, smoking, an improper diet of rich, spicy food, too much alcohol, too much multitasking, living in a dry environment (with central heating, for example), regular use of bronchodilator medication (as commonly used for asthma), or prolonged emotional stress.

An Explanation
The immediate pain or discomfort of a sore throat is from a local obstruction pattern affecting the flow of the river systems in your neck area. Heat is often present and comes in from outside your body as part of a climate pattern, usually accompanied by wind. It normally enters through your mouth or neck and can easily lodge itself in your throat. If this is the case, the sore throat would normally be more acute—red, sore, and swollen—and resemble that of an infection.

The heat in your throat can also be caused internally from the lung (due to smoking), from the stomach (due to an over-rich diet), or from the liver system (when there is a strong emotional component). Sometimes, this heat flares up to your throat and causes acute throat symptoms, as it does with external heat; instead, though, internal heat often smolders like the embers of a bonfire and leads to a slight inflammation that goes on for a long time.

Other internal causes are related more to weakness than to heat. When the pattern is chronic, it flares up when you are tired and never completely disappears. It can be due to lung and kidney *yin* weakness, which can come with age, overwork, and regular smoking. As with most *yin* weakness patterns, your throat may be worse in the evening.

The cause may also be a stomach and pancreas impairment from treatment with too many antibiotics. Antibiotics clear heat but not wind or damp, and their repeated use weakens the stomach and pancreas, causing the pattern to be complicated by even more damp/phlegm.

In all cases of sore throat, the earlier it can be treated the better. Lingering sore throats can cause damage to the tissues of the upper respiratory tract, and sometimes can develop into more troubling conditions, such as abscesses.

Food Therapy
Dietary Factors That Can Worsen a Sore Throat
Warming foods, such as coffee, alcohol, lamb, beef, and warm spices, such as cinnamon, ginger, and fennel, feed heat. See Heat and the list of Hot and Warm Foods for more details.

Dietary Factors That Can Improve a Sore Throat
- Moistening foods, such as apricots, lemons, limes, persimmons, strawberries, pears (especially pear juice), watercress, and

cucumbers (and their juice) can soothe the throat.

- Cooling foods such as radishes also expel phlegm and are particularly calming for a sore throat.
- Useful homemade recipes for sore throats include:
  ▸ Dice 3cm of daikon radish (with the peel), and soak it in a little honey. Leave for about an hour and then add a small amount of warm water and drink the mixture.
  ▸ Cook the flesh of a grapefruit with a little water and honey for around five minutes and then eat.

Manual Therapy

ON YOUR HEAD: Finger-circle outwards at the base of the skull, towards the ear and back again. Now use a tool or thumb-press along, focusing on the occipital areas (Gb-12, Gb-20, Bl-10, and Du-16). Hard-press and knead any tense areas.

ON YOUR NECK: Scrape down the muscles on the back and sides of your neck, avoiding the front of your neck. It is very common for *sha* to appear in this area, if you have a sore throat. Any areas of tension can be pressed and kneaded afterwards.

ON YOUR BACK: Scrape down the lung back *shu* region in your upper back. Include the areas above and below. You may need help to do so.

ON YOUR FRONT: Finger-circle or scrape down your sternum, and knead any areas of tension, especially around Ren-17.

ON YOUR ARMS: Thumb-press or scrape up the large intestine river from Li-5 to Li-15 at your shoulder and down the lung river from Lu-5 to Lu-9, and knead any areas of tension.

ON YOUR LEGS: Scrape down the stomach river from St-36 to St-41 and up the pancreas river from Pa-5 to Pa-10. Press and knead any areas of tension.

ON YOUR HANDS: Press the following areas, and knead if sore: the thenar eminence on your palm below your thumb (I-N); zone 1 – chest (F-H).

ON YOUR FEET: Press the following areas, and knead if sore: Zone 1 – cervical area (O); zone 2 – chest (S) and Lv-3.

ON YOUR EARS: Press the following areas, and knead if sore: Zone 1 – B; zone 5 – chest (M-N); support regions – relaxation (2) and *shenmen* (1).

Exercise Therapy

Do exercises 1, 2, and 5 of the Five Qualities of Nature stretches (see p. 101 ff.). Any changes in the integrity of the metal, earth, and wood systems can easily affect the throat.

Lifestyle Therapy

If possible, stay out of the elements and rest. Exposure to wind, cold, or heat can exacerbate the problem, with the potential for a climate pattern to appear. Sometimes, the sore throat is simply the body telling you to stop. This is particularly the case with someone who leads a *yang*-type lifestyle and is consistently doing too much.

Neck Pain

Symptoms

Pain in one or both sides of the neck—the pain can be acute or chronic; tense muscles and tendons; muscle spasms and stiffness.

Can Include or Lead to

Hernia of the cervical disc, whiplash, torticollis, osteoarthritis, degeneration of the cervical vertebrae, and cervical spondylosis.

When to See a Doctor

If the symptoms are severe and steadily getting worse; if there is swelling or bruising; if there are pins and needles in the arms and fingers when touching the neck vertebrae; or if there are any symptoms of shock from a neck injury, such as whiplash.

Common Causes

Exposure to the weather, bad posture, overuse, a trauma or injury, overwork, emotional stress, an inappropriate spinal manipulation or massage, a chronic illness, or an inappropriate diet.

An Explanation

Both acute and chronic neck pain are often related to wind, damp, and cold and the subsequent climate obstruction patterns that arise in the neck area. The most common way for wind, damp, and cold to get into your neck is through direct exposure to the elements. It could be something as simple as being outside on a windy day, not covering up after swimming or exercise, or sleeping without a blanket or warm covers.

Once these climates find their way into your neck tissue, they disrupt the river circulation through your neck area and cause pain, stiffness, and discomfort. They do this by attaching to an area of tissue in the river system that has become disconnected from circulation. All of the river systems come through your neck in some way, so it is an extremely important area to keep clear of obstruction.

These rivers can also be blocked as a result of some kind of local trauma. If improperly treated, the area can drastically weaken over time, and the muscles in your neck can tighten as they are no longer being nourished, resulting in stiffness and cramping. This is often the case with unresolved traumatic injuries, such as whiplash, which start off as acute, very painful, and difficult to move.

Emotional stress and depression can weigh heavily on the liver system and cause it to slow down, which then leads to a general river stagnation pattern in your body. This stagnation can sometimes find itself heading upstream in the gallbladder or bladder river systems, towards the back of the neck, which will then aggravate any neck pain by causing more local neck stagnation.

Any underlying weakness, as often found in stressed, overworked, or chronically ill people, means that the bones, muscles, and tendons in the neck area are undernourished, causing the whole area to become weaker and more susceptible to stagnation or climate patterns.

Food Therapy

Dietary Factors That Can Worsen Neck Pain

If the pattern is one of damp or cold in your neck, it is important not to add to it by eating too many damp-forming or cold-natured foods, such as bananas, dairy products, and wheat. See Damp/Phlegm and Cold for more details.

Dietary Factors That Can Improve Neck Pain

The weakness underlying neck pain can be helped by following a strengthening diet to build up the force of circulation. See General Weakness and Blood Circulation Weakness for more details.

Manual Therapy

CAUTION: Manipulating your neck when there is neck pain can sometimes produce the opposite result to the one desired, making it worse and then take longer to cure. If your neck is very stiff, inflamed, and movement is difficult, it is often best to use areas away from the neck to treat symptoms. Note, too, that if there is a sensation of pins and needles in your arms and fingers when the neck vertebrae are palpated, it could mean that there is a structural problem with the vertebrae, which will need professional medical attention.

ON YOUR NECK: Knead the back of your neck with four fingers together in a circular motion, from the base of the skull to where the neck meets the shoulders.

Pinch the neck muscles with your thumb and fingers from the base of the skull downwards, and keep repeating the pinch as you move your hand down the neck.

Press the neck muscles with flat fingers and rub up and down until you feel warmth in the tissue in your neck.

Press and knead the occipital areas (Bl-10, Gb-20, Gb-12, and Du-16) and any areas of tension at the base of the skull.

Heat can sometimes be beneficial. Use a hot water bottle, heat lamp, or heating pad, or soak a towel in very hot water, wring it out, and then place it on the affected area of the neck.

Use a Gua sha tool to scrape down the back and sides of your neck and into your shoulders. Avoid the front of your neck.

ON YOUR BACK: Treatment on your upper back can sometimes release a pattern that is causing the neck discomfort. Scrape down the back *shu* regions in your upper back (lung, heart, and diaphragm).

ON YOUR ARMS: Thumb-press up the *yang* rivers (triple burner, large intestine, and small intestine) on your arms from Tb-4, Li-5, and Si-5 to Tb-14, Li-15, and Si-10. Press and knead any areas of tension.

ON YOUR LEGS: Thumb-press or scrape down the *yang* rivers (gallbladder, stomach, and bladder) from the top of your legs to Gb-40, St-41, and Bl-60. Press and knead any areas of tension.

ON YOUR HANDS: Press the following areas, and knead if sore: All of zone 4 – cervical spine; C2 – neck (1-2).

ON YOUR FEET: Press the following areas, and knead if sore: Zone 1 – neck (B-D), cervical area (O); zone 2 – shoulder (T); zone 3 – thoracic area (P), liver/spleen (J-L).

ON YOUR EARS: Press the following areas, and knead if sore: Zone 5 – neck (M); zone 2 – cervical area (D); zone 4 – shoulder (J); support region – *shenmen* (1). Press on the area of the ear corresponding to where the pain is.

Exercise Therapy

The following are simple exercises to help strengthen your neck. They should ideally be done sitting down:

❶ *Head Turn Sideways*
Turn your head slowly to the right as far as possible. Turn it to the left slightly and then go even farther to the right. Repeat this several times on the left and right.

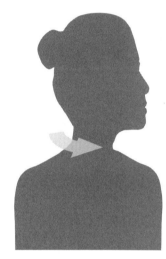

❷ *Head Turn Backwards*
Move your head backwards as far as possible. Return it a little and then move it farther back. Repeat several times.

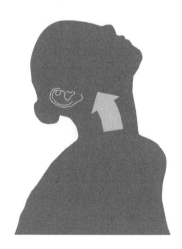

❸ Neck Resistance

Interlink the fingers of both hands, and place them behind your neck. Push your head backwards, and at the same time pull it forwards with your hands.

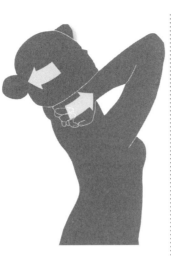

❹ Neck Circle

Relax your head and neck and then slowly move your head in a circular motion as far as possible. Do this several times—first, clockwise, then counter-clockwise.

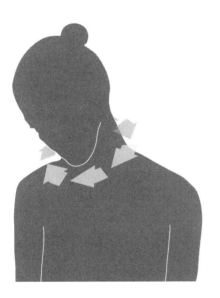

NOTE Be careful not to over-rotate your neck, to avoid injury.

❺ Bend Forwards

Stand with a straight back, feet close together and arms at your sides. Breathe in and then gently bend forward with your upper body. Stop when you reach resistance, and hold the position. As you breathe in, lift your head so you can see in front of you. Return slowly to the original position while breathing out.

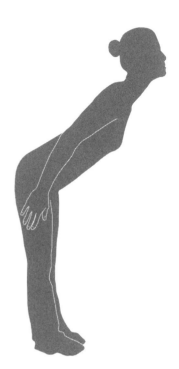

❻ *Do exercises 3 and 5 of the Five Qualities of Nature stretches (see p. 102 ff.).*

Lifestyle Therapy

1. Protect your neck as you engage in simple everyday activities, such as shopping or working at the office, and not just on windy days but from changes in temperature (usually due to air conditioning and artificial heating systems).

2. Do not hesitate to protect your neck from other people's well-meaning massaging fingers. Sometimes a massage can make the pain worse.

3. Be cautious when exercising. Any exercise, no matter how healthy it may seem (tai chi or yoga, for example), can cause damage if you go past your limits and overextend your neck.

To Ice or Not to Ice?

For acute injuries, most people automatically reach for the bag of frozen peas sitting in their freezer, but in order for the injury to heal well, you should not overuse ice. As a general guideline, the following may be helpful:

- If pain is from an acute injury, ice can be used to lessen the swelling during the first 24–48 hours.
- After a 24–48 hour period, or when the swelling has gone down, if sooner, the application of ice can sometimes harm the healing of the area. This is because cold usually causes obstruction by contracting the river systems, including the tissue, muscles, and tendons.
- Heat in the form of a heating pad, heat lamp, or hot towel that is replaced as soon as it cools down is often preferable to aid healing (provided of course the area is not red, hot, and inflamed).

Shoulder Pain

Symptoms

Pain or stiffness in one or both shoulders, including the shoulder joint, muscles, tendons, and the shoulder blade, and referred pain in the arm and back.

Can Include or Lead to

Frozen shoulder, periarthritis of the shoulder, synovitis of the shoulder joint, calcification of the shoulder joint, and tendinitis.

When to See a Doctor

If the symptoms are severe and getting worse, and if there is swelling, bruising, or you are unable to move the shoulder joint.

Common Causes

Overuse; an injury; exposure to the weather; emotional stress; and an improper diet of cold-natured, raw foods or greasy, sweet foods.

An Explanation

Pain in the shoulder area is usually an obstruction pattern. Locally, this may be caused by trauma, an operation, or overuse, or it may be connected to a body-wide pattern of lack of nourishment to the ligaments, tendons, and muscles that hold the shoulder joint in place.

Climatic patterns can often be involved. If the pain is related to a Cold pattern, it will normally be fixed and immovable and can be worse in the morning. This is because cold contracts your tissue structures and it takes time for the *yang* motion of breath to warm and loosen them up. Cold can easily become fixed in your shoulder if there is an existing weakness that allows it to attach to an area of tissue with poor circulation. This area of tissue is the "backwater" that is no longer connected to the main river flow, and which can remain disconnected indefinitely. Being out in cold, windy weather or swimming in the sea can be just enough for the cold to attach to these places.

Often appearing with cold is damp/phlegm. If the pattern is one of damp, then rainy weather can affect it, there may be little flexibility of movement, and it can usually be quite stiff.

With both cold and damp/phlegm, there can be further underlying internal causes. With cold, there can be a *Yang* Weakness pattern that causes an imbalance with the *yin* motion and makes your body more susceptible to cold. With damp/phlegm, it is more the case of an impaired digestive system, often from an improper diet of too many cold-natured, raw, or greasy and sweet foods, and poor eating habits. The stomach and pancreas systems become unable to process food efficiently and build up the accumulation of body fluids in the form of damp and, the more damp that collects, the greater the chance of obstruction.

Sometimes the shoulder pain is chronic, and with distending pain down your arm that worsens when you become stressed. This type of obstruction pattern is connected to a body-wide imbalance in how the liver system maintains smooth circulation. Emotional stress has a tendency to disturb the liver system in particular, and this usually results in stagnation and obstruction patterns wherever the areas of weakness in your body allow them.

Food Therapy

Dietary Factors That Can Worsen Shoulder Pain

- Inappropriate eating habits, such as overeating or eating late at night, can add to any general stagnation pattern in your body, and by definition in your shoulder, too.
- If cold, damp, or phlegm are present, it is very important to limit those foods in the diet that aggravate these conditions and remove a potential source of the problem. See Cold and Damp/Phlegm for more details.

Dietary Factors That Can Improve Shoulder Pain

- If a cold pattern is present in the shoulder, then adding more warming foods, such as garlic, ginger, black pepper, chestnuts, cherries, and red wine, to the diet will be beneficial. See Cold for more details.
- If damp/phlegm is present, eat more foods that reduce moisture, such as rye bread or rye crackers, watercress, adzuki beans, radish, onions, and pumpkins. See Damp/phlegm for more details.
- For any underlying Weakness of Blood Circulation, eat more blood-nourishing foods, such as dark leafy greens, beetroot, chicken soup, and legumes. See Blood Circulation Weakness for more details.
- Stagnation can be reduced by eating less, at regular times, and in a calm manner. The following foods can also help: spices such as turmeric, ginger, and cumin; turnip; the peel of citrus fruits; and radishes. See Stagnation for more details.

Manual Therapy

For treatment purposes with manual therapy, it is important to identify where the shoulder pain is located:

- Front: Lung river system
- Side: Large intestine river system
- Back: Small intestine and bladder river systems
- On top of the trapezius: Gallbladder river system

Movement is important. If you move your arm in different directions, note which direction worsens the pain.

- Forwards movement of your arm: *Yangming/taiyin* motion (stomach and lung).
- Sideways movement of your arm: *Yangming* motion (stomach and large intestine).
- Backwards movement of your arm: *Taiyang* motion (bladder and small intestine).
- If the pain is acute, it is best to use areas away from your shoulder so as not to potentially worsen the condition.

ON YOUR NECK AND SHOULDERS: Scrape downwards from your neck over the shoulder area. Be careful not to scrape over the bony structures towards your arm. Press and knead any sore areas you find.

ON YOUR FRONT: Scrape downwards at the Lu-1, Lu-2, and *jianqian* areas on the front of your shoulder, press and knead any tense areas.

Thumb-press or scrape down the sternum to Ren-17.

ON YOUR BACK: Scrape down the lung, heart, and diaphragm back *shu* regions and downwards and outwards to the side of these areas towards the side of your body.

ON YOUR ARMS: Thumb-press up any of the three *yang* rivers (triple burner, large intestine, or small intestine) or down one *yin* river, the lung, depending on which is most involved with the shoulder discomfort. Press and knead any areas of tension in the tissue.

ON YOUR LEGS: Thumb-press or scrape down whichever of the three *yang* rivers in your legs (gallbladder, stomach, or bladder) is most involved in your neck discomfort. Scrape or press to Gb-40, St-41, and Bl-60.

ON YOUR HANDS: Press the following areas, and knead if sore: All of zone 4 – neck; zone 5 – upper back area; fingers B and D – upper arm (1-2).

ON YOUR FEET: Press and knead zone 2 – shoulder and scapula (T), chest (S), thoracic area (P); zone 1 – cervical area (O).

ON YOUR EARS: Press the following areas, and knead if sore: Zone 4 – shoulder and arm (J-K): zone 2 – cervical area and thoracic area (D-E); support regions – relaxation (2) and *shenmen* (1).

Exercise Therapy

The following exercises can relax and strengthen your shoulders:

➊ *Shoulder Rotate*

Bend your waist slightly, stretch both arms out straight, and gently rotate the shoulder joint in a forwards direction.

➋ *Shoulder Stretch*

Stretch each arm upwards, while standing in front of a wall, and mark how high they go. Repeat this, and try to increase the height each time.

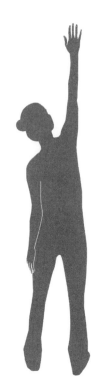

➌ *Arm Lift*

Stand with your arms at your sides and your feet shoulders'-width apart. Breathe in while gently bringing both arms out to the sides. Stop when your arms reach shoulder height. Breathe out, and let your arms fall. Repeat the sequence several times.

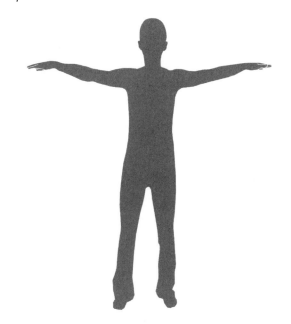

❹ *Twist Your Waist*

Stand with your arms at your sides and your feet shoulders'-width apart. Lift both arms to the sides. Using your waist as a pivot, twist the top half of your body until you feel resistance and then twist in the opposite direction. Repeat the sequence several times.

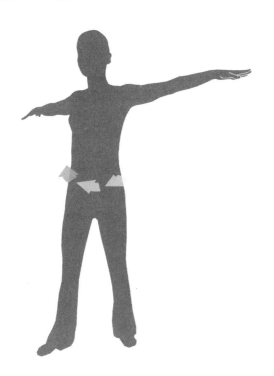

❺ *Do exercise Bend Forwards from Neck Pain as this gently moves the shoulder (see p. 192 f.).*

❻ *Do exercise Crouch Twist from General Weakness, as this involves twisting the shoulder joint (see p. 139).*

❼ *Do exercises 1 and 3 of the Five Qualities of Nature stretches daily (see p. 101 ff.). These can strengthen the river systems that run through your shoulder.*

Lifestyle Therapy

If possible, rotate the joint through its full pain-free range of movement daily (in other words, move it until it starts to hurt and do not go any farther). If the injury is acute, note the advice about putting ice on it in Neck Pain.

21

Chest Area

Colds and Flu

Symptoms
Runny nose, sore throat, cough, fever or chills, sneezing, tiredness, stiff and sore neck, muscle aches, and headache.

Can Include or Lead to
Common cold, influenza, upper respiratory infection, bronchitis, or pneumonia.

When to See a Doctor
If severe or symptoms last more than five days.

Common Causes
Tiredness, overwork, exposure to climates (wind, heat, and cold), air-conditioning, going in and out of heated or air-conditioned shops, not wearing appropriate clothing, or sitting in a draft.

An Explanation
Colds and flu are the classic symptoms of a body trying to defend itself from a climate pattern. While you might be more familiar with the idea of a virus that it is caught from being in close proximity to a carrier, the understanding of the ancient Chinese was that colds and flu result from a climate (wind) meeting the natural defences (*wei qi*) that surround your body. This means that you can develop the symptoms of a cold or flu from the simple motion of wind, whether it be air-conditioning, a draft, a breeze, a fan, or a windy day. And what you experience is *wei qi* fighting off the wind to prevent it from going deeper into the river circulation system.

Wind, however, is usually not alone. It acts as the carrier motion of a passenger climate into your body (cold, heat, or damp), and these find their way into the lung system via your mouth or nose. The immediate effect of this is to disrupt the downwards action of the lung system, causing sneezing and coughing. And then your body will react to the passenger climate—heat can cause a fever; cold may cause shivers; and damp may develop into phlegm and a cough. In many cases, more than one climate is present, and sometimes all of them—and with time, cold can develop into heat.

If the climate pattern can be expelled effectively within the first 24 hours, the symptoms usually go away fairly quickly. If left to take hold in the lung system without the right treatment, the pattern can often go deeper into the body and be harder to get rid of.

Food Therapy
Dietary Factors That Can Worsen Colds and Flu
- Overconsumption of damp-producing foods, such as cow's milk dairy products, fried foods, bananas, and cold drinks from the fridge, can lead to the accumulation of damp. See Damp/Phlegm for more details.

Dietary Factors That Can Improve Colds and Flu

Simple foods that are easy to digest are best. Choose vegetables or grains in the form of soups or broths, soft rice, and porridge (oatmeal). An important distinction to make is whether you feel more chilly (a cold pattern) or more hot and feverish (a heat pattern) as different types of foods help each pattern:

- If you feel mainly chilly: Parsnips, horseradish, cinnamon, garlic, and onions.
- If you have mainly a fever: Parsley, aubergines, carrots, peas, broccoli, turnips, lemon juice, grapefruit, and fruit.
- In both cases, tea can be beneficial, especially when made with sweat-inducing herbs, such as ginger (use fresh ginger root) or chamomile for a cold pattern and peppermint or elderflower for heat. Honey and lemon can be added to the tea to make it taste better.

Manual Therapy

ON YOUR HEAD: Knead, or scrape up and down, along the occipital area at the back of your head.

Hard-press any tension you feel, including Du-16, Gb-12, Gb-20, and Bl-11.

ON YOUR NECK: Scrape down the back and sides of your neck into your shoulders. Avoid the front of your neck.

ON YOUR BACK: Scrape down the lung back *shu* region on your upper back. Expect to see *sha* marks, as your body is dealing with the climate pattern.

ON YOUR ARMS: Scrape down the lung and thumb-press up the large intestine river in your arms. Knead any areas of tension, especially Lu-7 and Lu-10 and Li-4 and Li-11.

Thumb-press up the triple burner river on the back of your forearm, and knead any tense areas, including the Tb-5 area.

ON YOUR HANDS: Press the following areas, and knead if sore: Li-4 to Li-3 area; zone 1 – chest (S) and lung (F-H); C1 & C2 – throat, mouth, nose, head (1-4).

ON YOUR FEET: Press the following areas, and knead if sore: The whole of zone 1; zone 2 – lung (E-F), scapula and shoulder (T).

GINGER & DANDELION FOOT SOAK: Boil 50g (1.7oz) of ginger and 50g of dandelion in water, and simmer for 15 minutes. Add this liquid to the foot bath. The combination of ginger for cold and dandelion for heat makes this useful for colds and flu. For more information on foot soaks, see Heat Your Feet in *Yang* Weakness.

ON YOUR EARS: Press the following areas, and knead if sore: Zone 3 – head and face area (G-I); zone 1 – B.

Exercise Therapy

Do exercise 1 of the Five Qualities of Nature stretches (see p. 101) to help strengthen the lung system and prevent colds and the flu.

Lifestyle Therapy

1. If you are suffering from a cold or flu, the best place to be is at home resting. If you have to be outside, it is very important to wear clothing that covers and protects your neck.
2. The most effective solution to a cold or flu is usually to sweat it out. This literally means getting into bed, covering in a blanket or comforter, wearing extra clothes, and regularly drinking warm sweat-inducing tea (see earlier in this section). If sweating, any damp clothing or covers should be changed promptly.
3. If in the early stage of a cold or flu and not sweating, a hot bath can help to get it started. Afterwards, wrap yourself in a dressing gown or towels for 10 minutes, then take a warm shower.

4. It is important not to do any physical exercise and, if possible, stop working. The more rundown your body is, the greater the likelihood for the pattern to worsen.

5. Exercise is very important in the prevention of colds. A recent study concluded that the frequency of colds among people who exercised at least five days a week was half that of people exercising once a week or less.[61]

Cough

Symptoms
A cough that may be chronic or acute, dry or wet (brings up mucous), weak or barking, and with a tight chest.

Can Include or Lead to
Common cold, upper respiratory tract infection, bronchitis, pneumonia, pulmonary emphysema, and pulmonary tuberculosis.

When to See a Doctor
If you are coughing up blood, there is accompanying breathlessness, or the coughing lasts for longer than a week.

Common Causes
Overwork, emotional problems such as worry and frustration, too many dairy products and greasy foods, smoking, asthma medication, bad posture, or a long chronic illness.

An Explanation
A cough is a good example of a counterflow motion. The movement of the lung system is downwards, as it sends down the nutritive force from the air you breathe to mix with nutritive force extracted from digestion. This mixture is basically the fuel that runs your body. This downward motion sometimes becomes impaired, and instead of flowing downwards it rises, causing a cough.

The impairment is usually connected to a climate pattern, and coughs often occur due to wind entering the lung system, as described in the previous Colds and Flu section. They are usually accompanied by heat, with any mucous being thick and yellow or green, or by cold, in which case any mucous would be watery, white, or clear.

Coughs can also be caused by the accumulation of damp/phlegm in the lung system or from eating an improper diet. A distinctive sign of this is when phlegm is expelled with the cough and a rattling sound can be heard in the lungs, often worse at night or first thing in the morning. They can also be caused by stagnation from an impaired liver system due to stress and emotional issues. This agitation from below can then obstruct the downwards motion of the lung system. With this pattern, the cough usually becomes worse with stress and can result in a barking cough that is worse in the afternoon.

If the *yin* motion of the lung and kidney systems is impaired, there will not be enough moisture for either to function properly, as *yang* often generates too much heat and dryness. This dry pattern is usually worse in the afternoon or evening.

Dietary Factors That Can Worsen a Cough
- Hot-natured, spicy food and greasy food can worsen any kind of cough. See Heat for more details.
- Dairy products, peanuts, bananas, and other damp-forming foods should be avoided in coughs with lots of mucous. See Damp/Phlegm for more details.

Dietary Factors That Can Improve a Cough
- If the cough is dry and due to a weakness of *yin* in the lung system, the following foods may help moisturize the lungs again: Bananas, pears, tangerines, honeydew melons, almonds, sunflower and sesame seeds, milk, and honey.

- If the cough is barking and caused by too much heat, the following may be helpful in reducing the heat in the lung system: Apples, pears, asparagus, radish, carrots, tomatoes, mushrooms, mung beans, green tea, and peppermint tea.
- If there is a lot of phlegm with the cough, it is important to add the following foods to your diet: Grapefruit, tangerine peel, grapefruit peel, watercress, radishes, peppermint tea, and lemon juice.

Manual Therapy

ON YOUR FRONT: Finger-press or scrape down the middle of the sternum to Ren-17, and knead any areas of tension.

Scrape down the area around Lu-1 and Lu-2 and into the pectoral muscle, and press and knead any tense areas.

ON YOUR BACK: Scrape down the lung and diaphragm back *shu* regions on your upper back. Expect to see *sha* marks as your body deals with the climate pattern.

ON YOUR ARMS: Thumb-press or scrape down the lung and up the large intestine rivers. Knead any tense areas, especially around Lu-5 and Li-11, the root *shu* regions in the elbow area.

ON YOUR HANDS: Press and knead the following areas if sore: Li-3 to Li-4 area; Lu-10 to Lu-11 area; zone 1 – throat area, lung, and chest (F-H).

ON YOUR FEET: Press and knead the following areas if sore: Zone 2 – chest and lung (E-F); scapula and shoulder (T).

ON YOUR EAR: Press and knead the following areas if sore: Zone 1- B; zone 5 – chest (M-N); support region – *shenmen* (1).

Exercise Therapy

Do exercises 1 and 2 of the Five Qualities of Nature stretches (see p. 101 f.). These can strengthen the lung system and reduce damp/phlegm.

Lifestyle Therapy

1. Smoking is a major cause of coughs, and the use of all tobacco products should be stopped. The action of smoking is the inhaling of a heating substance into your physical lungs, which can damage the *yin* motion of the lung system. Often simply avoiding tobacco is enough to stop a cough.
2. The simplest remedies are often the best. A recent American study of children aged between two and 18 years of age concluded that the effects of buckwheat honey on night-time coughs was more soothing than an over-the-counter medication.[62]

Asthma, Breathlessness, and Wheezing

Symptoms

Shortness of breath, wheezing, difficulty in breathing, stuffiness in the chest, cough, and phlegm.

Can Include or Lead to

Asthma, chronic obstructive pulmonary disease (COPD), bronchitis, pulmonary tuberculosis, emphysema, pleurisy, and lung cancer.

When to See a Doctor

If the symptoms worsen or persist.

Common Causes

A constitutional weakness; an improper diet of greasy foods; a chronic illness; emotional stress; overwork; and a hectic lifestyle.

An Explanation

Asthma is a common problem, so common, in fact, that it is thought that more than 334 million people worldwide currently suffer from it, and that this number will increase by 100 million in the next decade.[63]

Asthma is usually caused by a climate pattern. It is often due to wind that has entered the lung system, usually because of a weakness in the body's defences, and stayed there in an area of tissue that is disconnected from the main circulation, disrupting how circulation patterns flow around the body. This, combined with a weak digestive process, often due to an improper diet or overuse of antibiotics, can cause damp/phlegm to accumulate and be stored in the lung system.

A combination of this accumulated phlegm at the bottom of your lungs, and the obstruction patterns caused by wind, can quickly transform into heat and burn up any moisture within the lung system. This then leaves it dry, weak, and susceptible to further climate obstruction.

Acute Asthma

HEAT IN THE LUNG SYSTEM: If an asthma attack is caused by wind and heat, any mucus is usually yellow or green and thick and sticky.

COLD IN THE LUNG SYSTEM: If an asthma attack is caused by wind and cold, it is often more difficult to exhale. Any mucus is normally watery, white, or clear, and there is usually a feeling of coldness. The pattern worsens with cold weather.

Chronic Asthma

In the young, old, and chronically ill, it is sometimes the case that breathing problems involve a breakdown of the relationship between the lung and kidney systems. There is a close partnership between the lung and the kidney when we breathe. The lung system sends a forceful downwards motion towards the kidney, and the kidney system continues this motion to the termination of the breath. If this relationship is stable, there is the smooth motion of breath, the same as the *yin/yang* base pattern of the universe. If the kidney system, however, is in any way impaired, then the smooth breathing process becomes interrupted.

With this pattern, it is usually more difficult to inhale than to exhale.

Ironically, prolonged use of the most common asthma medications can make this imbalance worse. Salbutamol or albuterol, commonly known as Ventolin, among others, gradually deplete the lung system, and inhaled corticosteroids like Pulmicort or Flovent can dry up both lung and kidney and the moisture in the *yin* motion.

Food Therapy

Dietary Factors That Can Worsen Breathing

- Cold-natured, raw foods can solidify the phlegm in the chest and generate more mucus by weakening the digestive process. See Cold for more details.
- Hot-natured, spicy food and seafood can cause heat to build up in the lung system. See Heat for more details.

Dietary Factors That Can Improve Breathing

- Follow a simple, bland strengthening diet to fortify your lung system. See General Weakness for more details.
- The following foods can help with asthma:
  - **IN GENERAL:** Green vegetables, pumpkins, carrots, and apricots can help strengthen and protect the lung system.
  - **FOR CHEST TIGHTNESS AND SPASMS:** Anchovies, salmon, mackerel, sardines and tuna, and pumpkin seeds, dark green vegetables, and blackcurrant can help.
  - **FOR PHLEGM PATTERNS:** The peel of citrus fruits, such as tangerines, lemons, and grapefruit, and horseradish and adzuki beans help expel phlegm from the lung system.
  - **FOR COLD PATTERNS:** Garlic, basil, ginger, oats, walnuts, almonds, and sunflower seeds.
  - **FOR HOT PATTERNS:** Radishes, lemons, and limes may be helpful.

Manual Therapy

ON YOUR FRONT: Finger-press or scrape down the middle of the sternum to Ren-17, and knead any areas of tension.

Scrape down the area around Lu-1 and Lu-2 and also into the pectoral muscle, and press and knead any tense areas.

ON YOUR BACK: Scrape down the lung and diaphragm back *shu* regions on your upper back. Expect to see *sha* marks, as your body is dealing with the climate pattern.

ON YOUR ARMS: Thumb-press down the lung and up the large intestine rivers. Knead any tense areas, especially around Lu-5 and Li-11 in the elbow area.

ON YOUR LEGS: Thumb-press or scrape down the stomach and bladder rivers, from your upper leg to St-41 and Bl-60. Press and knead any areas of tension, in particular the area between St-36 and St-40 and your calf muscles.

Thumb-press up your kidney river, from Kd-3 to Kd-10.

ON YOUR HANDS: Press and knead the following areas, if sore: Zone 1 – throat area, lung, and chest (F-H).

ON YOUR FEET: Press and knead the following areas, if sore: Zone 2 – chest and lung (E-F); zone 3 – kidney (I), scapula and shoulder (T). Thumb-press from Kd-1 to Kd-3, and Bl-67 to Bl-60.

ON YOUR EARS: Press and knead the following areas, if sore: Zone 1 – B; zone 5 – chest (M-N); support regions – relaxation (2) and *shenmen* (1).

Exercise Therapy

Do exercises 1–5 of the Five Qualities of Nature stretches to help open and strengthen the lung system and your chest (see p. 101 ff.).

Lifestyle Therapy

A variety of preventative measures can be taken to lessen the chances of problems with asthma:

1. Weather can affect your lung system. To avoid the climates entering your body and affecting the lung system, it is important to dress appropriately when outside, especially protect your neck from the wind and cold.
2. Asthma attack triggers include fumes, smoke, or dust. Minimize situations where you are likely to encounter these.
3. Posture can also affect the lung system, and habitually bad posture often creates weakness. A British study concluded that children who spend more than two hours a day sitting watching TV have double the risk of developing asthma.[64] Extended periods of inactivity, stooping over work, prolonged periods in front of a computer, and working without breaks should, therefore, be avoided.
4. The lung system can be strengthened by gentle exercise and fresh, clean air. Some form of outdoor activity, such as walking, is essential to support the lungs.

Chest Pain

Symptoms
Pain, stuffiness or heaviness in the chest, palpitations, and shortness of breath.

Can Include or Lead to
Heart problems, pulmonary embolism, pleurisy, angina, depression, hiatal hernia, peptic ulcer, pancreatitis, and hyperventilation.

When to See a Doctor
If the symptoms are severe, persistent, or with numbness, tingling, or pins and needles in the limbs. Seek immediate medical attention for a crushing chest pain that may extend to the arms and jaw.

Common Causes

An improper diet, which weakens the stomach and pancreas systems; emotional stress; old age; or repeatedly catching colds or coming down with flu.

An Explanation

Chest pain suggests that there is some kind of obstruction pattern present. The question is where and why. It often stems from the effects of stress, repressed emotions, or a sedentary lifestyle on the liver system, and is frequently connected to the muscular structures around your chest. For this reason, the pain can often feel worse when stressed and is more of a discomfort or stuffiness than pain. It often feels better when relaxing and after a big sigh.

Related to this is the pancreas system and how digestion can directly affect the feeling of the chest area. The "Great Collateral of the Pancreas" is a bird cage-like structure of blood vessels covering the inside of the chest area and influencing both the smooth breath motion of the chest and the circulation of blood through the tissue bed.

Should the chest pain be acute, and there is a stabbing, crushing, or sharp sensation, this suggests the obstruction is more localized within the chest and perhaps the heart system. This could feel worse at night and would normally signal the need for a rapid hospital visit to check on the condition of your heart.

Obstructions can also be caused by damp/phlegm, which can collect in your lungs as a result of an inappropriate diet or due to a climate pattern. Your chest can sound rattly when breathing, owing to the excess phlegm present in the lungs, and coughing can often produce phlegm. If heat is also present with the phlegm, your chest can feel congested, accompanied by a burning sensation.

Underlying the above conditions, some form of heart system weakness is normally present in cases of chest pain. This normally manifests as palpitations and an irregular heartbeat, and may be part of a General Weakness pattern. Unless this is resolved, the chest pain is likely to either continue or return at a later date.

Food Therapy

Dietary Factors That Can Worsen Chest Pain

- Overeating can cause stagnation in the digestive process and, therefore, add to any blockage in the chest.
- Salads, raw fruit and vegetables, dairy products, ice-cold drinks, and other cold-natured foods can also add to the stagnation pattern. See Cold for more details.

Dietary Factors That Can Improve Chest Pain

- A diet that strengthens can help rebalance the systems within the chest area. See General Weakness for more details.
- The peel of citrus fruits, such as tangerines, lemons, and grapefruit; horseradish; barley; and adzuki beans can help if the pattern is one of damp/phlegm in the chest. See Damp/Phlegm for more details.
- Herbs and spices, such as chives, cloves, marjoram, turmeric, and basil have a moving quality that is beneficial for stagnation patterns. See Stagnation for more details.

Manual Therapy

ON YOUR FRONT: Finger-circle or scrape down your sternum, and knead any areas of tension. If it feels relieving, hard-press Ren-17, as this can have a relaxing effect on the intercostal muscles.

ON YOUR BACK: Scrape down the back *shu* regions of your upper back behind your chest area. This means covering the lung, heart, and diaphragm areas. This is your upper back, so you will need the help of another person to treat you.

ON YOUR ARMS: Thumb-press the heart ruler and lung rivers, down to Hr-7 and Lu-9 at your wrist. Knead any tension you find, especially below Hr-3 and Lu-5.

ON YOUR LEGS: Scrape or thumb-press down the stomach and gallbladder rivers to St-41 and Gb-40. Check the two root *shu* regions, St-36 and Gb-34, for tension, and press and knead if tense.

Scrape or thumb-press up the pancreas and liver rivers from Pa-5 and Lv-4 to Pa-9 and Lv-8 (all of which are root *shu* regions), and press and knead any areas of tension.

ON YOUR HANDS: Press and knead the following areas, if sore: Li-4 area; zone 1 – chest, lung, and heart (F-H); zone 5 – upper back area.

ON YOUR FEET: Do the Foot Circulation sequence in chapter 13. Use your fingers or a Gua sha tool.

Also press the following areas, and knead if sore: Zone 2 – chest and lung (E-G); zone 3 – liver/spleen, heart, and kidney (J-H).

Thumb-press the root *shu* and source regions, from Pa-1 to Pa-5 and from Lv-1 to Lv-4.

ON YOUR EARS: Press the following areas, and knead if sore: Zone 5 – chest (M-N); zone 1 – B; support regions – relaxation (2) and *shenmen* (1).

Exercise Therapy

❶ *Five Qualities of Nature Stretches*

Do exercises 1–5 of the Five Qualities of Nature stretches to help open and strengthen the chest area (see p. 101 ff.).

❷ *Bend Backwards*

Stand with a straight back, feet shoulders'-width apart, and place your palms on your lower back. Breathe in, then gently bend backwards from the hips as you breathe out. Stop when you reach resistance, and hold it for a few seconds. Slowly return to the original position, and repeat the sequence several times.

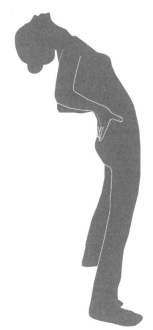

Lifestyle Therapy

1. Obstruction patterns in the chest can often be helped with light, regular exercise, especially exercise that involves twisting and stretching the upper part of your body.

2. If stress is part of the picture, reduce it with stress management techniques, such as managing your time better or just letting things go.

3. Breathing deeply and meditatively can help to train your lungs and focus your attention on the chest area. You can do this by just being aware of your breathing. We do it all the time but we rarely think about it. So take time out of your schedule, sit in a quiet, comfortable place, and breathe. Start by taking larger breaths in than normal, keeping it in your lungs for slightly longer, then releasing it for a longer time. Repeat until you reach a state of relaxation and breathe comfortably.

Palpitations and Irregular Heart Beat

Symptoms

A pounding heartbeat, a fluttering feeling in the chest, restlessness, anxiety, insomnia, shortness of breath, and tiredness.

Can Include or Lead to

Cardiac arrhythmias, hyperthyroidism, anaemia, menopausal complications, coronary artery disease, neurosis, angina, and depression.

When to See a Doctor

If the symptoms are severe and persistent, and if there is breathlessness, chest pain, or dizziness.

Common Causes

Emotional stress, depression, prolonged grief, sadness, overwork, medication side effects, and overexercise.

An Explanation

Palpitations and irregularities in your heart beat can be a symptom of a heart condition and should be investigated by a medical professional. Despite how it may feel, however, for many cases of palpitations, there is little actually wrong with the physical heart itself.

The problem often lies with an impairment of the heart system, and by definition, an impairment of the heart ruler, the system connected to the main blood vessels feeding your heart. The cause of this imbalance in the heart, in turn, can often be found elsewhere in the body.

As in nature, there is a close relationship between fire (heart) and water (kidney) in your body. Both have the ability to directly affect the other through their heating or cooling actions. The balance of motion with *yin* and *yang* in the kidney system is, therefore, directly linked with the balance of motion of heart *yin* and *yang*. If the kidney system is impaired, the heart system is too, and vice versa.

In practice, what this means is that when there is an impairment of kidney *yin* motion, it can no longer help contain heart *yang*. Without being controlled, heart *yang* motion can then become hot and agitated, which will affect the heart system and often lead to palpitations, sleeping problems, and a feeling of heat.

An improper diet and bad eating habits can often lead to a weakness and sluggishness in digestion. This means that the stomach and pancreas systems are no longer efficient in transforming food into the five flavours and sending the nutrition from the bitter flavour to the heart system. This then weakens heart *yang* motion, causing palpitations, sleeping problems, panic attacks, and dizziness.

A weakened digestive process can also contribute to the formation of phlegm in your chest, especially when accompanied by a diet of hot, phlegm-forming foods. The phlegm combines with heat to obstruct your heart, and causes restlessness, waking up before dawn, and digestive problems, in addition to palpitations.

Stagnation is often caused by the liver system and related to emotional stress or sedentary lifestyle habits. The stagnation creates an obstruction pattern in your chest and disrupts correct heart functioning, which can be accompanied by pain or congestion in the chest.

Dietary Factors That Can Worsen Palpitations

- Coffee, caffeinated soft drinks, alcohol, and other stimulants can agitate the heart system.
- Deep-fried foods, fatty meat, junk food, beer, and other hot-natured, damp/phlegm-producing foods will add to the phlegm, heat, and stagnation. See Heat and Damp/Phlegm for more details.
- Salads and other cold-natured, raw foods can contract and constrict circulation, adding to any stagnation pattern. See Cold for more details.

Dietary Factors That Can Improve Palpitations

- A general strengthening diet can improve the pancreas, kidney, and heart systems. Wheat, in particular, can be very nourishing for the heart system and quinoa for the heart ruler system. See General Weakness for more details.
- For cases of stagnation, add foods that will move circulation, such as turmeric, oregano, nutmeg, and ginger. See Stagnation for more details.

Manual Therapy

ON YOUR FRONT: Scrape down the middle of your sternum as far as Ren-17. Press and knead any areas of tension, especially at the attachments of the ribs to the sternum.

ON YOUR BACK: Scrape down the heart and diaphragm back *shu* regions on your upper back.

ON YOUR ARMS: Thumb-press or scrape down the heart and heart ruler rivers to Ht-7 and Hr-7 at your wrist. Press and knead any areas of tension, especially in the muscle below Hr-3 and Ht-3, and at Hr-6 near the wrist.

ON YOUR LEGS: Thumb-press up the kidney and pancreas rivers to Kd-10 and Pa-9, and hard-press around the Kd-7 area to help bring down the pulse rate.

Thumb-press or scrape down Crouching Rabbit on the stomach river, and continue down to the muscles around St-36 and St-40.

ON YOUR HANDS: Press and knead the following areas, if sore: Li-4 area; zone 1 – heart and chest (F-H); zone 5 – upper back area.

ON YOUR FEET: Do the Foot Circulation sequence in chapter 13. Use your fingers or a Gua sha tool.

Also press the following areas, and knead if sore: Zone 2 – heart, chest, and lung (E-G); zone 3 – liver/spleen, pancreas, and kidney (J-H).

ON YOUR EARS: Press the following areas, and knead if sore: Zone 1 – A & B; zone 5 – chest (M-N); support regions – relaxation (2) and *shenmen* (1).

Exercise Therapy

❶ *Do the Bend Backwards exercise from the Chest Pain section (see p. 205).*

❷ *Do stretches 1–5 of the Five Qualities of Nature stretches (see p. 101 ff.). When done regularly, they can strengthen the chest area and heart system.*

Lifestyle Advice

1. Exercise is essential to prevent stagnation, but it is important to avoid strenuous exercise like tennis, squash, and running, as excessive sweating can weaken the *yang* motion of your heart system.

2. Avoid smoking, as it can cause or add to an accumulation of phlegm and heat in your chest.

3. Sometimes, there is a strong emotional component to palpitations and heart irregularities and changes need to be made. One of the most important is letting your feelings out. This could be talking with someone close or just writing out how you feel on paper.

4. If dealing with stress is a problem, think about how this can be resolved. Actually asking for help is often a major step in a positive direction, as is being honest about what works or does not work and letting go of things you cannot change.

22

Stomach and Abdominal Area

Nausea

Symptoms

Nausea, bloating, acid reflux, loss of appetite, and tiredness.

Can Include or Lead to

Morning sickness, travel sickness, food intolerance, and gastritis.

When to See a Doctor

If the symptoms are severe or persistent.

Common Causes

Strong emotions, stress, overeating, an improper diet, overuse of antibiotics, medication side-effects, travel, pregnancy, or over-worry.

An Explanation

When you consume food, the process of digestion begins with the stomach and pancreas systems. The stomach system has a holding function, whereby it keeps the food within it and starts the fermenting process.

This is how the food is broken down into the five flavours and sent towards the related systems in your body: Sour to the liver, pungent to the lung, bitter to the heart, salty to the kidney, and sweet to the pancreas system. In order to hold the food in your stomach, and for it to go on through the digestive tract, there is a downwards motion within the stomach system. What happens with nausea is that this downwards motion is impaired, and the subsequent imbalance causes a counterflow upwards motion.

The cause of this could be an obstruction pattern. This for example is the case with morning sickness—the obstruction being the little person in the uterus. It can also be caused by emotional stress, which allows the liver system to stagnate. The muscles used to process food downwards in the stomach and intestines can easily then become tense and unable to function properly. The downwards motion then goes sideways instead of downwards and disrupts the stomach system. This is how a sudden outburst of anger can cause nausea.

The process of digestion can become sluggish with an irregular diet or if consuming too many damp/phlegm-forming foods. The stomach and pancreas systems, therefore, cannot process food efficiently, and as a consequence, overproduce damp, which further blocks the downwards motion and disrupts digestion.

Food Therapy

Dietary Factors That Can Worsen Nausea

- Overeating greasy and cold, raw foods can weaken the stomach and pancreas systems and lead to nausea. See Damp/Phlegm and Cold for more details.

Dietary Factors That Can Improve Nausea

- A diet of easily digestible bland food that strengthens the stomach and pancreas systems should be followed to prevent nausea. See General Weakness for more details.
- Drinks should be sipped frequently rather than drunk in a large amount at once.
- In cases of morning sickness or drug reactions, where regular nausea is experienced, it may be necessary to eat many small meals throughout the day.
- Pumpkin or squash seeds, millet, rice, ginger, and spiced teas can help manage nausea. Celery can also help, as it encourages the downwards motion of the stomach system.
- Several trials have confirmed the efficacy of ginger in significantly reducing nausea in pregnant women.[65] Read the Colds and Flu section for more about how to use ginger. One popular method is to drink ginger tea, which can be made by simply pouring boiling water on a small slice of fresh ginger and allowing it to soak. Drink the tea warm, not hot.

Manual Therapy

ON YOUR HEAD: Hard-press the midline of your chin, halfway between your lower lip and bottom of your chin. Use your forefinger to press into the chin, with your thumb pressing and stabilizing beneath the chin.

ON YOUR FRONT: Finger-circle or scrape down the middle of the sternum to Ren-17, and press any areas of tension.

Palm-circle in a clockwise direction around Ren-12. Repeat several times.

ON YOUR BACK: Scrape down the pancreas and liver back *shu* regions in your mid back.

ON YOUR ARMS: Thumb-press down the heart ruler river from Hr-3 to Hr-7, and press and knead any areas of tension. Hard-press Hr-6 near your wrist, and repeat several times, then gently knead the area.

ON YOUR LEGS: Thumb-press or scrape down the stomach river from St-36 to St-41, and up the pancreas river from Pa-5 to Pa-9. Press and knead any areas of tension, especially St-37, St-39, and St-40.

ON YOUR HANDS: Press the following areas, and knead if sore: Li-4 area; zone 2 – liver, pancreas, and stomach (K-I); zone 5 – mid-back area.

ON YOUR FEET: Use a Gua sha tool to scrape down your foot in the area of zone 3 – stomach, pancreas, liver/spleen, and gallbladder (J-H). Then press and knead any sore areas. Also hard-press Lv-3 area.

ON YOUR EARS: Press the following areas, and knead if sore: Zone 1 – A & B; zone 8 – ear; support regions – relaxation (2), sensorial (3), and *shenmen* (1).

Exercise Therapy

❶ *Whole Body Stretch*
This exercise is similar to the Relax the Whole Body exercise in Sleeping Disorders. In this case, it can help strengthen the stomach system and prevent nausea.

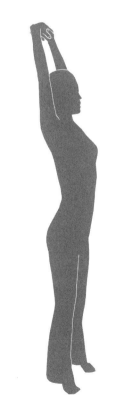

Stand with your arms at your sides and feet shoulders'-width apart.

Lift your arms slowly until they are straight above your head, palms upwards.

Link your fingers, and turn the palms. At the same time, lift your heels and look upwards while breathing in.

Slowly move your body into a squat position as your arms are lowered back to the sides of your body. Breathe out as you bring your elbows and knees together and your heels flat, exhaling at the same time.

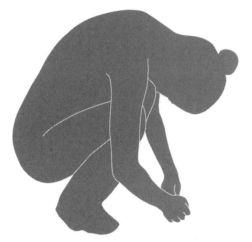

Repeat several times.

❷ Bend Backwards

Do the Bend Backwards exercise from the Chest Pain section, as this stretches the stomach river (see p. 205).

❸ Five Qualities of Nature Stretches

Do exercises 2, 3, and 5 of the Five Qualities of Nature stretches to help strengthen the digestive organs and reduce nausea (see p. 101 ff.).

Lifestyle Therapy

As a fisherman in Japan, I used to suffer periodic seasickness while out on the ocean, and more than my fair share of stomach contents would regularly empty into the East China Sea. I found that many of the techniques listed above greatly helped counteract the nausea. However, keep in mind the following:

1. Activity can worsen nausea, so it is very important to rest but let gravity help. Rest either in a sitting position or in a propped lying position.

2. Fresh air and being outside often relieve some of the symptoms. Avoid warm, stuffy places, especially if they are not well ventilated.

3. Long deep breaths can sometimes help. Adults often breathe with shallow breaths, usually due to stress and bad habits, using only the ribs to pull air in. Just using the upper portion of your lungs reduces the breath motion of your lung system.

To see if you are breathing correctly, place one hand on your chest and the other on your abdomen. Inhale slowly and deeply, visualizing the breath moving all the way down into the abdomenal area. If you are breathing as nature intended, you should feel this area push out first with the movement of the diaphragm and then afterwards the expansion of your chest, in one full inhalation breath.

Pause for a moment after inhaling, then slowly exhale upwards into the chest and out the mouth.

The exhale should be longer than the inhale, allowing the breath to fully expel from the lungs. Repeat this slowly and methodically several times.

Feeling Bloated

Symptoms
The abdomen feels full and tight and painful, and can appear uncomfortably swollen and gassy.

Can Include or Lead to
Gastritis, intestinal obstruction, hiatal hernia, coeliac disease, irritable bowel syndrome, colitis, and peptic/gastric ulcer.

When to See a Doctor
If the symptoms are severe or persistent.

Common Causes
Emotional stress, overeating, irregular eating habits, a diet of excess cold, raw, or processed

foods, overthinking and worrying, lack of exercise, or constipation.

An Explanation

Bloating often occurs when damp or an accumulation of food clogs up the stomach and pancreas systems. This can happen as a result of following an inappropriate diet and overeating at meal times. Digestion then slows down, and the stomach and pancreas systems become impaired.

Like a reservoir behind a dam on a river, fluids collect in the intestines and abdominal walls because your body lacks the digestive power to process them and send them onwards. This leads to discomfort and a sense of fullness. The abdomen often feels soft when pressed, and there is normally little actual pain.

A weakness in the stomach system contributes to the overflow by being unable to send enough downwards motion to the intestines to ensure that stools pass through smoothly during the evacuation process. There is a slowing of peristalsis, the involuntary relaxing and contracting motions in the intestines that allow food to pass through, and the resultant constipated backlog stagnates, which, in turn, furthers the stagnation in the stomach and pancreas systems.

With this pattern there is more likely to be weight fluctuations, swollen eyes and fingers, and bloating when tired or at the end of the day.

The relationship between the stomach and pancreas (the earth systems) and the liver and gallbladder (the wood systems) is a close one. Weakness in one brings out weakness or overactivity in the other. When the stomach and pancreas become impaired, the liver system has a tendency to overflow and flood the two earth systems when your body becomes stressed and agitated. The stomach and pancreas effectively act as the lid to a boiling kettle (the kettle being the liver system). If the lid stays on the kettle as it boils, then the steam can be released in a controlled way out of the spout and it can cool down quicker. If, however, the lid does not fit or is not there at all, the hot water bursts out the top and becomes uncontrollable. This spillage floods the stomach and pancreas systems and interrupts the digestive process causing bloating, which can worsen when emotionally affected.

Food Therapy

Dietary Factors That Can Worsen Bloating

- Overeating and irregular meal times can both add to the food stagnation and weaken the digestive process.
- Raw, cool-, and cold-natured foods will add to the general blockage of circulation and food. See Cold and the Cool and Cold food lists for more details.
- Dairy products, wheat, bread, bananas, alcohol, and other damp-forming foods can weaken the stomach and pancreas systems. See Damp/Phlegm for more details.

Dietary Factors That Can Lessen Bloating

- Steam or boil foods to make them easier to digest.
- In general, follow a strengthening diet that will support the stomach and pancreas systems. See General Weakness for more details.
- Carrots, leeks, fennel, garlic, coriander, pepper, and barley can get the digestive system moving again.

Manual Therapy

ON YOUR FRONT: Palm-circle with slight pressure around your navel.

ABDOMEN CIRCLE: Press nine areas equally spaced around your navel with the heel of your palm. Work *clockwise*, and push each area towards the navel. Press when breathing out, and hold for 10 seconds.

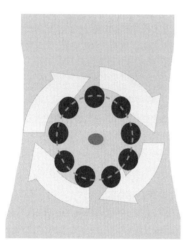

Press and knead Ren-12, St-25 and Ren-6 if you feel tension in the tissue.

ON YOUR BACK: Scrape down the pancreas and liver back *shu* regions in your mid back. Also scrape down the kidney region, and continue down to the water *shu* region on the sacrum area.

ON YOUR ARMS: Thumb-press or scrape along the large intestine river from Li-5 to Li-11 at your elbow. Knead any areas of tension.

ON YOUR LEGS: Scrape or thumb-press down the stomach and gallbladder rivers—the stomach from Crouching Rabbit to St-41 at your ankle, and the gallbladder from Gb-31 to Gb-40 at your ankle. Knead any tense areas, including St-37, St-39, and St-40, and Gb-34, Gb-37, and Gb-38.

ON YOUR HANDS: Press the following areas, and knead if sore: Zone 2 – stomach, pancreas, large intestine, and small intestine (K-I).

ON YOUR FEET: Do the Foot Circulation sequence in chapter 13. Press the following areas, and knead if sore: Kd-3; zone 3 – stomach, pancreas, liver/spleen, and gallbladder (J-H); zone 4 – small intestine and large intestine (K-M).

ON YOUR EARS: Press the following areas, and knead if sore: Zone 1 – B; zone 5 – abdomen (N); support regions – relaxation (2) and *shenmen* (1).

Exercise Therapy

1 *Do the exercise Bend Backwards from the Chest Pain section (see p. 205).*

2 *Do exercises 2 and 5 of the Five Qualities of Nature stretches (see p. 101 ff.), which can help strengthen the stomach system and increase circulation via the liver system.*

Lifestyle Therapy

1. Regular gentle exercise can be very beneficial, as it moves circulation and strengthens the main systems involved in bloating.

2. Be cautious about the claims of manufacturers of products connected with bloating, especially those mentioning gut flora, probiotics, and "food intolerance". These are usually looking at the problem in isolation of your eating habits, the type of food you are eating, the strength of your stomach and pancreas and, of course, the rest of your body. If your diet and eating habits are appropriate, there is normally no need to "help" your digestion with any supplements.

Stomach/Abdominal Pain

Symptoms

Pain or discomfort in the central part of the stomach, between the ribcage and the navel (stomach), or pain or discomfort around and below the navel (abdomen).

Can Include or Lead to

Gastritis, indigestion, gastrointestinal spasm, gastrointestinal dyspepsia, gastroenteritis, hyperchlorhydria, gastric ulcer, duodenal ulcer, intestinal neurosis, ulcerative colitis, irritable bowel syndrome, dysmenorrhoea, fibroids, ovarian cysts, and endometriosis.

When to See a Doctor

If the symptoms are severe, the pain is worse with movement, or there is abdominal rigidity.

Common Causes

A diet containing too many cold-natured, raw foods; stress; overwork; worry; repressed anger; exhaustion; or bad eating habits.

An Explanation

Discomfort in the region between the lower border of your rib cage and your navel can be termed "epigastric", or "stomach", pain. It can often involve the liver system and those systems related to digestion, such as stomach, pancreas, gallbladder, triple burner, and small/large intestines.

Discomfort in the region below your navel can be termed "abdominal pain", and while there could be a digestive component, as above, there can also be impairments in the systems related to female reproduction, especially the liver system.

Pain or discomfort in these areas suggests an obstruction pattern, which can take many forms. Cold can enter the body directly and attach within the intestines or uterus. This could be due to anything from being inappropriately dressed on a cold day to sitting on a concrete park bench.

It can also develop from a diet containing too many cold-natured, raw foods, which can lower the internal temperature of the stomach and cause severe, cramping pain as the cold pattern contracts the muscles of the stomach lining. This type of pain is often relieved by the application of heat but not with pressure.

A stagnation pattern often develops from emotional stress, as the liver system is hindered from regulating circulation. Obstruction patterns can find their way into the stomach and abdomen, causing pain that initially hurts with pressure, then lessens with continued pressure. The pain often worsens with emotional stress and improves with activity or exercise.

A diet containing too many processed, hot-natured, or spicy foods can increase the temperature of the stomach considerably. The pain is often accompanied by a burning sensation and other signs of heat and agitation.

A diet containing too many damp-forming foods, such as greasy foods, dairy products, and alcohol, can weaken the stomach and pancreas systems, causing them to overproduce thick body fluids that, in turn, weaken the stomach and pancreas further. The subsequent stagnation of fluids generates heat and often causes dull pain, a tight chest, and frontal headache. Heat dries up the moisture in the intestines or uterus and often combines with damp. It can develop from an existing pattern of stagnation or *yin* weakness or the transformation of a long-standing cold pattern. The pain is usually worse with pressure, there is often a burning sensation, and the skin can be hot to the touch. In women, there can be heavy periods, an irregular cycle, and vaginal discharge.

In some long-standing cases of obstruction, an actual physical blockage to circulation develops. These masses can sometimes be felt in the abdomen. The resultant pain is often very sharp and fixed, worse with pressure, and at night.

Poor eating habits, a diet that weakens digestion, an unhealthy lifestyle, a long-term illness, or a variety of depleting factors can lead to an underlying weakness of blood circulation and the stomach and pancreas systems. The accompanying pain is often dull and lingering, accompanies eating, and feels better with pressure, rest, and the application of heat.

Food Therapy

Dietary Factors That Can Worsen Stomach/Abdominal Pain

- Overeating at mealtimes is one of the most common causes, both in the short and long-term. Ideally, the stomach should be two-thirds full when you have finished eating.
- Excess damp-forming foods, such as bananas, wheat, processed foods, and foods containing concentrated sweeteners and nuts can weaken the stomach and pancreas systems. See Damp/Phlegm for more details.
- Deep-fried foods and other hot-natured, oily foods, and black pepper, chilli, ginger, cinnamon, and other pungent spices worsen heat in the body. See Heat for more details.
- Overeating cold-natured foods, such as raw fruit and vegetables, salads, dairy products, and soya products, can worsen cold in the body. See Cold for more details.

Dietary Factors That Can Improve Stomach/Abdominal Pain

- Follow the guidelines for good eating habits in chapter 9. If eating habits remain poor, the stomach and pancreas systems cannot strengthen and the pain will continue.
- A simple diet of broths and thick soups, which reduces the strain on digestion, is beneficial in strengthening the stomach and pancreas systems.
- Rice, barley, cucumber, spinach, lettuce, watercress, and yogurt help cool the body. See Heat for more details.

NOTE Too many cooling foods can easily lead to damp/phlegm, and any dietary changes should be in moderation.

Manual Therapy

CAUTION: Be cautious when manipulating around the stomach and abdomen, as it can worsen the pain. Only use the areas mentioned in the list if pressure feels comfortable there.

- Palm-circle with slight pressure around your navel.
- Do the Abdomen Circle sequence in Feeling Bloated (see p. 212).

ON YOUR BACK: Scrape downwards on or around the liver and pancreas *shu* regions. And then press and knead any sore or tender areas.

ON YOUR ARMS: Thumb-press up the large intestine river along your lower arm from Li-5 to Li-11. In particular, focus on the area below Li-11.

Also thumb-press down the heart ruler river from Hr-3 to Hr-7, and knead any tight areas, especially around Hr-6.

ON YOUR LEGS: Scrape or thumb-press down the stomach and gallbladder rivers—the stomach from Crouching Rabbit to St-41 at your ankle and the gallbladder from Gb-31 to Gb-40 at your ankle. Knead any tense areas, including St-37, St-39, and St-40, and Gb-34, Gb-37, and Gb-38.

ON YOUR HANDS: Press the following areas, and knead if sore: Li-4; zone 2 – stomach, pancreas, large intestine, small intestine, and liver (K-I).

ON YOUR FEET: Use a Gua sha to scrape down your foot in the area of zone 3 – stomach, pancreas, liver/spleen, and gallbladder (J-H); zone 4 – small intestine and large intestine (K-M). Press and knead any sore areas.

ON YOUR EARS: Press the following areas, and knead if sore: Zone 1 – A; zone 5 – abdomen (N); support regions – relaxation (2) and *shenmen* (1).

Exercise Therapy

❶ *Abdomen Imaging*

This exercise can be useful in relieving stomach/abdominal pain.

In a relaxed standing or seated position, imagine there is a mass of hot air in the stomach/abdomen. Put one hand on top of the other, and place it above your navel.

Imagine turning the mass of air as the hands circle clockwise up to 30 times and then the same anticlockwise. Be careful not to apply any pressure on the abdomen while doing this.

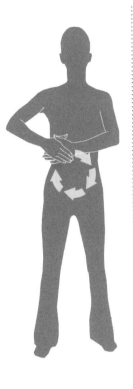

❷ *Five Qualities of Nature Stretches*

Do exercises 2, 4, and 5 of the Five Qualities of Nature stretches (see p. 101 ff.).

Lifestyle Therapy

1. Taking an overly long siesta in the afternoon can lead to the accumulation of damp/phlegm in the stomach and intestines and should be avoided. A short rest after lunch is, however, very beneficial to the stomach and pancreas systems.

2. To prevent any sluggish circulation in the stomach and abdominal areas, it is important to avoid sitting for long periods and do regular gentle exercise. Ideally, choose an exercise that will require you to twist your waist, such as swimming or tennis, or it can be an activity such as gardening, which can require considerable rotational movements depending on the task.

Constipation

Symptoms

Difficulty in passing stools, long gaps between passing stools (once a day or once every two days is considered normal), or inability to properly evacuate, despite a strong desire to do so.

Can Include or Lead to

Irritable bowel syndrome, diverticulitis, and ulcerative colitis.

When to See a Doctor

If the symptoms are severe, are accompanied by bleeding, are getting worse, or are accompanied by vomiting and abdominal bloating.

Common Causes

Lack of exercise, an improper diet, emotional stress, frustration, smoking, working in a dry office environment, overeating, excess caffeine, overwork, travel, and changes in routine.

An Explanation

The peristaltic movement of the intestines follows the contraction and expansion patterns of *yin/yang* breath motion in controlling body fluids. When the *yin* motion increases in the intestines, it cools and moistens them and helps the passage of stools. When the *yang* motion increases, the heat and dryness generated restricts the stool's movement. It is essential, therefore, to have sufficient levels of fluids in the intestines to prevent constipation and ensure the smooth motion of breath.

The following patterns can occur:

- Heat can originate from the stomach system as the result of a stagnation of food, bad eating habits, and an improper diet of heating, damp-forming foods.
- Heat can also derive from the liver system, often related to emotional disturbances or too much rich food and alcohol, resulting

in stools like rabbit droppings and a pattern that is usually worse when emotionally stressed.

- A climate pattern resulting from catching a cold or flu, if not properly expelled, can sink deeper into the body and transform into raging heat, often with an accompanying fever.
- Positioned in the midst of the intestines, if the *yin* motion of the kidney system becomes weak, the *yang* motion will heat up rapidly and burn up the moisture in the intestines around it.
- In all patterns of heat, the stools are normally dry and infrequent.
- Cold can develop from a *yang* weakness or enter directly through exposure to a cold environment and can act as an obstruction by constricting the intestines. With this pattern, the stools can only be expelled with effort but are quite often normal in appearance and moisture.
- Underlying any overflow pattern is normally a pattern of weakness, and in the case of constipation, there is sometimes not enough power to push the stools through the intestines. It is often necessary to strain, and the stools are normally soft and long. If blood circulation is weakened, it cannot moisten the intestines, and stools are usually small, round, and dry.

Food Therapy

Dietary Factors That Can Worsen Constipation

- Drinking during meals literally floods your stomach and can clog up the digestive process.
- Some foods, such as barley, dry up the moisture in the intestines, and others, such as string beans, increase the *yin* motion and add to constipation.

Dietary Factors That Can Improve Constipation

- It is important to chew food thoroughly before swallowing to trigger the digestive juices needed for digestion and help the passage of food through the intestines.
- Apples, apricots, bananas, pears, peaches, prunes, carrots, cauliflower, spinach, honey, sesame seeds, walnuts, and tofu moisten the intestines and can help the passage of a stool.
- Asparagus, cabbage, black sesame seeds, figs, papayas, sweet potatoes, and castor oil have laxative qualities.

Manual Therapy

ON YOUR FRONT: Palm-circle with slight pressure in a *clockwise* direction around the navel. Do the Abdomen Circle sequence in Feeling Bloated (see p. 212).

ON YOUR BACK: Scrape downwards on or around the pancreas, liver, and kidney back *shu* regions and then press and knead any tense areas.

ON YOUR ARMS: Thumb-press up the large intestine river along your lower arm from Li-5 to Li-11. In particular, focus on the area below Li-11.

ON YOUR LEGS: Scrape or thumb-press down the stomach river from Crouching Rabbit to St-41 at your ankle. Knead any tense areas, including St-37, St-39, and St-40.

ON YOUR HANDS: Press the following areas, and knead if sore: Zone 2 – large intestine, small intestine, stomach, and pancreas (K-I).

ON YOUR FEET: Use a Gua sha to scrape down your foot in the area of zone 3 – stomach, pancreas, liver/spleen, gallbladder (J-H); zone 4 – small intestine and large intestine (K-M). Then press and knead any sore areas.

ON YOUR EARS: Press the following areas, and knead if sore: Zone 1 – A, B & C; zone 7 – rectum; zone 5 – abdomen (N); support region – *shenmen* (1).

Exercise Therapy

The following exercises can help to loosen the intestines:

❶ *Arm Cross and Stretch*

Stand with your legs shoulders'-width apart. Relax, and hang your arms loosely at your sides. Clench both fists loosely, and slowly raise them up towards your chest while breathing in. Cross over your arms at chest level so that each fist comes to rest on the opposite shoulder.

Open your palms, bend your waist, and slowly swing your arms downwards and outwards in a fluid motion while breathing out. The arm movement should end by stretching outwards at right angles to your bent body. Repeat this several times.

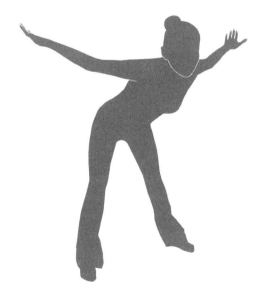

❷ *Arm Lift*

Lie face up on a bed, relax, and place both arms loosely at your sides. Slowly raise both arms while breathing in, and bring them down so that they touch the bed above your head. Then bring your arms slowly back, breathing out, until they reach the starting position. Repeat several times.

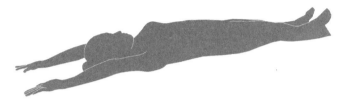

❸ *Twist Your Waist*

Do Twist Your Waist from Shoulder Pain, with the focus more on moving your waist than on your shoulders. Repeat the sequence several times (see p. 197).

❹ *Bend Your Hip*

Do the exercises Bend Your Hip, Crouch Twist and Swing Your Waist from General Weakness to encourage movement in the abdomen (see p. 139).

❺ *Five Qualities of Nature Stretches*

Do exercises 1, 2, and 5 of the Five Qualities of Nature stretches to help strengthen digestion (see p. 101 ff.).

Lifestyle Therapy

1. It is important to do regular exercise to promote river circulation – both to lubricate the intestines and to prevent obstruction patterns and areas of weakness.
2. Avoid taking laxatives regularly as they can damage the *yang* motion of your intestines and actually cause constipation as a side effect. Some people are caught in the vicious spiral of increasing the quantity and dosage of laxatives to combat constipation that the drug is itself causing.

3. Antibiotics are very cooling and can weaken the *yang* motion of the digestive systems. A balanced *yang* motion is needed for food to be pumped through the intestines efficiently and any impairment in this can cause constipation.
4. The body reacts well to routines. Have a toilet routine, and try to keep to it. Physiologically, the best time to open your bowels is between 5 and 7 am, as this is when the tidal circulation is most concentrated in the large intestine river system.

Diarrhoea

Symptoms
An increase in daily bowel movements; loose, watery stools; abdominal pain; lack of appetite; tiredness; fever; and gas.

Can Include or Lead to
Gastroenteritis, food poisoning, food allergies, irritable bowel syndrome, Crohn's disease, and ulcerative colitis.

When to See a Doctor
If the symptoms are severe or persistent, with blood or mucus, or if you feel dehydrated.

Common Causes
Weak digestion, stress, overwork, repressed emotions, an inappropriate diet, exposure to the weather, or a long chronic illness.

An Explanation
Diarrhoea involves all of the systems that control the digestive tract. Principally, this is the stomach, which includes the small and large intestine, triple burner, and gallbladder systems within its umbrella of influence.

Sometimes you eat something that causes an immediate reaction within your stomach and intestines, as might happen with food poisoning. This sudden and rather explosive reaction is caused by your body trying to process a climate pattern (heat, damp, or wind) that enters via the food and is often accompanied by symptoms of nausea and vomiting. Shellfish (clams, oysters, mussels) are notorious for containing the motion of wind within them, and when improperly prepared, the wind enters your circulation and attaches within your liver system, in some cases causing serious disease patterns.

The systems with the most influence on diarrhoea are the stomach and pancreas. Their main function is to transform food into the fuel the body runs on (via the five flavours) and also to send this fuel to wherever needed (via the five *zang* storage systems). If the stomach and pancreas systems become impaired, there can be a counterflow in the upwards movement they need for this process, so that the food rushes down through the intestines causing diarrhoea. This pattern is usually accompanied by undigested food in the stools, the desire to go to the toilet straight after eating, and sometimes abdominal pain afterwards. If the diarrhoea is early in the morning it may be an extension of this pattern but involve kidney *yang* weakness.

When weak, the stomach and pancreas systems accumulate damp as they slow down the processing of food. They then become more susceptible to dampness from external sources, such as catching a cold or flu. The damp sinks and often combines with either heat or cold to stay in the intestines on a long-term basis, causing periodic flare-ups of diarrhoea, sometimes accompanied by blood and mucus. This pattern can be acute, with abdominal pain. If the pattern is cold, the stools tend to be watery; if the pattern is heat, the stools are normally darker or yellowish, and the smell is usually worse.

When stagnation patterns develop in the liver system, it can also have a destabilizing effect on peristalsis, which moves food through the intestines during the digestive process. This can often result in alternating constipation and diarrhoea, and gas and bloating that may worsen with emotional stress.

Food Therapy

Dietary Factors That Can Worsen Diarrhoea

- Dairy products, tropical fruits, nuts, junk food, wheat, and other damp-producing foods weaken digestion. See Damp/Phlegm for more details.
- Spices, coffee, alcohol, and other heat-producing foods can add to any heat present. See Heat for more details.
- Cold-natured, raw foods, such as salads, soya bean products, and refrigerated drinks, aggravate cold conditions. See Cold for more details.
- Apricots, plums, prunes, walnuts, spinach, sesame seeds, and sugary foods, processed foods, and all types of oil aggravate diarrhoea.

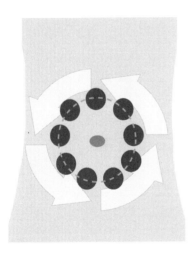

Dietary Factors That Can Improve Diarrhoea

- Ideally, drink lots of water or diluted juice, and eat small meals of easily digestible foods, such as soups and gruels made from rice, oats, and other grains.
- Persimmons, garlic, button mushrooms, carrots, leeks, apples, aubergines (eggplants), olives, string beans, adzuki beans, sunflower seeds,

blackberry juice, and rice broth can be generally beneficial in combating diarrhoea.

- For cold-type diarrhoea: Eat hot-natured foods, such as peppers, ginger, nutmeg, cinnamon, and chestnuts. See Heat for more details.
- For hot-type diarrhoea: Eat cold-natured foods, such as pineapples, tofu, and mung beans, and drink peppermint tea. See Cold for more details.

Manual Therapy

ON YOUR FRONT: Palm-circle with slight pressure in an *anticlockwise* direction around the navel.

ABDOMEN CIRCLE (ANTICLOCKWISE): Press nine areas equally spaced around your navel with the heel of your palm. Work *anticlockwise* and push each area towards the navel. Press when breathing out, and hold for 10 seconds.

Press Ren-12, Ren-6, and Ren-4, and knead, if tender.

ON YOUR BACK: Scrape downwards on or around the pancreas, liver, and kidney back *shu* regions and then press and knead any tense areas.

ON YOUR ARMS: Thumb-press up the large intestine river along your lower arm from Li-5 to Li-11. In particular, focus on the area below Li-11.

ON YOUR LEGS: Scrape or thumb-press down the stomach river from Crouching Rabbit to St-41 at your ankle. Knead any tense areas, including St-37, St-39, and St-40. Scrape or thumb-press up the pancreas river from Pa-5 to Pa-9. Knead any tense areas, including Pa-6.

ON YOUR HANDS: Press the following areas, and knead if sore: Zone 2 – large intestine, small intestine, stomach, and pancreas (K-I).

ON YOUR FEET: Use a Gua sha to scrape down your foot in the area of zone 3 – stomach, pancreas, liver/spleen, and gallbladder (J-H); zone 4 – small intestine and large intestine (K-M). Then press and knead any sore areas.

ON YOUR EARS: Press the following areas, and knead if sore: Zone 1 – A, B & C; zone 7- rectum; zone 5 – abdomen (N); support region – *shenmen* (1).

Exercise Therapy

❶ *Do exercises 1 and 2 of the Five Qualities of Nature stretches to help strengthen the stomach, pancreas, and large intestine systems (see p. 101 f.).*

❷ *Do the exercises Bend Your Hip, Crouch Twist, and Swing Your Waist from General Weakness to encourage circulation movement (see p. 139).*

Lifestyle Therapy

Avoid taking antibiotics for diarrhoea symptoms unless a clear bacterial cause has been identified, or if your immune system is weakened. Antibiotics can weaken the stomach and pancreas systems considerably (often the underlying cause in diarrhoea).

Painful Urination

Symptoms

Frequent, painful, or burning urination; pain in the lower back; urine could be clear, dark, or cloudy, or with stones, sand, or blood.

Can Include or Lead to

Cystitis, urethritis, vaginitis, herpes, urinary retention, menopausal complications, urinary calculi, prostatitis, and prostatic hypertrophy.

When to See a Doctor

If the symptoms are severe or persistent.

Common Causes

An improper diet of greasy, hot-natured food; emotional stress; repressed frustration or anger; overwork; lack of sleep; dehydration; and extended contact with cold surfaces, such as sitting outside, standing, or lifting excessively.

An Explanation

In making a diagnosis, you can make important distinctions between the types of symptoms of painful urination being presented.

Symptoms of acute, burning pain when urinating suggest the presence of heat. This is usually the result of a heavy diet of rich, greasy foods and alcohol, but it can also be from heat generated from a general stagnation pattern in circulation, or from a long-term imbalance in the *yin* motion of breath. The heat is usually accompanied by damp, which, as it is heavy and clinging by nature, causes the heat to sink into the bladder area. In patterns of heat, the urine is usually darker and more concentrated, and, if cloudy, suggests the presence of damp.

Sometimes there is blood in the urine, as the heat quite literally pushes out the blood from the blood vessels. Antibiotics can help reduce heat (they are cooling by nature), and therefore the symptoms.

This may sound contradictory, but not all heat symptoms are due to heat.

If the urinary symptom is either burning pain or more of a dragging discomfort and if it is relieved by pressure and warmth, it suggests that the symptoms are less connected with heat and more to a General Weakness or Stagnation pattern.

When the liver system is impaired, it can directly affect the urinary and reproductive areas because of the trajectory and subsequent influence of the liver river system as it comes up the body (it goes straight through the groin and lower abdominal area). This pattern can worsen with emotional stress and cause pain before urination.

Chronic pain that recurs and gets worse when tired indicates that there is an impairment in the kidney system. It is normally accompanied by other General Weakness symptoms, such as lower back pain, pale urine, and pain after urination. For this type of pattern, antibiotics may have a temporary relieving effect but can often make the condition worse.

The pain sometimes comes from urinary stones in the kidneys, ureter, or bladder. These are often the end result of long-term damp and heat, whereby the heat solidifies the damp. This could be due to lack of exercise and an inappropriate diet—in particular, a diet that includes a lot of dairy products, spinach, rhubarb, liver, kidney, sardines, and fish roe.

Food Therapy

Dietary Factors That Can Worsen Painful Urination

- Overeating and a diet of hot-natured, damp-forming food, such as hamburgers, pizzas, and other fast food; alcohol; and soft fizzy drinks (sodas) can directly lead to dampness and heat via the stomach or pancreas systems. See Heat and Damp/Phlegm for more details.
- Cheese, cow's milk, rhubarb, spinach, potatoes, liver, kidney, fish roe, sardines, tinned fish, plums, cranberries, chocolate, and alcohol have the effect of hardening phlegm, due to their acidity. This can lead to the formation of calculi, gravel, and stones, so it is important to avoid eating them.

Dietary Factors That Can Lessen Painful Urination

- Melon, watermelon, blueberries, radishes, cucumbers, celery, carrots, asparagus, mushrooms, barley, adzuki beans, mung bean sprouts, lemon juice, and cranberry juice can reduce dampness and heat in the bladder. See Damp/Phlegm and Heat for more details.
- For patterns of General Weakness and a weakened kidney system, eat a diet consisting of plenty of strengthening foods. The following foods specifically strengthen the kidney system: Smoked fish, lobster, salmon, shrimps, tuna, lentils, black soya beans, and walnuts. See General Weakness for more details.

Manual Therapy

ON YOUR FRONT: Hard-press Ren-4 and any tense area closer to the pubic symphysis bone, or farther out to the sides.

ON YOUR BACK: Scrape down the kidney back *shu* region in your lower back, and continue down to the sacral area and the water *shu* region.

ON YOUR LEGS: Scrape or thumb-press down the bladder river from your buttocks to Bl-40 at your knee and then onto Bl-60 at your ankle. Press and knead any areas that feel tense.

Thumb-press the area between Kd-3 and Kd-7, and hard-press any tension.

ON YOUR HANDS: Press the following areas, and knead if sore: Zone 3 – kidney and bladder (L-N); zone 6 – lower back area.

ON YOUR FEET: Press the following areas, and knead if sore: Zone 4 – bladder (M); zone 3 – kidney (I); zone 5 – cover any reactive areas.

ON YOUR EARS: Press the following areas, and knead if sore: Zone 1 – A; zone 7 – urethra; support regions – relaxation (2) and *shenmen* (1).

Exercise Therapy

❶ *Do exercise 4 of the Five Qualities of Nature stretches to help strengthen the kidney and bladder systems (see p. 102 f.).*

❷ *Do the exercises Bend Your Hip, Crouch Twist, and Swing Your Waist from General Weakness, all of which encourage movement in the lower abdomen (see p. 139).*

Lifestyle Therapy

Regular exercise is very important to prevent stagnation in the lower body. Avoid extended periods of standing, if possible.

23

Back Area

Backache

Symptoms
Pain in the upper, mid, lumbar, sacral, or coccyx areas of the spine.

Can Include or Lead to
Muscle spasm, herniated disc, spine curvatures, fibromyalgia, osteoporosis, spondylosis, and arthritis.

When to See a Doctor
If the symptoms are severe, are getting worse, and are accompanied by bowel or urinary symptoms, numbness, or tingling in the leg.

Common Causes
Overwork, stress, a lack of or too much exercise, exposure to the weather, pregnancy, childbirth, or trauma.

An Explanation
Backache affects most people at some time in their lives. Often, we presume that back pain must originate from the spine. As a result, it is all too easy to find a slight spinal abnormality and undergo a spiral of sometimes extremely invasive treatments and investigations to "cure" it, only for the pain to continue or even worsen afterwards.

Sometimes, back pain is due to spinal disorders or other conditions, such as heart disease, kidney stones, or a bladder infection, but often, back pain sufferers remain in the dark and frustrated as to the real cause of their backache.

When back pain is acute, in that it is sudden and very sharp, there is an obstruction pattern present. It is like a tree falling into the stream and blocking its flow. This could be from an accident or sudden trauma, but can often appear after an apparently trivial event like a sneeze or a stretch. The symptoms of this type of pattern are normally much more acute and feel worse with movement.

While the initial pain of this obstruction pattern can go, the actual pattern itself can remain unresolved well after the initial incident and be periodically triggered by emotional stresses or simply keeping the same posture for extended periods. This is one of the most common patterns in backache. Instead of removing the tree that is blocking the stream, a water channel has been dug around it, so the stream can continue on but the tree is still there. So, whenever the water channel becomes silted up and blocked, it will naturally radiate to this area, and you feel the effects of the blocked tree again.

One of the ways to determine if a backache is due to an obstruction pattern is whether it is relieved by doing exercise. If it feels worse after doing exercise, the condition is more likely to be one of a weakness pattern.

Most people with chronic lower backache have an underlying weakness. This is usually in the kidney system, which gives support and strength to the back area, especially the lower back.

When a weakness exists, it is much easier for a climate pattern to attach within the tissue of the back area and create an obstruction. In most cases, it is cold and damp that fix themselves in tissue in a back obstruction pattern, and this condition often worsens when the weather becomes cold and wet. It can also usually feel better with the application of heat.

In practice, most people seem to have a combination of each of the above patterns causing their backache. There is usually a stagnation pattern, accompanied by a climate pattern (damp, cold, or heat) and, underlying it all, a weakness pattern originating in the kidney and pancreas systems.

Food Therapy

Dietary Factors That Can Worsen Backache

- Eating late at night or overeating can add to stagnation.
- Cold-natured, raw, or damp-forming foods, such as dairy products, bananas, tomatoes, wheat, and tofu, aggravate those patterns. See Cold and Damp/Phlegm for more details.

Dietary Factors That Can Improve Backache

- Radishes, adzuki beans, turnips, pumpkin, and seaweed help remove dampness. See Damp/Phlegm for more details.
- Herbs and spices, such as cloves, chives, garlic, turmeric, marjoram, and basil, and citrus peel help warm up cold and move any stagnation. See Stagnation for more details.
- Smoked fish, oysters, lobster, salmon, shrimps, tuna, lentils, oats, millet, black soybeans, walnuts, and black sesame seeds strengthen the kidney system. As the kidney system has a strong influence over the back, it is very important to maintain it through diet.

Manual Therapy

CAUTION: Treating the back when there is acute pain can often produce the opposite result to the one desired. If in any doubt, avoid manipulating around the area of pain, and use areas that are further away.

ON YOUR BACK: Despite the caution on treating the back directly, it can sometimes be appropriate; for example, treating the upper back for a lower back problem, or if the back pain is chronic and receptive to pressure. In general, when treating the back, use the back *shu* regions as your guide. Start in an area away from the symptomatic area, and slowly come closer. Scrape or thumb-press on your back, but always work in a downwards direction.

ON YOUR ARMS: Thumb-press or scrape up the small intestine river from Si-5 to Si-8 and then up the back of your arm on the triceps. Press and knead any areas of tension.

ON YOUR LEGS: Scrape or thumb-press down the bladder river from your buttocks to Bl-40 at the back of your knee and then onto Bl-60 at your ankle. Press and knead any areas of tension.

ON YOUR HANDS: Press the following areas, and knead if sore: Si-1 to Si-4; Li-3 to Li-4 (next to the metacarpal); all of zone 4 – cervical spine; zone 5 – thoracic spine; zone 6 – lumbar spine; zone 3 – kidney (M).

ON YOUR FEET: Thumb-press or use a Gua sha tool to scrape down the inside of the foot from Kd-3 at the heel to the toe joint. Knead any sore areas, including cervical, thoracic, lumbar, sacral, and coccyx areas across all zones (O-R). Hard-press the kidney area on the sole of your foot.

ON YOUR EARS: Press the following areas, and knead if sore: Zone 2 – cervical, thoracic, or lumbar-sacral areas (D-F); zone 6 – buttocks (P); zone 1 – A; support regions – relaxation (2) and *shenmen* (1).

Exercise Therapy

The following exercises can strengthen the lower back:

❶ Pelvic Stretch

Lie face up on a comfortable flat surface, and relax with your arms at your sides and legs out straight.

Stretch your left leg outwards, away from you, as far as is comfortable, and at the same time, bend and raise your right leg straight up. This assymetrically stretches the pelvic muscles holding the hip bones in place, with the left hip bone low and the right hip bone high.

Repeat this on the other side, and alternate up to 20 times.

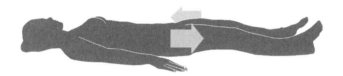

❷ Leg Stretch

Stand sideways next to a wall, and use the hand closest to the wall to steady the body while you lift the opposite leg.

Keeping your knee straight, lift your leg sideways as high as possible while breathing in.

When you reach the highest point, stretch and hold it for a few seconds. At the same time bend your body forward until you can feel strain on the back of your thigh and hip. Then slowly lower the leg while breathing out. Repeat with the other leg and then continue a total of five times.

❸ Leg Lift

Using the support of a wall or a solid object, lift your leg as high as it will comfortably go, and rest it on a chair, table, or other object. Ideally, lift the leg to a 90° angle (but do not overstretch).

Stretch both arms forward, and try to touch your toes. Hold for a few seconds.

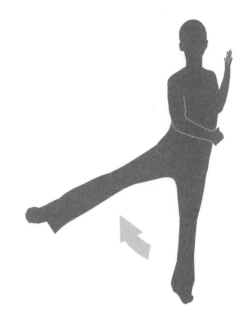

Slowly lower the leg, and repeat with the other leg. Repeat a total of five times.

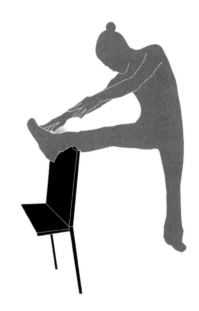

❹ Draw a Fishing Net

Stand with one foot in front of the other, bend the body forwards, and imitate the action of drawing in an imaginary fishing net with both hands.

As you are bending forward, bring the heel of the back foot off the ground, and breathe in while drawing the net up.

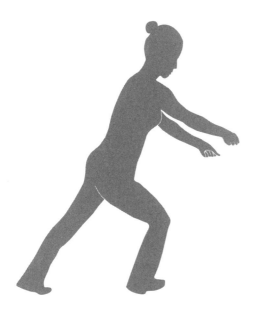

❺ *Leg Contraction*

Lie face up, and raise one leg with the knee bent.

Kick the leg out straight in the air, then contract the muscles of the leg for a few seconds before bringing it down.

Repeat with both legs up to 20 times.

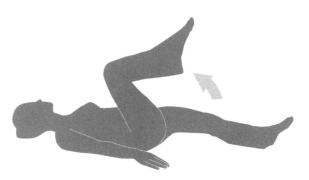

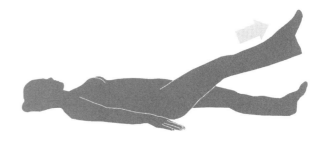

Then draw the net back and slowly straighten the body. At the same time, breathe out.

Continue, so that the body is leaning backwards slightly, and bring the heel of the front foot off the ground.

❻ *Body Back Twist*

Lie face down and, keeping your legs relaxed, lift your body with both arms, as if starting to do a press-up.

Lift the head and upper body, and stick out the chest. Rest and repeat five times.

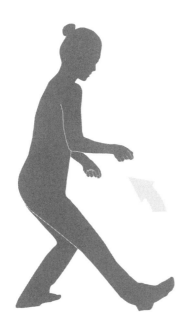

Repeat up to 10 times on either side.

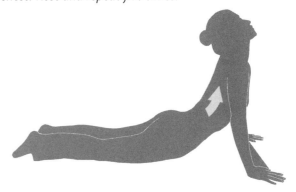

❼ *Body Rocking Chair*

Lie face down with arms relaxed at your sides.

Stretch both arms backwards and both straight legs upwards. This movement raises the upper body and legs simultaneously and resembles the bottom of a rocking chair.

Do not overstretch, and only go as far as is comfortable.

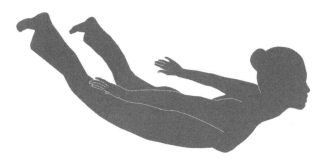

Hold this position for as long as possible, rest, and repeat up to five times.

❽ *Bend Backwards*

Do the exercise Bend Backwards from the Chest Pain section (see p. 205). This can be very strengthening for the back.

❾ *Five Qualities of Nature Stretches*

Do exercise 4 of the Five Qualities of Nature stretches to help strengthen the kidney and bladder systems (see p. 102 f.).

Lifestyle Therapy

1. In most chronic cases of backache, using an ice pack or ice spray on the affected area can do more harm than good (unless there are obvious signs of heat). In many cases of back pain, cold is actually a feature of the painful obstruction pattern and adding more cold to an already cold situation will not improve it. Instead, heat therapy, such as a hot water bottle or a hot towel, normally has a relieving effect and can help the muscles relax and increase blood circulation.

2. While it is important to keep the area warm, it is best to avoid hot baths as, although it may relieve the pain, it can worsen afterwards as the back cools down. Hot showers are preferable.

3. Posture is important. Sit in a chair with a backrest that supports your back. Adjust the height so that your knees are level with your hips. Both feet should be flat on the floor or resting on a foot rest. If you look at a screen ensure that the top of the screen is about eye level.

4. Protect your back from the elements. Dress appropriately, and be very cautious of exposure to wind. After any exercise, change quickly out of sweaty clothing.

5. Emotions can sometimes be an underlying issue in back pain. The obvious emotions are fear, which can weaken the kidney system, the main storage region of the back, and anger, aggression, and irritability, which can tighten muscles and tendons, causing pain.

6. Regular stretching and gentle exercise are usually beneficial. Avoid strenuous exercise or exercise with fast, jerky movements. The most important thing is to keep the back moving and prevent any stagnation patterns.

7. If the injury is acute, note the advice about putting ice on it in Neck Pain.

Sciatica/Leg Pain

Symptoms
Numbness, pins and needles, stabbing, tingling, or burning pain radiating down the upper or lower leg usually with lower back pain.

Can Include or Lead to
Muscle sprain, nerve pain, disc hernia of the spine, and osteoporosis.

When to See a Doctor
If the symptoms are severe.

Common Causes
A diet of too many cold-natured and raw foods, exposure to the weather, long-term back pain, or bad posture.

An Explanation
The pain or uncomfortable sensation felt in what is often diagnosed as sciatica, but which is essentially leg pain, is almost always due to a climate pattern. And this is usually a combination of wind, cold, and damp, which literally obstruct the rivers of the leg.

While they can be the result of an internal disorder such as *yang* weakness or impairments in the stomach or pancreas systems, which can generate cold and dampness in the back, they are more likely to be due to climate patterns. These climates can enter from outside via exposure to cold, damp, or wind, in situations such as swimming, cold showers, or inappropriate clothing on a windy day.

Although this type of leg discomfort can appear independently, it is normally part of a wider area of pain that includes the lower back. Cold is constrictive, and damp is heavy and obstructive. When these become attached to your lower back, it is common for them to sink and affect the *yang* rivers of the leg.

The two river systems normally affected are the bladder, when the pain radiates mainly down the back of the leg, and the gallbladder, when the pain radiates mainly down the side. It can also be located in the area in between, in which case both may be involved.

Food Therapy

Dietary Factors That Can Worsen Leg Pain
- Concentrated orange juice, wheat, bananas, dairy products, peanuts, and other cold-natured or damp-forming foods can add to the stagnation in the *yang* river systems. See Damp/Phlegm for more details.

Dietary Factors That Can Improve Leg Pain
- Radishes, rye, celery, turnips, and pumpkin improve dampness. See Damp/Phlegm for more details.
- Cold can be warmed by spices like ginger, black pepper, and nutmeg, also by garlic, onions, and turnips. See Cold for more details.

Manual Therapy

CAUTION: Treating leg pain when it is acute can sometimes make it worse, especially when treating on or near the area of pain. If in any doubt, avoid manipulating around the area of pain and use areas further away.

ON YOUR BACK: Scrape down the kidney back *shu* region in your lower back. Scrape down into the sacral area and down and outwards in the buttock area. Feel the other back *shu* regions, and if you feel tension in the tissue under the skin, treat those, too.

ON YOUR LEGS: Sometimes, treating the leg with the pain can be counterproductive, so always start with the leg without the pain. For pain radiating down the back of the leg, scrape down the centre of the back of the thigh to

Bl-40. From Bl-40, scrape down over the calf muscle to Bl-58 and onto Bl-60 at the lateral side of the ankle.

For pain radiating down the side of the leg, scrape down the side of the thigh over Gb-31 and onto Gb-34. Then down the lower leg over Gb-37 and Gb-38 to Gb-40.

ON YOUR ARMS: For pain radiating down the back of your leg, thumb-press or scrape up the small intestine river from Si-5 to Si-8 and then up the back of your arm on the triceps. Press and knead any areas of tension.

For pain radiating down the side of your leg, thumb-press or scrape up the triple burner river from Tb-4 to Tb-10, then up the side of your arm to Tb-14. Press and knead any areas of tension.

ON YOUR HANDS: Press the following areas, and knead if sore: All of zone 4 – cervical spine; zone 5 – thoracic spine; zone 6 – lumbar spine; zone 3 – kidney (M); fingers A and E on the joints of your little finger and thumb (1-4).

ON YOUR FEET: As for Backache, thumb-press or use Gua sha on the inside of the foot from the heel to the big toe to cover the spine area (O-Q). Knead any sore areas.

Also knead or Gua sha along and around the Achilles tendon in the ankle.

ON YOUR EARS: Press the following areas, and knead if tender: Zone 6 – leg area, hip, and buttocks (O-P); zone 2 – lumbar-sacral area (F); support regions – relaxation (2) and *shenmen* (1).

Exercise Therapy

As there is often a close relationship between sciatica and back pain, many of the exercises in Backache can be practiced here (see p. 224 ff.).

Lifestyle Therapy

Much of the advice given in Backache is also relevant here. It is also very important to avoid sitting for long periods, to take regular exercise, and to keep your legs and lower back warm, dry, and protected from the wind.

24

Upper Limbs

Elbow Pain

Symptoms
Pain in one or both elbow joints, with limited movement.

Can Include or Lead to
Tennis elbow, a traumatic injury to the elbow joint, rheumatoid arthritis, rheumatism, and muscle strain.

When to See a Doctor
If the symptoms are severe, and there is swelling, bruising, or an inability to move the joint.

Common Causes
Overuse, overwork, an inappropriate operation, exposure to the elements, or an accident.

An Explanation
Pain in your elbow is almost always due to an obstruction pattern. This could be due to the effects of an accident, a trauma, an operation, or it could be due to just doing too much, such as too much work or overdoing sports.

One or more of the rivers that run across the elbow area (*yang*: Large intestine, small intestine, and triple burner; *yin*: Lung, heart, and heart ruler) and the muscles and tendons around them can become impaired. The circulation of blood cannot flow freely over this damaged area and becomes stuck, causing pain in the elbow. If there is a weakness in the elbow area and an area of tissue that is separated from the main circulation patterns, any of the climates (wind, cold, heat, or damp) can establish themselves there. Cold contracts the muscles and tendons around the elbow and causes sharp pain and stiffness. It will often feel better with the application of heat. Damp lingers and feels fixed in one place, often feeling worse in wet weather. Heat can cause swelling, a burning sensation, and redness. It will often feel better with an ice pack or a cold towel. If wind is present, the symptoms can easily change location, either around the elbow to another joint and the other side of your body.

Food Therapy

Dietary Factors That Can Worsen Elbow Pain

- Overeating and irregular meal times can add to stagnation in the body.
- Cow's milk, cheese, tofu, bananas, and other cold-natured, damp-forming foods can slow digestion and weaken blood circulation. See Damp/Phlegm and Cold for more details.

Dietary Factors That Can Improve Elbow Pain

- Ideally, follow a diet that is supportive and that will nourish the muscles and tendons. See General Weakness and Blood Circulation Weakness for more details.

Manual Therapy

> **CAUTION:** If the pattern is acute, avoid manipulating directly on or around the elbow.

ON YOUR ARMS: For chronic pain, it can be appropriate to treat locally, either in the area of pain or on the other arm, the one without symptoms.

Effective treatment depends on identifying which of the rivers that flow through the elbow are affected.

For this reason, move the elbow into different positions to locate where the pain is located and then identify which river(s) are implicated by their proximity to the area of pain.

LATERAL SIDE: Large intestine or triple burner rivers

BACK: Triple burner or small intestine rivers

MEDIAL SIDE: Small intestine river

FRONT: Lateral – lung river; middle – heart ruler; medial – heart river

The key is to use your knowledge of the trajectories of the river systems to understand the pattern. They go through the root *shu* regions at your elbow (Ht-3, Hr-3, Lu-5, Tb-10, Si-8, and Li-11). And these are areas that can be pressed if not acute and inflamed and pressure is tolerable.

Treatment starts on the rivers above and below the elbow, and the idea is to encourage circulation if there are any obstruction patterns. If you find any areas of tension in the tissue upstream or downstream, press and knead them.

Use Gua sha to scrape in the appropriate direction, and look for areas of soreness and tightness. Press and knead these areas with your fingers.

ON YOUR LEGS: Press and knead the equivalent root *shu* areas around your knee: Kd-10, Lv-8, Pa-9, Gb-34, Bl-40, and St-36. Also thumb-press upstream and downstream to any of the rivers affected.

ON YOUR HANDS: Press the following areas, and knead if sore: D and B on the second joints of your index and ring Fingers (2-3).

ON YOUR FEET: Press the following areas and knead if sore: Zone 3 – elbow and arm (U).

ON YOUR EARS: Press the following areas and knead if sore: Zone 4 – arm and elbow (K); support regions – relaxation (2) and *shenmen* (1).

Exercise Therapy

The following exercises can help maintain the elbow joint:

❶ *Cover Your Ears*

Stand with your feet shoulders'-width apart and your arms relaxed at your sides.

Keeping your arms straight, slowly lift them in front of you as you breathe in.

When your arms reach chest level, bend your elbows towards you, and swing your forearms towards your ears.

Both open palms should end up facing your ears, as if you were about to cover them.

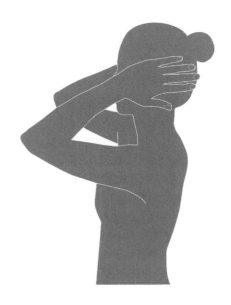

While breathing out, swing the forearms back down, and when they reach chest level, straighten your arms, and bring them down slowly to your sides. Repeat for five minutes.

❷ *Do exercises 1 and 3 of the Five Qualities of Nature stretches, which can strengthen the rivers flowing over the elbow (see p. 101 f.).*

Lifestyle Therapy

Avoid exposing your elbow to the outside elements, especially wind and cold. For chronic pain, if it feels better with warmth, put something warm (like a hot pack or warm towel) on it every now and again; if it feels better with cold, use a cold towel.

Immobilizing the elbow is a common treatment, but ideally, moving the elbow joint through its full pain-free range of motion at least once a day helps ensure that the circulatory patterns do not stagnate and the problem becomes worse.

If the injury is acute, note the advice in Neck Pain about putting ice on it.

Wrist Pain

Symptoms
Pain, swelling, numbness, and tingling in the wrist, limitation of movement of the wrist, weakness in the hand, a heavy sensation, possible soft nodules.

Can Include or Lead to
Muscle or tendon sprain, carpal tunnel syndrome, rheumatoid arthritis, rheumatic pain, and tenosynovitis.

When to See a Doctor
If the symptoms are severe.

Common Causes
Overwork, overuse, a traumatic injury, emotional stress, exposure to the weather, or a chronic disease.

An Explanation
Pain in the wrist is usually due to an obstruction pattern. This could be due to a local injury in the wrist area from trauma or overuse. It could also have an underlying cause of Blood Circulation Weakness, which has been unable to nourish the muscles and tendons of the wrist effectively (often felt as a numb, tingling sensation in your hand). Or it could be a climate pattern whereby wind, cold, or damp have attached themselves in the tissue or joint, and are causing pain and blocking free movement.

Stagnation in the liver system can cause the obstruction pattern to affect other joints, and ironically, any stagnation can often worsen with the frustration that comes with not being able to use the wrist normally. An inability to work, do chores, or do daily activities without pain or discomfort can in itself be so frustrating that it can disrupt the smooth circulation flow around the body, causing even more stagnation in the wrist.

Food Therapy

Dietary Factors That Can Worsen Wrist Pain
- Irregular eating habits and overeating can add to the stagnation pattern.
- Too many damp-forming, oily foods can weaken your digestion and increase the likelihood of damp settling in the wrist. See Damp/Phlegm for more details.
- Too many cold-natured, raw foods can slow digestion and weaken circulation. See Cold for more details.

Dietary Factors That Can Improve Wrist Pain
Ideally, follow a diet that supports and nourishes the muscles and tendons. See General Weakness and Blood Circulation Weakness for more details.

Manual Therapy

> **CAUTION:** Direct treatment on your wrist can sometimes worsen acute conditions.

ON YOUR ARMS: Locate the river systems that may be involved in the wrist discomfort from their proximity to the pain area. Once located, treat the river system in the arm. Use Gua sha to scrape in the appropriate direction, and look for areas of soreness and tightness. Press and knead these areas with your fingers.

Radial (Thumb) Side

BACK AND SIDE: Large intestine river
FRONT: Lung river
MIDDLE: Triple burner river; front: Heart ruler river

Ulnar: (Little Finger) Side

BACK AND SIDE: Small intestine river
FRONT: Heart river

ON YOUR HANDS: Do the Hand Circulation sequence in chapter 13. Use your hands or a Gua sha tool.

Press any sore areas, especially the root *shu* regions. Also the top segments of the five fingers, as all of these river systems run through the wrist (A-E 1).

ON YOUR LEGS/FEET: Use your knowledge of the parent river system to treat the paired river in your legs. Image your ankle as your wrist, and scrape or thumb-press along the lower leg area. Press the root *shu* or junction regions around your ankles (Kd-3, Pa-5, Lv-4, Gb-40, Bl-60, and St-41), and knead any that feel tight. Treating the ankle can often benefit the wrist, and vice versa.

ON YOUR EARS: Press the following areas, and knead if sore: Zone 4 – arm, wrist, and hand (K-L); support regions – relaxation (2) and *shenmen* (1).

Exercise Therapy

The following exercises can help maintain the wrist joint:

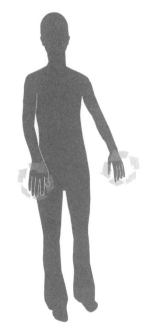

❶ Wrist Shake
Stand with your hands relaxed at your sides.

Loosen the muscles of your arms, wrists, and hands, and gently shake both wrist joints. Ensure that your wrists and hands are limp.

Continue until you feel a slight numbness or pins and needles sensation in the hands.

❷ Wrist Rotation
With one hand supporting the wrist of the other hand, rotate your wrist joint in a clockwise direction 10 times, then do the same number anticlockwise.

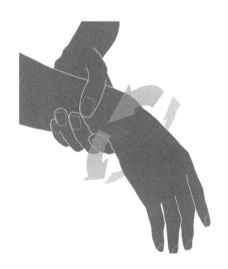

Lifestyle Therapy

1. It is essential to avoid all activities that may aggravate the pattern, if possible. Your wrist usually cannot heal without taking the time to rest it.
2. It is also important to adapt any work or home situation to lessen any strain in the future. This could mean making major life-changing job decisions, or it could be just a matter of buying a wrist support for clicking on a computer mouse. It depends on the severity of the condition.
3. If the injury is acute, note the advice about putting ice on it in Neck Pain.

Pain in Your Hand and Fingers

Symptoms
Pain, discomfort, or swelling in the hand or one or more fingers.

Can Include or Lead to
Osteoarthritis, rheumatoid arthritis, rheumatic fever, chilblains (perniosis), nerve pain, paralysis or injury of the nerves, and a local injury of the muscles or tendons.

When to See a Doctor
If the symptoms are severe.

Common Causes
Overuse, trauma, exposure to the weather, a diet of too many hot-natured, damp-forming, or raw cold-natured foods.

An Explanation
Obstruction patterns in your hand or fingers can be climate related. Damp and cold climates can come via a *yang* imbalance in your body or your hands being repeatedly exposed to cold water. The cold can contract the muscles and tendons in your hand and cause severe pain, swelling, or numbness. It is often worse in cold, wet weather.

Damp and heat patterns also have external and internal causes. Damp can be generated by an inappropriate diet or exposure to water, and heat as a development from damp or stagnation, or from weakness or *yin*. The presence of damp and heat can lead to redness and swelling, and it can often make it difficult for your hand to grasp things.

Any local injury can cause stagnation, as well as damp, heat, or cold. The obstruction to circulation often causes pain that feels better with movement but is worse at night and can lead to deformities of the bone.

If your body does not have enough circulation strength to maintain itself, it often cannot nourish the body parts farthest away. This can result in stiff, weak hands or fingers.

Food Therapy

Dietary Factors That Can Worsen Hand or Finger Pain

- Irregular eating habits and overeating, too many damp-forming, oily foods, and too many cold-natured, raw foods can slow digestion, weaken *qi* and blood, and add to stagnation in the body. See Damp/Phlegm and Cold for more details.

Dietary Factors That Can Help Hand or Finger Pain

- As with other joint and bone pain, it is best to follow a diet that is supportive and that will nourish the muscles and tendons. See General Weakness and Blood Circulation Weakness for more details.

Manual Therapy

> **CAUTION:** If the condition is acute, inflamed, or painful to the touch, avoid treating the hand or fingers directly.

ON YOUR HANDS: If acute, you can treat the other hand with the following (otherwise treat the same hand):

Do the Hand Circulation sequence in chapter 13. Use your fingers or a Gua sha tool.

Press the following areas, and knead if sore: B and D at the top of the index and ring fingers (4); Li-3, Li-4, Tb-3, Tb-5, Si-3, and Si-5.

ON YOUR FEET: Do the Foot Circulation sequence in chapter 13. Match the area of discomfort in your hand or fingers with the equivalent part on your foot, and treat that area.

ON YOUR EARS: Press the following areas, and knead if sore: Zone 4 – hand and fingers (L); support regions – relaxation (2) and *shenmen* (1).

Exercise Therapy

❶ *Do exercises 1 and 3 of the Five Qualities of Nature stretches to increase circulation in the hand river systems (see p. 101 f.).*

❷ *Do the Relax Your Fingers and Toes exercise from Sleeping Disorders (see p. 172).*

Lifestyle Therapy

1. When doing daily chores, such as washing dishes, wear protective gloves to minimize external damp, cold, or heat on the hands.

2. Avoid certain actions that may make the pain worse, such as making a fist or gripping objects. Instead of a clutch bag, take a shoulder bag. Instead of holding a book while reading, use a book stand. When writing, typing, or using your hands, take a break every 15 minutes, or when your hand feels tired or painful.

3. If the injury is acute, note the advice about putting ice on it in Neck Pain.

25

Lower Limbs

Knee Pain

Symptoms

Pain, swelling, or stiffness in either one or both knee joints or the muscles and tendons around the knee area.

Can Include or Lead to

Synovitis of the knee, rheumatic arthritis, fibrositis, local ligament damage, and local nerve damage.

When to See a Doctor

If there are severe symptoms, or the joint is immovable.

Common Causes

Overuse, overexercise, an improper diet with too much greasy food, an injury, an inappropriate knee operation, chronic illness, or old age.

An Explanation

Your knee joint takes the weight of your whole body and twists and turns at all angles, and as such, it can be susceptible to obstruction patterns—this is especially true if the knee has been subjected to overexercise or too much activity. The obstruction pattern impairs the circulation flow within the knee and often leads to pain and swelling.

If your knee is swollen, affected by damp and cold weather, and the pain is more on one side, then damp or cold patterns could have become attached within your knee. The cold motion contracts the muscles and tendons around the knee, causing severe pain, and the damp motion causes swelling and numbness. It can be easy for any of these climate patterns to attach to your knee when an existing weakness within the tissue structure allows them to do so.

Sometimes, the pain can mysteriously jump from place to place, or even from one knee to the other. This can be difficult to explain without the knowledge of climate patterns. This type of movement is normally caused by wind, which tends to move within the body as it does outside the body. It can often develop from long-term patterns of weakness of circulation or from exposure to the weather.

If wind, cold, or damp patterns remain stuck in your knees for too long, they can transform into damp and heat, which can cause swelling, inflammation, and a burning sensation. This condition is often found in people who drink too much alcohol or eat a diet containing too many greasy foods. In these cases, the damp and heat in the knee are being fuelled by the damp and heat coming from the stomach and pancreas systems and the digestive process.

Most knee problems involve an underlying weakness in the kidney system. This is because both water river systems (kidney and bladder) run behind the knee and the kidney system protects the integrity of bones and joints. Any long-term weakness in the kidney system is, therefore, implicated if the pain develops gradually and is located in both knees. It is frequently behind many of the overflow patterns, and either existed before the obstruction pattern in your knee or developed afterwards as a result of the blockage.

Food Therapy

Dietary Factors That Can Worsen Knee Pain

The patterns of weakness and overflow above can often originate from an improper diet:

- Processed, junk foods, such as pizzas and hamburgers, soft fizzy drinks (sodas), and alcohol, can lead to damp and heat in the body, which can then sink to the knees. See Damp/Phlegm for more details.
- Salads, grapefruit, melons, mangos, tomatoes, watermelons, cucumbers, lettuce, ice cream, and other raw, cold-natured foods weaken the stomach and pancreas systems, and damp can collect in joints. See Cold for more details.

Dietary Factors That Can Improve Knee Pain

- Radishes, rye bread, celery, and pumpkin improve dampness in the knees. See Damp/Phlegm for more details.
- A strengthening diet that allows the stomach and pancreas to digest food properly will allow better nourishment of the knee. See General Weakness for more details.

Manual Therapy

CAUTION: If the the condition is acute and the knee is inflamed or painful to the touch, avoid massaging it directly.

ON YOUR LEGS: As with any obstruction pattern causing pain or discomfort, it is important to identify which rivers are affected in order to provide relief. To do this, you need to locate the pain and the river(s) in close proximity to it. The following is a simple association:

Front
MEDIAL SIDE: Pancreas river
MIDDLE: Stomach river
LATERAL SIDE: Stomach or gallbladder rivers

Back
MEDIAL SIDE: Kidney or liver rivers
MIDDLE: Bladder river
LATERAL SIDE: Bladder or gallbladder rivers

Local treatment can consist of using your palm to gently rub the knee area in a circular motion to create warmth, then pressing and circling around the kneecap at the front.

The focus should be on whichever rivers are implicated in the knee pattern and associated areas. The root *shu* regions in the knee area act like local areas for the knee, so St-36, Gb-34, Bl-40, Pa-9, Lv-8, and Kd-10 can be hard-pressed, kneaded, and scraped.

For pain above your knee, scrape down Crouching Rabbit on your thigh.

For pain on the inside of the knee, explore the river systems coming up the inside of the leg (kidney, pancreas and liver).

For pain on the outside of the knee, explore the river systems coming down the outside of the leg (gallbladder, stomach and bladder).

For pain at the back of your knee, explore the bladder river.

Provided the knee is not hot and swollen, heat can be applied (a hot pad or towel) to encourage blood circulation.

ON YOUR FEET: As your ankle is the next joint down, treat the river(s) affected on and around the ankle to affect the river(s) on the knee. The equivalent root *shu* or junction regions in the ankle are St-41, Gb-40, Bl-60, Pa-5, Lv-4, and Kd-3.

ON YOUR ARMS: The equivalent joint to your knee in the upper body is your elbow, so apply the same approach to the elbow joint as with the ankle above using Ht-3, Hr-3, Lu-5, Tb-10, Si-8, and Li-11 and their rivers.

ON YOUR HANDS: Press and knead the following areas, if sore: A and E on the second joint of the little finger and thumb (2-3); zone 3 – kidney (M).

ON YOUR EARS: Press and knead the following areas, if sore: Zone 6 – leg area and knee (O-P); support regions – relaxation (2) and *shenmen* (1).

Exercise Therapy

The following exercises can strengthen and loosen the knee joint:

❶ *Knee Rotation*
Stand with both legs together.
Keeping your legs together, bend from the waist, and place one hand on each knee for support. Bend your knees slightly, and rotate your legs in a clockwise circular motion for 10 rotations, then for 10 rotations in an anticlockwise direction.

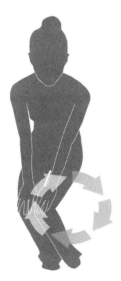

❷ *Do exercise 2 and 5 of the Five Qualities of Nature stretches (see p. 101 ff.). This strengthens the earth (stomach and pancreas) and wood (liver and gallbladder) river systems, all of which flow on or near the knee.*

❸ *Do exercise Swing Your Bottom in General Weakness, as this involves gentle movement of the knees (see p. 138).*

❹ *A good way to encourage flexibility and strength in your knee is to use an exercise bike. Position the seat high, so that the knee is only partially bent, and keep the resistance level low. As this becomes comfortable, the seat can be lowered and resistance increased.*

Lifestyle Therapy

1. If possible, avoid keeping the knee joint in the same position for any prolonged length of time. While watching television, for example, get up, stretch, and move around every half-hour.
2. At work or home, adjust the height of your chair to reduce the stress on the knees when getting up. Higher is generally better.
3. If the injury is acute, note the advice about putting ice on it in Neck Pain.

Ankle Pain

Symptoms

Pain or discomfort in one or both ankles, with possible restricted movement and swelling.

Can Include or Lead to

Sprain or dislocation of the ankle, gout, tarsal tunnel syndrome, synovitis, and rheumatoid arthritis.

When to See Your Doctor

If the symptoms are severe.

Common Causes

A traumatic injury; overuse; exposure to the elements; an improper diet of too many greasy foods; an inappropriate operation; standing for too long; strong emotional problems; or a chronic illness.

An Explanation

A great deal of strain is put on your ankle as it supports your body weight and rotates at different angles. Indeed, ankle sprain is one of the most common musculoskeletal injuries in people at any age, and this often manifests as damage to the lateral ankle ligaments, when your foot involuntarily rolls inwards.

Weakness is the main underlying issue to ankle pain. This is especially true with anyone who regularly engages in sports or exercise. If there is a weakness pattern in your body, the river systems that run over your ankle may no longer be able to give enough nourishment to the soft tissue structures of the ankle area. This will lead to an underlying weakness in how your ankle is held in place and can make it much easier to injure.

Any injury to the ankle, whether from an accident, or overuse, will cause an obstruction pattern in the ankle. This can often linger well after the ankle itself appears to mend, and can make the ankle more susceptible to climate patterns through direct exposure to cold, damp, and wind, or generated internally from an impairment in the digestive system or the balance of *yin/yang* motions. Wind moves the pain from place to place; cold contracts the tendons and rivers around the ankle and leads to severe pain; and damp numbs and swells the ankle with a fixed, heavy pain. Any one of these, if left long enough, can transform into heat and inflame your ankle.

Food Therapy

Dietary Factors That Can Worsen Ankle Pain

Patterns of weakness and patterns of overflow like those above can originate from an improper diet:

- Hot-natured, damp-forming foods, including processed foods, can lead to damp and heat in the body. This can then sink to the ankles. See Damp/Phlegm for more details.
- Too many cold-natured, raw foods can cause the stomach system to weaken and cold and damp to collect in the joints. See Cold for more details.

Dietary Factors That Can Improve Ankle Pain

- A strengthening diet that allows the stomach and pancreas systems to digest food properly help nourish the ankle. See General Weakness for more details.

Manual Therapy

CAUTION: Avoid treating the ankle itself when it is inflamed and the pain acute.

ON YOUR FEET: Knowing where the river systems flow over the ankle area can help identify which of the systems are implicated in any given obstruction pattern:

Front

Stomach river

Lateral Side

ANTERIOR TO (in front of) the lateral malleolus (outside ankle): Gallbladder river

POSTERIOR TO (behind) the lateral malleolus (outside ankle): Bladder river

Medial Side

ANTERIOR TO the medial malleolus (inside ankle): Pancreas or liver rivers

POSTERIOR TO the medial malleolus (inside ankle): Kidney river

The root *shu* and junction regions in the ankle area act like local areas for the ankle so Kd-3, Pa-5, Lv-4, Gb-40, Bl-60, and St-41 can be hard-pressed, kneaded, and scraped.

- For pain on the medial (inside) ankle, explore the river systems coming up the inside of the leg (kidney, pancreas, and liver) above and below the ankle.

- For pain on the anterior (front) of the ankle, explore the stomach river superior (above) and inferior (below) to the ankle.

- For pain on the lateral (outside) part of the ankle, explore the gallbladder and bladder rivers above and below the ankle.

- For pain at the posterior (back) of the ankle, explore the bladder river above and below the ankle.

- Provided the ankle is not hot and swollen, heat can be applied (a hot pad, a heat lamp, or hot towel) to encourage blood circulation.

ON YOUR ARMS: The equivalent joint to your ankle in the upper body is your wrist, so apply the equivalent areas and rivers (parent river relationships) to the wrist joint and the following areas: Ht-7, Hr-7, Lu-9, Tb-4, Si-5, and Li-5.

ON YOUR HANDS: Press the following areas, and knead, if sore: A and E at the last joint of the little finger and thumb (3-4).

ON YOUR EARS: Press the following areas, and knead, if sore: Zone 6 – leg area and ankle (O-P); support regions – relaxation (2) and *shenmen* (1).

Exercise Therapy

The following ankle exercises can help chronic ankle pain:

❶ *Ankle Rotation*
Rotate the ankle by supporting it with one hand and guiding your foot in a circular motion with the other hand. Repeat in both directions 10 times.

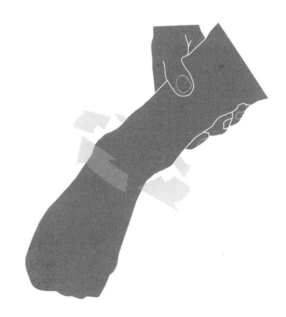

❷ *Do the Knee Rotation exercise from Knee Pain, as this also gently rotates the ankles (see p. 237).*

❸ *Do the exercise Swing Your Bottom from General Weakness, if possible, as it gently moves the ankle joint (see p. 238).*

❹ *Do exercises 2, 4, and 5 of the Five Qualities of Nature stretches (see p. 101 ff.). These can strengthen the river systems that run through the ankle.*

Lifestyle Therapy

1. It is important to rest the ankle as much as possible. No amount of bandaging, stretching, and taping to allow you to continue use will replace simple resting the ankle.
2. After exposure to wet or cold conditions, dry and warm the ankle area quickly and thoroughly.
3. Ideally, moving the ankle joint through its full, pain-free range of motion at least once a day will maximize circulation patterns.
4. If the injury is acute, note the advice about icing in Neck Pain.

Foot and Toe Pain

Symptoms
Pain or discomfort in the heel, sole, or toes of one or both feet.

Can Include or Lead to
Osteoarthritis, rheumatoid arthritis, bunions, tenosynovitis, gout, soft tissue injury, metatarsalgia, plantar fibrositis, plantar fasciitis, and heel spurs.

When to See Your Doctor
If the symptoms are severe.

Common Causes
Living in a damp environment, wading through water, overwork, stress, overuse, a chronic illness, a local traumatic injury, and an improper diet with irregular eating habits.

An Explanation
Obstruction patterns in your feet and toes are your body's perfectly normal reaction to a traumatic event, such as stubbing your toe. Problems can arise, however, after the trauma seems to have disappeared but may be hiding an obstruction pattern, which can linger long after an injury appears to have "healed" and continue to cause pain. With this pattern of unresolved obstruction, the pain is often worse at rest and feels better with movement.

Climate patterns involving wind, cold, or damp can settle in an area of tissue, causing it to become disconnected from the main circulation patterns, which then further block circulation, resulting in swelling and heaviness that can be worse in cold or wet weather. As with any climate pattern, over time, the wind, cold, and damp in your foot can develop into heat, which will dry up the rivers, tendons, and muscles of the foot. This can lead to an acute, hot, swollen condition.

General Weakness in your body means that it does not have enough force to maintain itself and often cannot effectively nourish the body parts farthest away. This will result in stiff, weak feet or toes. The accompanying pain is often worse after walking and standing, and when tired.

When your body ages, the balance between *yin* and *yang* motions in the kidney system shifts. People who develop *Yin* Weakness often display general low heat due to unbalanced *yang* motion. This can mean that any obstruction pattern causing pain in the foot or toe can involve a feeling of heat, especially at night.

Food Therapy

Dietary Factors That Can Worsen Foot or Toe Pain
Weakness patterns and overflow patterns like those above can originate from an improper diet:

- A diet of hot, damp-forming foods, such as processed, junk food high in saturated fats, sugary soft drinks, and alcohol, can lead to damp and heat in the body. This can then sink to the feet. See Damp/Phlegm for more details.
- A recent Canadian study strongly associates sweetened soft drinks with an increased risk of gout (damp and heat in

the foot) in men. Researchers looked at tens of thousands of men with no history of gout and monitored them over 12 years.

They found that the risk was 85 percent higher among men who drank two or more servings of sweetened soft drinks per day, compared to those who consumed less than one serving per month.[66]

- An excess of dairy products, tropical fruits, concentrated orange juice, and other cold-natured, damp-forming foods cause the stomach and pancreas systems to weaken, so that cold and damp collect in the lower joints. See Cold for more details.

Dietary Factors That Can Improve Foot and Toe Pain

Ideally, follow a strengthening diet that allows the stomach and pancreas systems to digest food properly and ensure that the foot can be nourished. See General Weakness for more details.

Manual Therapy

CAUTION: If the condition is acute and the foot or toes are inflamed or painful to the touch, avoid treating them directly.

ON YOUR FEET: Treating your foot and toe depends on where the pain or discomfort is located and which rivers are implicated by being in close proximity.

Foot
TOP: Stomach river
MEDIAL SIDE: Pancreas, kidney, or liver rivers
LATERAL SIDE: Gallbladder or bladder rivers

Toes
Each of your toes is the starting point or terminating point of a river system.
BIG TOE: Pancreas, liver, or gallbladder rivers
SECOND TOE: Stomach river

THIRD TOE: Stomach river
FOURTH TOE: Gallbladder river
LITTLE TOE: Bladder river (kidney is on the sole, at the base of the little toe)

Physiological differences in individual toes are connected to the river system associated with that toe. So if one toe bends a certain way or is longer than others, this is useful information about that particular river in your body. Once the affected river(s) has been determined, base your treatment on that, and treat the root *shu* regions of that river.

If the condition is acute, treat the other foot using the following protocol (otherwise treat the same foot):

- Do the Foot Circulation sequence in chapter 13. Use fingers or a Gua sha tool.

ON YOUR LEGS: Thumb-press or scrape up or down the affected river systems on your legs.
ON YOUR HANDS: Do the Hand Circulation sequence in chapter 13. Match the area of discomfort in your foot or toes with the equivalent part on your hand, and treat that area. Also, press and knead the tips of A and E on the little finger and thumb (4).
ON YOUR EARS: Press the following areas, and knead if sore: Zone 6 – leg area and toes (O-P); support regions – relaxation (2) and *shenmen* (1).

Exercise Therapy

The following foot exercises can help chronic foot or toe pain:

❶ *Do the Ankle Rotation exercise from Ankle Pain (see p. 239).*

❷ **Foot Scrunch**
Begin seated, with your legs shoulders'-width apart. Five rolled-up socks should be prepared and positioned next to your right foot.

Each pair of socks needs to be moved from the right side to the left side with the toes of your right foot.

Once completed, the socks can be pushed to the outside of your left foot, and then the process is repeated with the other foot.

The sequence can be repeated up to five times.

3 *Do exercises 2, 4, and 5 of the Five Qualities of Nature stretches to help strengthen the foot river systems (see p. 101 ff.).*

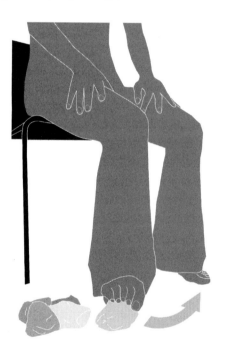

Lifestyle Therapy

1. For pain originating from cold and damp external conditions, it is very important to keep your feet warm and dry. This is especially the case after doing exercise, swimming, or any activity that encourages your feet to sweat.
2. If possible, avoid exercising while you are experiencing pain. If your tendons are undernourished they will easily tire and begin to hurt.
3. If the injury is acute, note the advice about putting ice on it in Neck Pain.

Conditions Affecting Men

Prostate Disorders

Symptoms
Pain or discomfort in the perineum and lower back, increased frequency of urination (especially noticeable at night), poor urine flow, pain on urination, and a bloated abdomen.

Can Include or Lead to
Prostatitis, prostatic hypertrophy (enlarged prostate), urinary retention, and prostatic cancer.

When to See Your Doctor
If the symptoms are severe.

Common Causes
Lack of exercise; a diet of hot-natured, damp-forming foods; emotional stress; and exposure to the weather.

An Explanation
Prostate disorders do not just appear overnight; they are the result of sustained patterns in your body that have often been going on for a long time. A climate pattern is often involved. It can be either externally generated or internally generated, and attaches in the prostate area where a part of the river has lost its connection to the main circulation.

Sitting on a cold seat or in a draft for any length of time can sometimes be enough for a cold pattern to attach itself. And the contracting and sinking nature of the motion of cold will cause it to stay and result in an uncomfortable and often painful condition in the prostate area.

A sustained diet of rich, damp-forming food that weakens the stomach and pancreas systems and causes an accumulation of damp to sink in the body can add to the cold. It can be accompanied by a heavy, dragging feeling and bloating, and also either a feeling of heat or cold.

Emotional stress causes muscles and tendons to tense up and creates blockages in the smooth movement of circulation around the body. With a lack of regular exercise, this blockage can easily worsen the pattern in the lower abdomen area.

Weakness usually underlies these patterns, causing the rising motion of the pancreas system to instead sink in the direction of the prostate, and also affect the balance of *yin* and *yang* motions in the kidney system, which can have a direct weakening effect on the prostate area.

Food Therapy

Dietary Factors That Can Worsen Prostate Problems
Limiting damp- and hot-natured foods is essential in the managing of most prostate conditions:
- Dairy products and processed foods containing high levels of saturated fats, such as donuts, chocolate, cookies, cakes, and deep-fried foods, produce damp in the body. See Damp/Phlegm for more details.

- Heat-producing foods include red meat, particularly lamb; oily fish, such as tuna, mackerel, salmon, herrings, sardines, and pilchards; and drinks containing caffeine or saccharin, such as coffee, fizzy soft drinks, fruit juice, and alcohol, especially beer. See Heat for more details.

Dietary Factors That Can Improve Prostate Problems

- In general, a simple, bland diet will strengthen and benefit the stomach and pancreas systems. See General Weakness for more details.

  In addition the following foods help to maintain the prostate:

  ▸ **FRUIT:** Pomegranate, raspberries, blackberries, papayas, cherries, watermelon, and grapefruit.
  ▸ **VEGETABLES:** Tomatoes (cooked), carrots (cooked), red or green peppers, cabbage, turnip, cauliflower, broccoli, and Brussels sprouts.
  ▸ **LEGUMES, SEEDS, AND NUTS:** Pumpkin seeds, Brazil nuts, and lentils.
  ▸ **GRAINS:** Rice and quinoa.
  ▸ **MEAT:** Chicken and white fish.
  ▸ **DRINKS:** Green tea.
  ▸ **OTHER:** Miso, soy sauce, and seaweed (especially kelp).

Manual Therapy

ON YOUR FRONT: Palm-circle with slight pressure in a large *clockwise* circular motion around your navel.

Do the Abdomen Circle sequence in Feeling Bloated (see p. 212).

Hard-press Ren-4 and Ren-6 areas.

ON YOUR BACK: Scrape down the kidney back *shu* region in your lower back, and continue farther into the buttocks and on the sacrum.

ON YOUR LEGS: Explore the balance of the rivers that flow into the groin area. This includes the *yin* rivers (kidney, pancreas, and liver), which flow up your leg. Thumb-press along the rivers, and knead any areas of tension, paying particular attention to the kidney river.

ON YOUR HANDS: Press and knead the following areas, if sore: Ht-7 to Ht-9; zone 3 – kidney, bladder, and reproductive organs (L-N).

ON YOUR FEET: Press and knead the following areas, if sore: Kd-1 to Kd-4; zone 5 – prostate and any reactive areas in the whole zone (N-R); zone 3 – kidney, pancreas, stomach, and liver/spleen (J-H); zone 4 – bladder (M).

ON YOUR EARS: Press and knead the following areas, if sore: Zone 6 – prostate (P); zone 1 – A; zone 7 – genitals, urethra, testes; support region – *shenmen* (1).

Exercise Therapy

❶ *Do exercises 2, 4, and 5 of the Five Qualities of Nature stretches to help strengthen the river systems in the pelvic area (see p. 101 ff.).*
❷ *Do exercises Bend Your Hip and Swing Your Waist from General Weakness, as both of these help to reduce stagnation in the lower abdomen (see p. 139).*
❸ *Do the Body Twist exercise from Constipation (see p. 217).*

Lifestyle Advice

To prevent stagnation in the lower abdomen, it is very important to take regular exercise, which will stretch and twist the muscles in this area.

27

Conditions Affecting Women

Premenstrual Tension

Symptoms
Pre-period irritability; depression; changeable moods; swollen breasts, hands, face, or feet; bloating and abdominal pain; nausea; chest tightness; lack of concentration; constipation or diarrhoea.

When to See Your Doctor
If the symptoms are severe.

Common Causes
Emotional stress, especially when emotions are repressed; a diet of too many hot-natured, damp-forming foods; overwork; lack of exercise; bad posture; and excessive sexual activity.

An Explanation
On a monthly basis, the force of a woman's body is redirected downwards to the uterus to prepare for menstruation. The liver system ensures that this process happens smoothly, as it controls how your circulation moves throughout your body.

If, however, the liver system has been impaired, such as by emotional stress or an obstruction pattern, it cannot prevent stagnation in this flow. As a result, the circulation is no longer smooth and tends to get clogged up and cause muscle tension, pain, and discomfort.

This obstruction pattern can affect the accumulation of fluids and how the digestive system works but also on an emotional level. If there is a tendency to be stuck in your body, it can limit the normal range of emotions as they move through the breath cycle. As a result, it can become very difficult to snap out of feeling depressed or irritable.

Underlying this pattern of stagnation and obstruction is often a general weakness in blood circulation which cannot meet the demands of the menstrual process, much like a river whose source has dwindled. If so, there can be a tendency to be depressed and tearful and feel tired and achy.

Food Therapy
Dietary Factors That Can Worsen Premenstrual Tension
- Overeating, eating too fast, eating too late at night or at irregular eating hours, and eating greasy, processed foods, including foods high in saturated fats, such as red meat, junk food, and dairy products, can cause a sluggish digestion that will add to stagnation. See Stagnation for more details.

Dietary Factors That Can Improve Premenstrual Tension
- Ideally, follow a simple, strengthening diet that nourishes and prevents stagnation. See General Weakness for more details.

- Beetroot, spinach, and sardines strengthen blood circulation. See Blood Circulation Weakness for more details.
- Spices and apple cider vinegar can help move stagnation. See Stagnation for more details.
- Brazilian research suggests that essential fatty acids may be helpful for the symptoms of premenstrual syndrome. In the study, women who received pills containing a few grams of essential fatty acids reported an improvement in symptoms such as sore breasts and depression.[67] Essential fatty acids in the form of soybean oil, safflower oil, walnuts, sunflower, sesame, and pumpkin seeds, flaxseed, fatty fish such as tuna and mackerel, and dark green vegetables may, therefore, have a useful blood circulation moving quality in PMT.

Manual Therapy

ON YOUR FRONT: Using a circular motion, rub your palm around your navel until you feel warmth on your skin.

Do the Abdomen Circle sequence in Feeling Bloated (see p. 212).

ABDOMEN LINE: Hard-press six equally spaced areas with the thumb or fingers on both sides of the stomach muscles—the first two are above your navel, the second two are in line with your navel, and the third two are below.

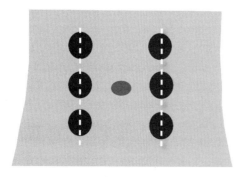

Rub the abdomen as noted in the first step.

ON YOUR BACK: Scrape down the liver, pancreas, and kidney back *shu* regions in your mid to lower back.

ON YOUR LEGS: Thumb-press up the liver and pancreas rivers, the liver from Lv-4 to Lv-5, then up to Lv-10 and the pancreas from Pa-5 to Pa-9. Press and knead any tense areas you find.

Scrape down the gallbladder and stomach rivers, the gallbladder from Gb-31 to Gb-40, and the stomach from St-36 to St-41. Press and knead any areas of tension, especially the Gb-34 and St-40 area.

ON YOUR HANDS: Do the Hand Circulation sequence in chapter 13. A moving action is needed, so this is best with a Gua sha tool. Press the following areas, and knead if sore: Li-4; zone 2 – liver, pancreas, and stomach (K-I); zone 6 – lower back area (Q-R).

ON YOUR FEET: Do the Foot Circulation sequence in chapter 13. Use a Gua sha tool. Press the following areas, and knead if sore: Lv-2 to Lv-3; zone 5 – uterus (N-R); zone 3 – liver/spleen, kidney, and pancreas (J-H); zone 2 – heart and chest (E-G).

ON YOUR EARS: Press the following areas, and knead if sore: Zone 1 – A; zone 7 – uterus and ovaries; zone 5 – abdomen (N); support region – *shenmen* (1).

Exercise Therapy

❶ *Do exercises 1–5 of the Five Qualities of Nature stretches. Particularly focus on exercise 5, as this helps to circulate the liver and gallbladder system (see p. 101 ff.).*

❷ *Do the Bend Your Hip exercise from General Weakness (see p. 139).*

Lifestyle Therapy

Correct posture can help reduce stagnation, especially in work situations. When seated, the ideal height for a work surface is about 2 inches below your bent elbow. Your back and feet should be well supported, with your forearms and upper legs resting parallel to the floor. Hunching is to be avoided, whenever possible.

Menstrual Flow Disorders

Symptoms
A period that initially gushes with blood and requires frequent changes of sanitary protection and can continue for a prolonged time; light bleeding during periods that is of short duration (two days or under) or periods absent altogether.

Can Include or Lead to
Fibroids, endometriosis, amenorrhea, polycystic ovarian syndrome, anorexia nervosa, and meno-pausal problems.

When to See Your Doctor
If the symptoms are severe, and if accompanied by abdominal pain.

Common Causes
Strong emotional issues, such as resentment, anger, and worry; an improper, irregular diet; a diet with too many hot-natured, spicy foods; overexercise; a competitive work atmosphere; a chronic illness; overwork; long-term use of oral contraceptives; post-surgery, or post-childbirth conditions.

An Explanation
Like any river that should be comfortably abundant with water, we often have to look upstream to see why there are changes in flow patterns. This is also true of menstrual disorders.

If the flow is too strong and the river is flooding, there may be heat. One of the main causes of heavy bleeding is that there is too much heat within the blood circulation, and it literally spills over, much like boiling water in an unattended cooking pot. Signs of this pattern would be bright or dark red thick blood and headaches, restlessness, and thirst. This could also be caused by diet (too much hot, greasy food) or a long-term pattern of *Yin* Weak-ness, which has developed into heat.

Stagnation patterns also cause heavy bleeding. This is a common pattern in people under stress or with unresolved emotional issues, and is often accompanied by musculoskeletal pain and discomfort, especially in the neck and shoulders. This obstruction pattern can form a blockage much like a dam. When fresh blood enters the uterus, the level of the blood rises above the height of the dam and overtops it and the flow cannot be controlled. This pattern would normally show as dark, thick blood, with clots and strong pain.

Sometimes blocks are created by a sticky damp or phlegm buildup in your abdomen, either from an improper diet or from exposure to cold. This pattern is more likely to occur in someone who is overweight and can be accompanied by discharge and heaviness.

If the pancreas system becomes impaired, often because of an improper diet, it no longer has the force to hold the blood in the blood vessels. The result is that blood quite literally leaks out. In this case, the accompanying blood would normally be pale, and there would be other signs of General Weakness, such as tiredness and a pale complexion.

If the flow is too weak and the river is reduced to a trickle, it could be an underlying cause of a lack of strength. The absence of periods can be because of a blood circulation weakness, arising from insuf-ficient life force to pump it around the body. This can be accompanied by other signs of weak blood circulation, such as dizziness, insomnia, and heart palpitations.

Sometimes the balance of *yin* and *yang* motions in the kidney system has swung too much in one direction. An impairment in the kidney *yang* motion can mean there is not enough *yang* force to move blood circulation. This can also be accompanied by lower back and knee pain.

Food Therapy

Dietary Factors That Can Worsen Menstrual Disorders

- Cold or cool-natured, raw foods impair the digestive process, weaken the stomach and pancreas systems and lead to a lack of control of blood flow. See Cold for more details.
- Overeating, alcohol, fatty food, and junk and processed foods may impair the liver system and lead to stagnation. See Stagnation for more details.
- Hot-natured and spicy foods, such as red meat, coffee, and alcohol, will cause more heat. See Heat for more examples.
- Raw and frozen foods, or foods that taste bitter and sour, have properties that interfere with the circulation of blood and cause weakened blood circulation. See the Bitter and Sour lists and Blood Circulation Weakness for more details.
- Dairy products; processed, fatty foods; and other raw, cold-natured, and damp-forming foods aggravate damp and cold patterns. See Damp/Phlegm for more details.

Dietary Factors That Can Improve Menstrual Disorders

- An overall strengthening diet to maintain the stomach and pancreas systems will help all patterns, but particularly help retain blood circulating in the blood vessels. See General Weakness for more details.
- Parsnips, fennel, leek, oats, quinoa, adzuki beans, pine nuts, black beans, and kelp and other seaweeds generally strengthen and help the holding function of blood.
- Mung beans, aubergines (eggplants), spinach, celery, cucumber, and seaweed can help cool heat in the blood circulation.
- Dark, leafy greens; carrots; chives; turmeric; nutmeg; garlic; and chamomile tea improve stagnation associated with damp/phlegm patterns. See Stagnation for more details.
- Egg yolk, almonds, dried fruit such as figs and currants, apricots, spinach, oats, fish, and high-quality red meat build up weakened blood circulation. See Blood Circulation Weakness for more details.
- Barley, rye, pumpkin, button mushrooms, and adzuki beans improve patterns of damp and phlegm. See Damp/Phlegm for more details.

Manual Therapy

ON YOUR FRONT: Only do the following if putting pressure on your abdomen feels comfortable:

- Finger-press down the centre line of the abdomen, and knead any areas of tension, including Ren-12 and Ren-6.
- Palm-circle with slight pressure in a clockwise direction around your navel.
- Do the Abdomen Line sequence in Premenstrual Tension.
- Using your palm, rub in a circular motion around Ren-4 to create warmth.

ON YOUR BACK: Scrape down the heart, pancreas, liver, and kidney back *shu* regions. Press and knead any areas of tension.

ON YOUR ARMS: In general, feel for any areas of tension in the tissue, and press, knead, or scrape them. Feel along both the *yin* and *yang* rivers in the upper and lower arms.

ON YOUR LEGS: Thumb-press up the pancreas river to the groin. Knead any areas of tension, including Pa-6, Pa-9 (and just below) and Pa-10.

ON YOUR FEET: Press the following areas, and knead if sore: Zone 5 – uterus, reproductive organs, and any reactive areas within the zone (N-R); zone 3 – liver/spleen and kidney (J-H). Foot soaks can help in the regulation of blood flow. A good agent to use for this is mugwort. See the Mugwort Foot Soak in Depression and Heat Your Feet in *Yang* Weakness for more information.

ON YOUR HANDS: Press the following areas, and knead if sore: Zone 3 – reproductive area and kidney (L-N); zone 2 – pancreas, liver, and stomach (K-I).

ON YOUR EARS: Press the following areas, and knead if sore: Zone 1 – A; zone 7 – uterus, ovaries; zone 5 – abdomen (N); support region – *shenmen* (1).

Exercise Therapy

Do exercises 2, 4, and 5 of the Five Qualities of Nature stretches; these can help harmonize the pancreas, liver, and kidney systems. The exercises in the Period Pain section can also be helpful here (see pp. 101 and 251).

Lifestyle Therapy

1. With patterns of General Weakness, it is very important to rest. Avoid standing for long periods, as it may make the condition worse.
2. Regular gentle exercise for all patterns can be beneficial, but especially for patterns of stagnation.
3. It is also important to keep your legs and feet warm and dry as much as possible. Watch where you sit, especially when outside.

Period Pain

Symptoms

Abdominal and/or back pain before, during, or after a period.

Can Include or Lead to

Dysmenorrhoea, pelvic inflammation, uterine fibroids, and endometriosis.

When to See Your Doctor

If the symptoms are severe or accompanied with heavy bleeding.

Common Causes

Emotional stress, overwork, an inappropriate diet, exposure to the weather, or excessive sexual activity.

An Explanation

If the accumulation of blood becomes blocked during your menstrual cycle, the build-up of pressure causes pain. This obstruction pattern can often happen after cold and damp enter your uterus by exposure to the cold, commonly from wearing inadequate clothing or sitting on a cold surface. The resulting pain is normally cramping, before or during a period, and there is usually a low quantity of blood. It can feel better with the application of heat (and worse with cold).

An impairment in the liver system causes a body-wide stagnation that leads to obstruction . This can often happen after emotional stress, as the circulation flow begins to clog up in certain weakened areas of the river system, where it is vulnerable. The pain in stagnation is often severe on one or both sides of the lower abdomen prior to the onset of a menstrual period. Dark purple blood clots and swollen, painful breasts often accompany this pattern, and the painful area is normally worse with pressure. It could also be more of a fixed, stabbing pain a few days before the start of the period. It is often located in the central part of the abdomen, the blood shows as dark purple clots, and can be worse at night.

Long-term cold and damp, accumulation or stagnation can also gradually transform into heat. This can result in heavy, dark-coloured blood, discharges, small clots, and a strong burning sensation.

Heat that originates from *yin* weakness often does not present with the severe symptoms of many of the other patterns. In this case, a burning sensation is involved, and the pain usually comes a few days after the period. The difference here is that the heat and subsequent pain results from weakness in your body.

Blood Circulation Weakness commonly underlies these patterns. If the force of blood itself is weak, it cannot support the menstrual cycle and can result in duller pain, which is better with pressure and heat and occurs during or after the period. It can be accompanied by low blood loss and tiredness.

Food Therapy

Dietary Factors That Can Worsen Period Pain

- Raw, cold-natured foods, such as bananas, lettuce, and cucumbers, aggravate a cold pattern. So can citrus fruits, such as grapefruits and lemons, due to their cooling nature. See Cold for more details.
- Red meat, dairy products, eggs, sweet and sugary foods, and other heat-forming foods aggravate a heat pattern. See Heat for more details.
- Fatty meat, concentrated fruit juice, bread, milk, and other damp-forming foods aggravate a damp pattern. See Damp/ Phlegm for more details.

Dietary Factors That Can Improve Period Pain

- For all patterns, it is important to strengthen the underlying weakness with simple, nutritious foods. See General Weakness and Blood Circulation Weakness for more details.
- Oats, black beans, dill, caraway, basil, black peppercorns, and other warming foods improve cold patterns. See Cold for more details.
- Spinach, lettuce, celery, carrots, mung beans, tofu, parsley, and other cooling foods improve heat patterns. See Heat for more details.
- Pumpkin, radishes, lemons, and other drying foods improve damp patterns. See Damp/ Phlegm for more details.

Manual Therapy

CAUTION: Abdominal massages can be of great benefit for period pain, but they should be discontinued during the period itself.

ON YOUR FRONT: Using your palm, rub in a circular motion around your navel until warm.
- Do the Abdomen Circle sequence in Feeling Bloated (see p. 212).
- Do the Abdomen Line sequence in Premenstrual Tension (see p. 246).
- Return to rubbing the abdomen.

ON YOUR BACK: Rub your lower back up and down with an open palm, either side of the spine.

Scrape down the pancreas, liver, and kidney back *shu* regions in your mid and lower back.

Press and knead the sacral area with the knuckles of a clenched fist.

ON YOUR ARMS: Thumb-press or scrape up the large intestine and triple burner rivers in the lower arm from Li-5 to Li-11 and from Tb-4 to Tb-10. Press and knead any areas of tension.

ON YOUR LEGS: Thumb-press up the three *yin* rivers (kidney, liver, and pancreas) to your groin. Press and knead any areas of tension, especially Pa-6.

Scrape down the stomach and gallbladder rivers in the lower leg from St-36 to St-41 and from Gb-34 to Gb-40. Press and knead any areas of tension.

A recent German study reported improved pain scoring in women with painful periods. They suggest applying pressure twice a day to Lv-3, Pa-6, and Li-4 from five days before menstruation, and on painful days during menstruation.[68]

ON YOUR HANDS: Press the following areas, and knead if sore: Li-4; zone 3 – reproductive organs (L-N); zone 2 – liver (K-J).

ON YOUR FEET: Do the Foot Circulation sequence in chapter 13. Use a Gua sha tool to encourage movement.

Press the following areas, and knead if sore: Lv-3; zone 5 – uterus and reproductive organs (N-R); any reactive areas in zones 4 and 5; zone 3 – liver/spleen and kidney (J-I).

ON YOUR EARS: Press the following areas, and knead if sore: Zone 1 – A; zone 7 – uterus and ovaries; zone 5 – abdomen (N); support region – relaxation (2) and *shenmen* (1).

Exercise Therapy

The following exercises can help to enhance circulation in the lower abdomen:

❶ *Air Cycling*

While lying on your back, lift your legs high into the air, then bend your knees and slowly simulate riding a bicycle in the air with your legs. Put your hands at your waist to support your back. Do this for a minute or until tired, then rest.

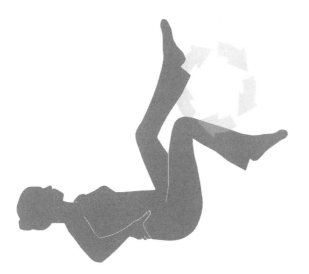

❷ *Leg Circles*

Lie face up, with both legs straight. Raise one leg, and make a circle in the air with the foot. The leg should remain straight, and the movement should come from the hip joint.

The circle should begin small but increase in size. Continue for 20 rotations, if you can, then repeat with the other leg.

Repeat the sequence several times.

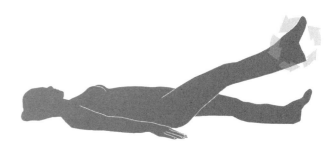

❸ *Do the Body Twist exercise in the Constipation section (see p. 217).*

❹ *Do exercises 2, 4, and 5 of the Five Qualities of Natures stretches, which can help to improve the circulation in the pancreas, liver, and kidney systems (see p. 102 ff.).*

Lifestyle Therapy

1. Keep your body as warm and dry as possible, and avoid regularly swimming in cold water.
2. Heat helps blood circulate better, so applying something warm to the abdomen can relieve pain. This could be a hot water bottle, a heating pad, or even your pet cat.

Menopausal Disorders

Symptoms
Hot flushes, tiredness, irritability, insomnia, aching joints, vaginal irritation, irregular bleeding, palpitations, sweating at night, headaches, stiff shoulders, depression, lower back pain, low libido, bone and muscle pain.

Can Include or Lead to
The onset of early menopause and perimenopause.

When to See Your Doctor

If there are severe mental or emotional symptoms.

Common Causes

Emotional stress, worry, anxiety, an improper diet and eating habits, overwork, a chronic illness, and multiple pregnancies.

An Explanation

The natural changes in menopause often reflect the imbalances that existed before the onset of menopause. If the imbalances are minor, the symptoms will be, too. However, imbalances of many years' standing do tend to lead to stronger symptoms as a woman goes through menopause, and Chinese medicine can help prevent or relieve some of the more unpleasant symptoms.

The kidney system is implicated strongly in menopause. It is basically the battery of your body. It stores all of the life force that has sustained you throughout your life and will sustain you in the future, until the kidneys eventually run out of power. It is here, at the very source of life, that an imbalance in breath motion can trigger menopausal symptoms. While both motions can be weak, the most common pattern is that the *yin* motion of the kidney system, which has been chipped away slowly over the years, gets so imbalanced that it can no longer contain the rising motion of *yang*. Yang then rises to your head from the kidney system, bringing heat with it.

This imbalance of kidney *yin* has other knock-on effects at menopause. One of these is the relationship between the qualities of fire and water. In nature, their relationship is obvious: To put out a fire, you need to pour water over it. If there is not enough water because the source of the water has dried up, the fire will get hotter and spread.

In the body, the kidney system represents water and the heart system represents fire, and the imbalance between the two can often be the source of heat. Resultant symptoms include palpitations, insomnia, and sweating at night. The *yin* imbalance in the kidney system can also affect the liver system and cause *Yin* Weakness symptoms, such as dizziness, irritability, and dryness.

Food Therapy

Dietary Factors That Can Worsen Menopausal Disorders

- Overconsumption of coffee, black tea, hot chocolate, caffeinated soft drinks, and alcohol can all cause heat and agitation.
- Avoid roasting, deep-frying, and other warm methods of cooking.
- Warming bitter and pungent foods, such as chilli, basil, cinnamon, cloves, ginger, prawns, and shrimps, can weaken *yin*. See *Yin* Weakness for more details.

Dietary Factors That Can Improve Menopausal Disorders

- A generally strengthening diet benefits the kidney system. See General Weakness for more details.
- Oats, adzuki beans, kidney beans, asparagus, eggs, sweet potato, walnuts, raspberries, quinoa, shrimps, lobster, mussels, and parsley strengthen the kidney system.

Manual Therapy

ON YOUR HEAD: For a pattern of heat rising to the head, treat the heat *shu* region. Using Du-20 as the anchor point, use a Gua sha tool to scrape downwards using short strokes. Go in several different directions, but always start at Du-20. This covers the heat *shu* regions on the top of your head.

ON YOUR FRONT: For heat rising to your chest, scrape outwards, above and below your clavicle, and the sides of your neck into your shoulder (the area of Open Basin), downwards from Lu-2 to Lu-1, and the area around *jianqian*.

ON YOUR BACK: For heat in the chest area, scrape down Bl-11 and the lung back *shu* region. Also scrape down the other back *shu* regions, especially the kidney region in your lower back.

ON YOUR ARMS: Thumb-press or scrape down the heart and heart ruler rivers from Ht-3 to Ht-7 and Hr-3 to Hr-7. Press and knead any areas of tension.

ON YOUR LEGS: Thumb-press up the kidney river to Kd-10. Hard-press on Kd-3, Kd-4, Kd-7, and any areas of tension.

ON YOUR HANDS: Press the following areas, and knead if tender: Zone 3 – reproductive area and kidney (L-N); zone 2 – liver, pancreas, and stomach (K-I); zone 1 – heart (G).

Using a Gua sha tool, scrape down each of your fingers on the front and back. Use short scrapes, and focus on the joints as you move downwards.

ON YOUR FEET: Do the Foot Circulation sequence in chapter 13.

Press the following areas, and knead if sore: Any reactive areas in zone 5 (N-R); zone 3 – liver/spleen and kidney (J-I); zone 2 – heart (G).

ON YOUR EARS: Press the following areas, and knead if sore: Ear apex (5); zone 1 – A; zone 7 – uterus and ovaries; zone 5 – abdomen (N); zone 3 – head area (G); support region – *shenmen* (1).

Exercise Therapy

Do exercises 3, 4, and 5 of the Five Qualities of Nature stretches to strengthen the kidney, heart, and liver systems (see p. 102 f.).

Lifestyle Therapy

Symptoms associated with menopause vary from woman to woman. However, it is very common to come across women who have been diagnosed with a certain condition on the basis of a slight abnormality on a medical test, been medicated, then developed a more complicated condition.

It is standard in mainstream medicine to diagnose a woman at menopause with a "hormonal imbalance", and many women are encouraged to have pharmaceutical hormone replacement therapy (HRT), despite sometimes not even showing symptoms. The argument is usually made that it will protect against heart disease and osteoporosis.

A much better approach is to see menopause as a natural process. After all, a woman's body is supposed to stop ovulating and reduce its oestrogen level once it reaches a certain age. It has been designed to do this; it is a natural transition in life. From a Chinese medicine viewpoint, both motions of *yin* and *yang* should naturally decline in the kidney system. It is the basis of the three "injuries" in the stages of life discussed in chapter 10, when the major rivers and reservoirs of the uterus gradually go offline from the ages of 35, 42, and 49 in women.

Rather than keeping these oestrogen levels artificially high, thereby forcing the body to use up more life force from the kidney system, a woman should be supporting the motions of *yin* and *yang* in her changing body by making shifts in lifestyle, work, diet, exercise, and general state of mind to support what is a natural and powerful passage in her life. Doing this offers a much safer and effective way of protecting a menopausal woman against heart disease and osteoporosis.

If you are undergoing HRT treatment, you need to be aware that while your hormones are being regulated by this treatment your kidney system is not being strengthened, so you need to take measures (with regard to diet and lifestyle) to preserve it in order to prevent potential health problems in the future.

Negative lifestyle factors can no longer be ignored at menopause. It is after all a transition from the summer to autumn of your life, and a *yang* lifestyle should be replaced by one more appropriate to the life stage you have reached and involve overworking less and slowing down and resting more.

Regular gentle exercise is also very important at menopause to strengthen the kidney system. Do not exercise later in the day, though, as this can draw on your *yin* stores and make menopausal symptoms worse.

Some factors, such as smoking, have been shown to bring on early menopause in women. According to research in Turkey, the likelihood of this happening correlates with the number of cigarettes a woman smokes daily. Women who smoke more than 10 cigarettes a day have an increased risk of going into menopause early, indicating that heat generated in the lung system has severely weakened the *yin* motion of breath.[69]

28

Conditions Affecting the Whole Body

Blood Pressure Disorders

Symptoms
High blood pressure – headaches, dizziness, palpitations, sleep problems, numbness, pins and needles, pressure in the head, tinnitus.

Low blood pressure – tiredness, dizziness, difficulty getting up in the mornings, fainting, lack of appetite, tinnitus, cold hands and feet, diarrhoea, and palpitations.

Blood pressure readings normally have two sets of numbers. The first number is the **systolic** rate (referring to the contraction of the heart muscle), and the second is the **diastolic** (referring to the relaxation of the heart muscle). Blood pressure is considered to be normal when the reading reads within the range of 90–120/60–80.
Blood pressure is considered to be higher than normal when it reads 120–140/80–90. High blood pressure is categorized as any reading above 140+/90+. Note, however, that this should be an average of several blood pressure readings at different times and on different days.Unlike high blood pressure, low blood pressure is not usually defined by a specific blood pressure number but purely on signs and symptoms.

Can Include or Lead to
Hypertension, hypotension, stroke, peripheral arterial disease, cardiac insufficiency, and Shy-Drager syndrome.

When to See Your Doctor
The symptoms are severe.

Common Causes
Emotional stress; overthinking; work stress; overwork; a diet of too many hot-natured, spicy, greasy foods; too much alcohol; a shock or accident; being overweight; a constitutional imbalance; heavy bleeding; side-effects of medications; smoking; or old age.

An Explanation
Blood pressure is all about rivers—literally. The regulation of the force of blood within the river systems has been impaired, and for this, we need to look at how breath motion is working in the key systems that control the flow of blood.

High blood pressure suggests that the river flow is coming too fast and with too much force, and in your body this suggests heat. If heat is going to come to the fore in the breath motion, it will be from the *yang* expansive motion of moving upwards and outwards.

High blood pressure normally has a strong component of *yin* weakness. What happens is that any long-standing low heat pattern in the body from *yin* weakness can gradually limit how *yin* moves in the kidney system. This can affect other systems, especially the liver (which controls the regulation of blood), and can cause further imbalances in both.

Once the motion of *yin* in both the kidney and liver systems has reached a certain point, strong signs of *yang* appear from the liver, as it is no longer controlled by the strength of *yin* motion. Hyperactive *yang* can rise in the body, go straight to the head, and cause a rise in speed and blood pressure. Often accompanying this imbalance is weakness in the area below the navel, and the chest can feel warm. For some people with this pattern, any fluctuations in blood pressure cause stress and worry, and there can be almost an obsession in maintaining a constant blood pressure.

Sometimes the opposite pattern is present. If the balance of kidney *yang* motion weakens, *yin* cannot be contained and damp can accumulate and prevent the movement of *yang*. Without the force of *yang* motion, the connective tissue through which your blood vessels flow will remain tense and the smooth flow of blood can then be restricted. This can add to or cause an impairment in the liver system and be accompanied by emotional stagnation, in the form of depression and physical discomfort and pain. Any long-standing stagnation will build up a counterflow heat, and this heat can rise and disturb blood flow in the river system.

With low blood pressure, the force of *yang* is unable to move upwards and outwards to warm your body and move blood circulation. This *yang* weakness often originates in the pancreas system, particularly if the tiredness worsens after meal times and there is difficulty finding the energy to speak.

The pancreas system helps ferment and transform the five flavours and sends nutrified blood as far as your four limbs, but when weakened by an improper diet or worry and stress, it no longer has

the power to do so. This can result in circulatory symptoms such as cold hands and feet, lack of strength, and dizziness, as not enough circulation force can travel to your head. The resulting cold pattern can also create stiff and sore muscles, as they contract more than usual.

Food Therapy

Dietary Factors That Can Worsen Blood Pressure Disorders

HIGH BLOOD PRESSURE

- Hot-natured, spicy, and warm foods, such as ginger, cinnamon, and lamb, fuel the fire. See Heat for more information.
- Too much table salt can thicken the blood and raise blood pressure.
- It is the same with processed, packaged food and junk food. A British report claims that as much as 75 percent of the salt we eat is surreptitiously hidden in our food. One takeaway pizza, for example, was found to contain an entire day's recommended allowance of salt (the report found one that was more salty than sea water!).[70] See the Salty Foods list for more details on salty food.
- Over time, coffee and alcohol can impair the *yin* motion and cause dryness in the riverbeds. To lower blood pressure, *yin* needs to be strong and balanced, so both coffee and alcohol should be reduced or avoided. See *Yin* Weakness for more details.
- Caffeinated drinks, such as coffee, black tea, fizzy soft drinks, and energy drinks, also agitate *yang* and can adversely affect blood pressure.

LOW BLOOD PRESSURE

- Too many cold and cool-natured foods, such as salads, raw foods, dairy products, and fruit juice, slow down digestion. See Cold for more details.

Dietary Factors Which Can Improve Blood Pressure Disorders

HIGH BLOOD PRESSURE

- Sour foods, such as citrus fruit, can be beneficial to the liver, and so to blood flow. See the list of Sour Foods for more details.
- Apples, pears, oranges, wheat, mung beans, spinach, green tea, and milk help bring down heat. See Heat for more details.
- Crab, octopus, blueberries, lemons, dandelion, spinach, celery, tomatoes, water chestnuts, and green tea help keep circulation moving smoothly. See Stagnation for more details.
- Duck, pork, chicken, grapes, spinach, celery, tomatoes, black soybeans, pine nuts, black sesame seeds, and sunflower seeds improve *yin* and blood circulation. See *Yin* Weakness and Blood Circulation Weakness for more details.

LOW BLOOD PRESSURE

- Eating regularly is very important, especially breakfast, which should be substantial. Food should be stewed, grilled, or lightly fried.
- In general, follow a strengthening diet consisting of lots of easy-to-digest grains and sweet-natured foods that promote digestion: Duck, chicken, beef, salmon, tuna, eel, cherries, peaches, fennel, carrots, dates, short-grain rice, corn, millet, oats, chilli, ginger, garlic, pepper, cinnamon, chestnuts, and walnuts.
- A little of the following salty-natured food can help raise kidney *yang*: Venison, lamb, mussels, oysters, sardines, raisins, cherries, corn, honey, and fennel.

Manual Therapy

ON YOUR HEAD: Put both hands on your head with your fingers bent and separate. Press and massage the whole head for a few minutes.

Gua sha over the top of your head. Start at Du-24 at the hairline above your forehead, and scrape backwards past Du-20 towards the nape of your neck. Use short scraping motions, and follow parallel lines so that you cover most of the head above your ears.

Rest the fingers of both hands on the midline of the forehead at Du-24, and finger-knead outwards to your temples. Repeat this several times.

Press and knead with four fingers together from the temples around the back of the ear to the occiput. At the occiput area, either thumb- and hard-press or use a Gua sha tool to scrape up and down along the area below the bone (Gb-12, Gb-20, Bl-10 and Du-16).

ON YOUR NECK: Raise your chin slightly. Put your left palm on the right side of your neck. Knead and rub from your jaw to your clavicle several times. Then swap sides and repeat.

ON YOUR FRONT: Using your palm, rub in a circular motion around your navel until warm. Do the Abdomen Circle sequence in Feeling Bloated (see p. 212).

Do the Abdomen Line sequence in Premenstrual Tension (see p. 246).

ON YOUR BACK: Scrape down the back *shu* regions on your back.

ON YOUR ARMS: Thumb-press or scrape down the heart and heart ruler rivers from Ht-3 to Ht-7 and Hr-3 to Hr-7. Press and knead any areas of tension.

ON YOUR LEGS: Thumb-press up the *yin* rivers on your leg (kidney, pancreas, and liver), and knead any areas of tension.

ON YOUR HANDS: Press the following areas, and knead if sore: Zone 1 – heart (G); zone 2 – liver (K-J); zone 3 – kidney (M).

Using a Gua sha tool, scrape down each of your fingers on the front and back. Use short scrapes, and focus on the joints as you move downwards.

ON YOUR FEET: Do the Foot Circulation sequence in chapter 13.

Press the following areas, and knead if sore: Zone 3 – liver/spleen and kidney (J-I); zone 2 – heart and chest (E-G, S); zone 1 – head/face (A).

A recent Indian study reported promising results from the use of foot soaks with warm red ginger to reduce blood pressure in elderly people with hypertension.[71] For more information about foot soaks see Heat Your Feet in *Yang* Weakness.

ON YOUR EARS: Press the following areas, and knead if sore: Zone 1 – A-B; zone 3 – head area (G); support region – *shenmen* (1).

Exercise Therapy

Do exercises 3, 4, and 5 of the Five Qualities of Nature stretches (see p. 102 f.). This can help strengthen the heart, kidney, and liver river systems.

Lifestyle Therapy

1. In the USA, studies have clearly linked dietary changes and exercise with a reduction in blood pressure. It is very important, therefore, to take regular exercise in combination with any dietary changes made above.[72]
2. Some medications, such as beta-blockers (often prescribed for heart conditions) and antidepressants can cause low blood pressure as a side effect.
3. Be aware of how you move if you suffer from low blood pressure. There is very little *yang* rising motion inside, so actions such as standing up should be done gradually.

Painful or Aching Joints

Symptoms
Pain or discomfort of the joints and the muscles and tendons around them, swelling, limitation in movement, bony lumps, redness, and numbness.

Can Include or Lead to
Osteoarthritis, rheumatoid arthritis, osteoporosis, and fibromyalgia.

When to See Your Doctor
If the symptoms are severe and getting worse.

Common Causes
Overuse; exposure to the elements; overexercise; accidents; emotional stress, especially when repressed; an improper diet.

An Explanation
In many cases of joint pain, the main source of discomfort is one of five patterns. They can be distinguished by the distinctive symptoms each produces:

WIND: The pain seems to move from joint to joint.

DAMP: The pain is fixed and often accompanied by numbness, swelling, and heaviness. It can worsen in wet, rainy weather.

HEAT: The joint may feel hot to the touch and be swollen and inflamed. The pain is usually severe.

COLD: The pain is fixed in one joint and is very painful. It may also worsen in cold weather.

PHLEGM: The joint may be swollen with bony lumps and deformities.

Underlying these overflow patterns, there is normally a weakness pattern that needs to be redressed.

Food Therapy

Dietary Factors That Can Worsen Painful Joints

- Cold foods, such as raw vegetables, fruit, and cold drinks, aggravate cold patterns. See Cold for more details.
- Dairy products, concentrated fruit juices, and other damp-forming foods aggravate damp and phlegm. See Damp/Phlegm for more details.
- Seafood, such as shrimps, prawns, lobster, and crab, and spinach and mushrooms aggravate wind. See Wind for more details.
- Lamb, beef, alcohol, and hot spices aggravate heat in the body. See Heat for more details.

Dietary Factors That Can Improve Painful Joints

- In general, a strengthening diet will support digestion. See General Weakness for more details.
- Meat, ginger, eggs, garlic, and alcoholic spirits such as brandy (but only in small amounts) can be helpful. See Cold for more details.
- Chicken, rice, and carrots nourish the blood and help wind conditions. See Blood Circulation Weakness for more details.

Manual Therapy

For specific details see the section related to the corresponding pain area:

NECK: p. 190
SHOULDER: p. 194
ELBOW: p. 229
WRIST: p. 231
HAND AND FINGERS: p. 233
BACK: p. 222
KNEE: p. 235
ANKLE: p. 238
FOOT AND TOES: p. 240

Exercise Therapy

Choose from exercises 1–5 of the Five Qualities of Nature stretches (see p. 101 ff.) and many of the specific exercises in each section, according to symptoms and the location of the river systems and the joint. See the relevant section for more details.

Lifestyle Therapy

1. Regular gentle exercise is essential to keep the joints supple.
2. If the pain is from an acute, and not a chronic, injury, note the advice about putting ice on it in Neck Pain.

Fatigue

Symptoms
Tiredness, lack of concentration, heaviness, depression, and aching muscles.

Can Include or Lead to
Chronic fatigue syndrome/myalgic encephalomyelitis, Addison's disease, hypothyroidism, glandular fever, and narcolepsy.

When to See Your Doctor
If the symptoms are severe.

Common Causes
Stress, overwork, irregular eating patterns, an improper diet, overeating, constitutionally weak, anxiety, worry, overthinking, long-term illness, trauma or shock, and overuse of antibiotics.

An Explanation
The most important distinction that needs to be made with the symptoms of fatigue is how much of the fatigue is from a weakness pattern and how much from an overflow pattern.

It might seem almost counterintuitive to consider that fatigue is not due to weakness, but if we go back to the river and how it flows down the mountain, the force of water does not reduce without good reason. An object might fall into the river, the banks might collapse, or it may silt up farther upstream, causing a blockage—this is what the overflow pattern is doing. You feel fatigue not because you cannot generate enough energy to move, but because you are obstructed from doing so. The problem is, therefore, usually one of obstruction and less of weakness.

This pattern is often seen with an impairment in the liver system and caused by emotions, especially when repressed, or when you are under stress. Smooth circulation through the river systems is consistently maintained by the liver, and when that works inefficiently, areas of stagnation and obstruction appear. A clear indicator of this pattern is often when you feel better after doing exercise.

Fatigue is intricately connected with the digestive process, as it is through digestion that we generate the power we need to thrive on a daily basis. The pancreas is very important in this, because after extracting the nutrients of food into the five flavours, it sends this generated life force to your arms and legs, which will become heavier and more difficult to move when this action is impaired. Also, together with the stomach system, it will be unable to process food efficiently and tend to store damp. This is heavy and sticky and can weigh you down, thereby increasing fatigue. Signs of damp include a feeling of heaviness, especially after eating or in the morning, and sometimes a strong desire to lie down.

Wind entering the body may cause symptoms, such as a cold, for example. If not cleared properly, it can go deeper into the layers of the body, where it can remain for a long time and transform into heat. The heat will eventually burn outwards and come to the surface, causing sudden weakness and hot, feverish symptoms.

Food Therapy

Dietary Factors That Can Worsen Fatigue

- Eating too much, too quickly or irregularly especially while not being in a relaxed state will create stagnation.
- Damp-forming foods such as oily foods, processed foods that are highly sweetened, dairy products, bananas, and fatty meat like lamb slow down the body. See Damp/Phlegm for more details.

Dietary Factors That Can Improve Fatigue

- The stomach and pancreas systems need to be nourished with a simple diet of easily digestible, freshly cooked food. See General Weakness for more details.
- Pears, cherries, grapes, and other warming and drying foods help counteract fatigue with damp patterns. See Damp/Phlegm for more details.

Manual Therapy

Do the Dry Towel Friction sequence detailed in General Weakness.

ON YOUR HEAD: Put both hands on your head with your fingers bent and separate. Press and massage the whole head for a few minutes.

Rest the fingers of both hands on the midline of the forehead at Du-24, and finger-knead outwards to your temples. Repeat this several times.

Gua sha over the top of your head. Start at the hairline above your forehead, and scrape backwards past Du-20 towards the nape of your neck. Use short scraping motions, and follow parallel lines so that you cover most of the head above your ears.

Press and knead with four fingers together from the temples around the back of the ear to the occiput. At the occiput area, either thumb- and hard-press or use a Gua sha tool to scrape up and down along the area below the bone (Gb-12, Gb-20, Bl-10, and Du-16).

ON YOUR NECK: Raise your chin slightly. Put your left palm on the right side of your neck. Knead and rub from your jaw to your clavicle several times. Then swap sides and repeat.

ON YOUR FRONT: Scrape down your sternum to Ren-17, and also the sides of your sternum, where the ribs attach. Press and knead any areas of tension.

Hard-press any sore areas on the centre line of the abdomen including Ren-6, Ren-12, and Ren-15.

ON YOUR BACK: Scrape down the back *shu* regions. Start gently, and slowly increase pressure. Press and knead any areas with tension.

ON YOUR ARMS: With fatigue, motion is important, so use Gua sha on your arm rivers to scrape down the *yin* and up the *yang*. First check your arms by circling and kneading, so that you can locate areas with tension, and then concentrate on them with Gua sha and the rivers associated with them.

ON YOUR LEGS: As above with the arms, encourage circulation in the leg rivers. Scrape down the *yang* and up the *yin*, and press and knead any areas of tension.

ON YOUR HANDS: Do the Hand Circulation sequence in chapter 13. Use your fingers or a Gua sha tool.

Press and knead any sore areas in zones 1, 2, and 3 on the palm of your hand.

ON YOUR FEET: Do the Foot Circulation sequence in chapter 13. Use a Gua sha tool to encourage movement.

Press the following areas, and knead if sore: Zone 2 – lung and heart (E-G); zone 3 – pancreas, stomach, liver/spleen, and kidney (J-H).

ON YOUR EARS: Press the following areas, and knead if sore: Zone 1 – A & B; zone 2 – spinal column (D-F); support regions – *shenmen* (1), relaxation (2), sensorial (3), and cerebral (4).

Exercise Therapy

❶ *Do exercises 2 and 5 of the Five Qualities of Nature stretches to help strengthen the earth and wood systems (see p. 101 ff.).*

❷ *Do the Body Twist exercise from the Constipation section (see p. 217).*

Lifestyle Therapy

Light physical exercise is very important for the circulation patterns in your body. It is, however, equally important not to do too much. The end result should be a feeling of more energy and rejuvenation, not further tiredness or exhaustion. Learning to pace yourself on a daily basis is one of the most important aspects of managing a fatigue condition.

Diabetes

Symptoms
(see below for an explanation of the groupings):
Usually a combination of the following although the key symptoms are in bold:

UPPER: *Thirst* and copious drinking, dry mouth and tongue, mouth ulcers, lack of appetite, and a red tongue tip.

MIDDLE: Increase in appetite, *weight loss*, restlessness, stomach discomfort, sweating, constipation, thirst and *weakness.*

LOWER: *Frequent and profuse urination*, dry mouth and tongue, dizziness, blurred vision, red cheeks, hunger but poor appetite, lower back and knee pain, and weakness.

Can Include or Lead to
Type 1 or Type 2 diabetes mellitus, gestational diabetes, atheroma, infections, arteriosclerosis,

ketoacidosis, peripheral neuropathy, and retinal damage.

When to See Your Doctor

Increasing severity of symptoms, rising blood sugar levels, hypoglycaemic episodes (dizziness, fainting, or seizures), and the presence of ketones in urination.

Common Causes

In the case of Type 2 diabetes: An improper diet of too many processed, fried, oily, or hot-natured and spicy foods; smoking; overconsumption of alcohol; emotional stress, especially when emotions are repressed; overworry; overweight; lack of exercise; old age; too much sexual activity. Type 1 is usually more related to a constitutional weakness.

An Explanation

Diabetes is a massive worldwide health problem. In the USA alone, diabetes affects 34.2 million people, and an astonishing 7.3 million of these are thought to be undiagnosed.[73]

In conventional terms, a diagnosis of diabetes mainly consists of either being insulin-dependent (Type 1) and requiring regular injections of insulin, or non-insulin-dependent (Type 2), which tends to appear later in life and requires lifestyle changes and medication.

The ancient Chinese had an understanding of diabetes and described a pattern of heat and dryness (known as *xiaoke*, or "wasting thirst") based on the "three excesses and one loss": Excess drinking liquids, excess food consumption, excess urination, and weight loss.

While you can apply this to diabetes as a condition, the life we lead now and the bodies that carry us around are significantly different from two thousand years ago, when these ideas were formulated. So, while a pattern of heat and weakness of *yin* in the lung system, the stomach system, and the kidney system is the end result, much as *xiaoke*

describes, we have to start elsewhere to find out how the body gets there.

The underlying pattern that can eventually lead to the symptoms of diabetes often has its origins in structural impairments long before the disorders of metabolic processes begin. This is why it is so important to approach your body within its three-dimensional matrix and acknowledge that potential obstruction patterns will develop into wider system disorders wherever they are in your body.

For example, you may have scar tissue impairing the stomach river system on your leg, which, if left untreated, can cause further impairments along the river, other rivers, and given the right circumstances and time, in the storage system itself.

As far as metabolic disorders are concerned, for many people, this starts in impaired stomach and pancreas systems and weakened digestion. As the stomach and pancreas systems become more sluggish, heat builds up, drying up moisture, and creating intense hunger and thirst. This pattern is normally associated with eating a lot and being overweight.

Other body-wide patterns can worsen the heat in the stomach or lung systems. Emotional stress, for example, can impair the smooth circulation maintained by the liver system and lead to blockages and obstruction patterns in the tissue anywhere around your body. Over time, these blockages create counterflow heat, which can then rise along the river systems and add fuel to the fire that is drying the body fluids of the stomach system.

The heat burning in the stomach system can also rise to the lung system and consume the moisture there. In a regular smoker, the lung system is often already weak and dry, so the pattern will be exaggerated. This pattern is normally associated with the desire to drink lots of liquids.

The heat in the stomach, lung, or liver systems can also have a domino effect on the kidney system causing the balance of the *yin* motion to weaken considerably. The resulting hyperactivity of *yang* can create even more heat, which rises upwards. This pattern is normally associated with both drinking and urinating a lot.

Insulin is taken by some diabetics, which is very cooling and moisturizing to the body. Over time, however, it can create further impairments in the stomach and pancreas systems and cause the build-up of dampness, bloating, and digestive symptoms.

Food Therapy

It is standard practice for diabetic sufferers to be assessed, diagnosed, and treated with Medical Nutrition Therapy. In this way a personalized diet is prepared that involves a focus on calories and the balance of carbohydrates, protein, sodium, fat, and other categories of food, and a plan of action is enacted. That being said, advice from Chinese medicine can be very helpful.

Dietary Factors That Can Worsen Diabetes

- Overeating and irregular eating habits weaken digestion and increase stagnation.
- Eating a lot of greasy, fatty foods, such as processed and dairy products, vegetable oils, meat, nuts, refined sugar and sugar products, and overly salty or spicy foods, and drinking alcohol and caffeineated drinks, weakens the stomach and pancreas, and by default the lung system, too.

Dietary Factors That Can Improve Diabetes

- The stomach and pancreas function best with regularity, so eating at the same time every day and not skipping meals will help optimize digestion.
- Slow-burning, high-fibre, complex carbohydrate foods, such as whole grains, fruits, and vegetables, are usually recommended for people diagnosed with

diabetes. The theory is that these foods are broken down into blood sugar, or glucose, slowly and steadily in the body and prevent unpleasant blood sugar spikes that exhaust insulin supplies and break down the body. In fact, the recommended diet for diabetes is remarkably similar to the standard healthy diet in Chinese medicine (high in unrefined carbohydrates, low in protein and fats) that appears frequently in this book to strengthen the stomach and pancreas systems. See General Weakness for more details.

- As the digestive system is severely weakened in people with diabetes, it makes sense that the stomach and pancreas cannot function properly when large meals are eaten; hence small frequent meals are recommended to help process food better and stimulate the production of the blood sugar-controlling hormone insulin.
- For conditions of dryness and heat in the stomach system, cooling and moistening foods, such as rice, avocado, cucumber, watercress, tofu, and yogurt can help. Eat these in moderation, as too many of such foods can weaken digestion. See Heat for more details.
- Foods like garlic, radishes, the peel of oranges and tangerines, and carrots move *qi* and can reduce stagnation in the liver system. See Stagnation for more details.
- Strengthening foods for kidney *yin* include black beans, kidney beans, black sesame seeds, and pork. See *Yin* Weakness for more details.
- The following foods can help regulate blood sugar and the level of fluids in the body:
  ‣ **FRUIT:** Plums, pears, blueberries, avocados, and any fruit with a sour taste, such as lemons, limes, strawberries, and grapefruit.
  ‣ **VEGETABLES:** Carrots, radishes, turnips, spinach, asparagus and dark, leafy greens.

▸ **GRAINS:** Rice, oats, and whole wheat.
▸ **BEANS:** Chickpeas (garbanzos) and mung beans.

- Research in China reported that a daily mixture of 60 g (2 ounces) of Chinese yam and 200 ml (6.5 ounces) of milk decreased the blood glucose level significantly in elderly participants with type 2 diabetes.[74]
- Another Chinese study looked at nutritional therapy for elderly participants who had a *Yin* Weakness presentation of diabetes, characterized by fever, large appetite, and hunger. The participants were put on a diet of rice porridge with winter melon, vegetables, and a little *yuzhu* or Solomon's seal plant, pine pollen, and wolfberry, resulting in a decrease in participants' fasting blood glucose.[75]

Manual Therapy

ON YOUR FRONT: Palm-circle with slight pressure in a clockwise direction around your navel.

Do the Abdomen Circle sequence in Feeling Bloated (see p. 212).

Press and knead Ren-12, Ren-6, and Ren-4. With your palm, rub in a circular motion around Ren-4 to create warmth.

ON YOUR BACK: Scrape down the lung, heart, pancreas, liver, and kidney back *shu* regions. Press and knead any areas of tension.

ON YOUR LEGS: Thumb-press up the pancreas river from Pa-5 to Pa-10, and scrape down the stomach river from St-36 to St-41. Knead any sore areas, especially Pa-6 and Pa-9, and St-40.

Press and knead around the area of Kd-3 to Kd-7.

ON YOUR HANDS: Press and knead any sore areas in zones 1, 2, and 3 on the palm of your hand.

ON YOUR FEET: Do the Foot Circulation sequence in chapter 13. Use a Gua sha tool to encourage movement.

Press the following areas, and knead if sore: Zone 2 – heart and lung (E-G); zone 3 – pancreas, stomach, liver/spleen, and kidney (J-H).

Although foot soaks can be problematic with diabetes, due to a lack of sensation in the feet, they can be very beneficial.

An Iranian study found that dissolving 250g (9oz) of powdered common mineral salt into the water of a foot bath with a temperature between 40 and 45°C (104 and 113°F) and soaking for 15 minutes, has positive effects on reducing pain in sufferers of diabetic peripheral neuropathy.[76]

For details of how to do a foot soak see Heat Your Feet in *Yang* Weakness. Warm foot baths can usually be tolerated by people with diabetes provided that the pulse in their feet is strong and the water is less hot. Nevertheless, seek advice from your medical professional before soaking.

ON YOUR EARS: Press the following areas, and knead if sore: Zone 1 – A-C; support region – *shenmen* (1).

Exercise Therapy

Exercises 1, 2, and 4 of the Five Qualities of Nature stretches can help strengthen the lung, stomach, and kidney systems (see p. 101 ff.).

Lifestyle Therapy

1. Lifestyle therapies are key in any diabetes treatment. An unhealthy lifestyle with a lack of physical activity and excessive eating patterns often lies behind many cases of type 2 diabetes.
2. If you have developed the symptoms of diabetes, your body is telling you to stop and take stock of your health. You should regulate not only your diet and eating habits but also your sleeping times, levels of stress, and exercise regime.

3. Regular gentle exercise—at least 30 minutes a day, five times a week—can increase circulation patterns and help lower blood sugar levels.

4. Losing weight is essential. US research has shown that weight loss in combination with exercise is more effective than medication in preventing or delaying the development of Type 2 diabetes.[77]

Obesity and Losing Weight

Symptoms

Overweight, excessive or no appetite, low energy, sleep problems, a bland taste in the mouth, scanty or no periods, impotence, chest and abdominal pain, dizziness, and palpitations.

Can Include or Lead to

Cushing's syndrome; orthopedic problems, such as back or joint pain; osteoarthritis; hypertension; diabetes; and heart disease.

When to See Your Doctor

If very or morbidly obese.

Common Causes

Lack of exercise, improper diet and eating habits, overeating, constitutional tendency, emotional stress; a medical condition, such as diabetes, or a glandular malfunction.

An explanation

Obesity can be graded by measuring body mass index (BMI). To find your BMI requires simply dividing your weight (kg) by your height (m). The result can be classified below:

WHO Class	BMI (kg/m^2)
Underweight	Below 18.5
Normal Weight	18.5-24.9
Overweight	25-29.9
Obese	30-35
Very Obese	35-40
Morbidly Obese	40 and above

A study in *The Lancet* offers a grim reminder of what carrying excess body fat does to health. According to the research, people with a BMI of 30–35 can expect to die 2–4 years earlier, and people with a BMI of 40–45 will live 8–10 years less than someone of normal weight. The study goes on to list the causes of early death, including heart disease, stroke, diabetes, liver disease, kidney disease, cancer, and lung disease.[78] Obesity is a medical condition that is becoming all too common, and for many people arises from a lack of understanding about how the body functions.

After eating, the stomach and pancreas systems are hard at work fermenting and transforming the food you consumed into the fuel that powers your body. The stomach system actually incorporates all of the other digestion-related systems, such as the small and large intestine, the triple burner, and the gallbladder, and is the root of how your body functions. When it becomes impaired, this means that a core part of how your body works goes offline, and the whole process can get clogged up and run inefficiently. A common cause of this is the result of a combination of bad eating habits and an improper diet of damp-forming, fatty foods.

Being unable to properly process food often leads to an accumulation of damp, which will then further impair the digestive process. The damp builds up in the form of fat, which is stored around the body, and a resulting lack of circulation to your arms and legs can create additional systemic weakness and feelings of fatigue.

Imagine your stomach and pancreas systems as a garden where occasional light drizzle allows plants and flowers to grow abundantly. When someone is overweight, the garden has become waterlogged, and the fresh grass has become a muddy patch. Not much can grow well in this environment. Symptoms such as discomfort in the stomach area, body heaviness, and scanty urine are often associated with this pattern.

Heat is a pattern that often accompanies damp. It can originate in the stagnation of circulation created by an impaired liver system and worsened by emotional stress. Over time, this stagnation can create heat, which can manifest as an insatiable hunger and subsequent overeating. It can also generate phlegm patterns, such as a tight and phlegmy chest and a bitter taste in your mouth.

Any attempt to reduce weight needs to take into account the importance of the stomach system, the effect of stagnation, and the presence of damp and phlegm. If not, at best the weight reduction, if any, may be only temporary. The way to do this is to follow simple guidelines in eating habits and exercise.

Food Therapy
Dietary Factors That Can Worsen Obesity
- Raw foods can put a strain on the stomach and pancreas systems by forcing them to work harder in digestion. Raw food should, therefore, be avoided, unless the cooling nature of raw food is needed in patterns of heat.
- Dairy products can be damp-forming in the body, especially when it has a pattern of weakness, as they are often too rich in nutrients for the stomach system to digest well. This can encourage some people's bodies to do the exact opposite of losing weight. See Damp/Phlegm for more details.
- Highly processed, artificially sweetened foods are deficient in the nutrients needed to strengthen digestion.

- Man-made hydrogenated fats and cheap, refined vegetable oils contain too many damaging fats—common in manufactured margarine spreads and frying oils in restaurants and supermarkets—which lead to damp and heat in the body.
- Very sweet fruits, such as figs, dates, and dried fruit, contain concentrated sugars that do not aid weight loss.
- Bananas, avocados, and coconut are damp-forming fruits and prevent weight loss.
- Meat is very nutritious, and for this reason should be eaten in moderation or it will lead to stagnation of the digestive system and an impairment of the stomach and pancreas systems. It is important, therefore, to dramatically reduce the amount of meat consumed if you want to lose weight.
- Salt should be used very sparingly.

Dietary Factors That Can Improve Obesity
- Regular meal times are important. Your digestion needs regularity to function well.
- An ideal diet is a strengthening diet of cooked foods in the form of soups or stews, which are easy to digest and include vegetables, whole grains, and legumes, and only a small amount of good-quality meat (less than 10 percent).
- Emphasize bitter and sour foods. Choose from the following list of useful foods:
  - GRAINS: Rye, amaranth, quinoa, and oats are bitter, and therefore drying and beneficial to digestion. Corn also helps to expel fluids, so can be useful in reducing fat.
  - FRUIT: Emphasize bitter fruits, such as lemons and grapefruits. Eat apples, plums, peaches, berries, oranges, and pears in moderation.
  - VEGETABLES: Lettuce, celery, asparagus, scallions, and other bitter vegetables, and turnips, radishes, and other pungent vegetables.

▸ **HERBS AND SPICES:** Pungent spices, such as cumin, ginger, cloves, cayenne, fennel, peppermint, chamomile, and white pepper. (Be cautious about eating too many of these herbs and spices if also suffering from a heat pattern.)

▸ **DRINK:** Chinese green tea.

▸ **OTHER:** Dairy products made from goat or sheep's milk are a viable alternative to cow's milk products. Use cold-pressed extra-virgin olive oil or unrefined sesame oil as an alternative to oils high in fatty acids.

Manual Therapy

Do the Dry Towel Friction sequence detailed in General Weakness.

ON YOUR FRONT: Using your palm, rub in a circular motion around your navel until warm.

Do the Abdomen Circle sequence in Feeling Bloated (see p. 212).

ON YOUR BACK: Scrape down the pancreas and liver back *shu* regions on your mid back. Press and knead any areas of tension.

ON YOUR LEGS: Thumb-press up the pancreas river from Pa-5 to Pa-10, and scrape down the stomach river from St-36 to St-41. Knead any sore areas, especially Pa-6 and Pa-9, and St-40 areas. Thumb-press up the liver river from Lv-4 to Lv-8, and scrape down the gallbladder river from Gb-31 to Gb-40. Knead any sore areas, especially Lv-5 and Gb-34.

ON YOUR ARMS: Thumb-press up the large intestine and triple burner rivers, and knead any areas of tension, especially around Li-6 and Li-11, and Tb-6.

ON YOUR HANDS: Press the following areas, and knead if sore: Zone 2 – stomach, pancreas, liver, large intestine, and small intestine (K-I).

ON YOUR FEET: Do the Foot Circulation sequence in chapter 13. Use a Gua sha tool to encourage movement.

Press the following areas, and knead if sore: Zone 3 – pancreas, stomach, liver/spleen, and kidney (J-H); zone 4 – small intestine and large intestine (K-M).

ON YOUR EARS: Press the following areas, and knead if sore: Zone 1 – A-C; support region – *shenmen* (1).

Exercise Therapy

❶ *Do exercises 1–5 of the Five Qualities of Nature stretches to generally harmonize and strengthen your body (see p. 101 ff.).*

Do these specific exercises for losing weight:

❷ *Twist And Roll Your Body*
Lie face up with your knees bent up to your chest and both arms stretched out to the side, level with your shoulders.

Breathing in and, keeping your shoulders tightly on the ground, turn your buttocks slowly to one side. Try to bring both knees to the ground, and meanwhile, turn your head to the opposite side, and breathe out.

Slowly twist back, breathe in, and repeat on the other side.

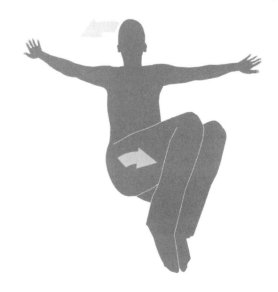

❷ *Raise Your Pelvis*

Lie face up, with both arms relaxed at your sides. Bend your knees, keeping your feet on the ground.

Breathe in, contract the buttock muscles, and raise the buttocks slowly to allow the whole back to lift off the ground supported by the shoulders. Hold for a few seconds, then breathe out, and slowly return to lying flat. Repeat five times or until tired.

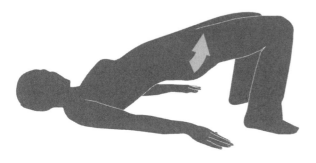

❸ *Dry Swimming*

Lie face down, arms bent, and palms flat pushing downwards.

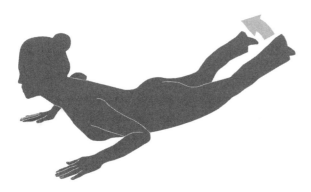

Lift both legs at the same time slightly. Contract your buttock muscles, and move your legs up and down as a fish might swim.

❹ *Kick in Arched Position*

Begin on all fours, and breathe in.

Keep your back perpendicular with the ground, and hang your head so you can see your knees. Then lift one knee towards your forehead.

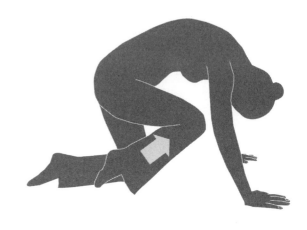

Breathe out, and contract your buttock muscles. Then lift your head, and stretch your right leg backwards at the same time.

Repeat this several times. The movement should be quick and continuous. Then repeat with the other leg.

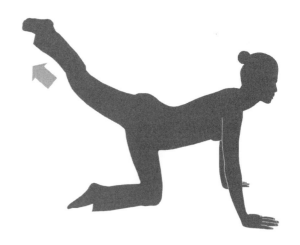

Lifestyle Therapy

1. Moderate, regular exercise, in addition to a change in diet, is esssential; without it, long-term change can be difficult. The aim should be to gradually build up to two hours of moderate-intensity activity per week, doing activities like brisk walking, doubles tennis, bike riding (avoiding hills), and water aerobics.

2. Weight loss achieved as a result of an awareness of the negative effects of weight gain is important. Weight loss for more superficial reasons will lead you to put on weight again because your motivation and long-term commitment to change are not as strong as they are when your health is at stake. This is why any lifestyle changes you do make should be realistic and appropriate, otherwise, they will not last.

Epilogue

Despite the term "self-healing", the title of this book does not mean that all the suggestions contained within should be restricted to treating yourself. They are designed to give you the foundation for helping yourself and those around you either in preventing ill-health or in helping to change patterns when they have become more established. This can be a valuable lifeline in treating a family-member or loved-one for something like a cold or cough when you know that the options of standard care are limited and in doing so can actually help prevent a worsening of symptoms. For many of the therapy suggestions this is the case. And remember that I did not choose these suggestions out of thin air, they come from firmly established nature-based principles in Chinese medicine and from observing real situations over decades of trial and error.

For me the main impetus of the approach taken by this book has been in the world of Gua sha, not because it holds special powers of healing that fixes everything, but because it uniquely embodies a front-line therapeutic technique used historically to treat febrile disease and with the potential for adaptation to be used on a world healthcare stage. Part of what we do through the institute I started (the Komorebi Institute), is promote this approach and foster the use of Gua sha in countries with underdeveloped healthcare systems. The difference being that rather than a top-down approach of standard healthcare, we go straight to the bottom part of the picture. The history and development of Gua sha has been at a community and family level and has a distinct tradition from other Chinese medicine components such as acupuncture and herbs in that it is rooted within the community. It is, therefore, in the community that we start. And it is within this bottom-up context that this book is firmly placed. It is not aimed at honing the skills of professionals but at laying out effective tools of health to individuals, families, friends, and loved-ones.

One of the goals of this text was to remove a barrier artificially placed on Chinese medicine and perpetually self-reinforced within it, and show that, rather than the exclusive use of the few, it is accessible to people everywhere exactly because it is not mysterious and otherworldly but grounded in the world around us. The world right outside our doors and that we see and feel every day. The magic and wonder of Chinese medicine are the same magic and wonder as that of our natural world which many people's daily lives have become so disconnected from. As I mentioned earlier in the book, I am lucky enough to actually live within a forest in a natural park but I did not always live here and have spent most of my life away from nature in big cities. I now quite literally spend every day spellbound at what happens around me with the trees, plants, creatures, and insects and not only has the life of the forest become an integral part of my life, but how I understand the body so much better from what I see. This was exactly what ancient Chinese thinkers at the time of the Huangdi neijing wanted to convey to us but over time their message became so diluted and the closer we come to our present, the further removed from the original ideas we have come.

The importance of the message they gave us – looking at the body not in terms of separation from nature but as an integral part of it – cannot be overstated. This is not something recent but what the ancient Chinese understood over two thousand years ago. And when we acknowledge that the same motions which formed the world around us actually formed us, and continue to influence how our bodies function throughout our lives, then our perceptions have to change. Not only of how our bodies function but so much more. In fact, everything else you thought you knew can easily topple over like some majestic domino tumble. In a flash you have a context with which you can not only understand the workings of health and ill health but you can make sense of wider life in general. If our bodies are an integral part of the natural world then so are our daily lives, our hopes, and our dreams. And this makes perfect sense in what the ancient Chinese were telling us. It was always about an approach to life, not about which point to press or which illness to treat. It was to tell you how to live up to your inner potential and shine like the stars.

You are probably familiar with 'natural' approaches and products in health and wellness and they usually involve products like detoxifying cleanses, organic oils and creams, and natural ingredients. Multinationals know this well and a huge industry is devoted to a superficial worship of all things natural. According to the Washington Post, in food alone the word 'natural' helps sell $40 billion worth of products and add to that the many supplements, herbs, oils, creams, and potions with the same 'natural' stamp on them and it is considerably more. The trouble is, apart

from the fact that much of what is being sold is far from what many people think is natural, the approach itself is a superficial one. What we have been exploring here in this book is not this cursory approach to nature. It is something totally different. We have taken a step back to show you how the ancient Chinese saw us literally as an integral part of nature. They saw rivers and forests and patterns and motions and climates and all the things you see and feel outside in the natural world, but they saw them as inside your body too and they spent generation upon generation perfecting their ideas around this.

This is using nature as the starting point, not adding it in later with 'natural' potions, diets, and therapies. It is acknowledging a revolutionary approach in how we see the body and one which we so desperately need right now. If I were to tell you that your backache was due to a cold obstruction pattern within the kidney river system, I would not need to delve deep into Western medicine explanations nor those of modern TCM to treat you. I could use the principles of nature and how they are applied to the body to both understand and treat it. This is not in any way denying other explanations. With the back pain, I would not be denying that there may be an injury to the ligaments that support the spine or to a muscle or tendon or degenerative herniated or ruptured discs, or inflammatory conditions, or osteoporosis, or fibromyalgia, or any number of potential causes within Western medicine. I would instead be looking at the same thing from a perspective based on the universal demonstrative rules of nature and when these rules are applied to the body, a radically different thought process and treatment procedure then ensues.

Linguistically, the demystification approach of Chinese medicine that I show in this book aims to give you a more realistic idea about what the ancient Chinese intended, so rather than repeating the overused simplifications of the energetic model of modern TCM, which sound so alien with their talk of invisible energy meridians, I want you to be firmly grounded with what this actually is within nature.

It makes sense to look at what we know to be true because we can see it, feel it, and experience it within natural science and it is ironic that when you go deeper along this scientific path and analyze how the natural world behaves both in our environment and that of the universe then the language and, in fact, the whole picture becomes far more enchanting and magical than before. Think about those nature programs you may have seen on TV, the ones where they take you into the life of plants or animals or microscopic organisms and how magically beautiful these strange worlds appeared. It is the same beauty when you realize that yin and yang are the motions of breath and we can apply this motion of the universe to everything everywhere around us, or when you realize that the shenming flowing in your blood is essentially a form of stardust and this links us in life and death to the stars.

And so from this viewpoint on nature and the body, we have clarity in understanding the effect of changing climate patterns and the approaching time of great upheaval. If our inherent interconnectedness to the climate is part of how we see ourselves, we can clearly see that any dramatic change to our environment means that our health will deteriorate in equal measure. We are designed to thrive within the seasonal changes around us, and when those seasons break down, so too will our internal well-being. The sooner people recognize the nature within us, the sooner dramatic systemic changes can happen to save us all.

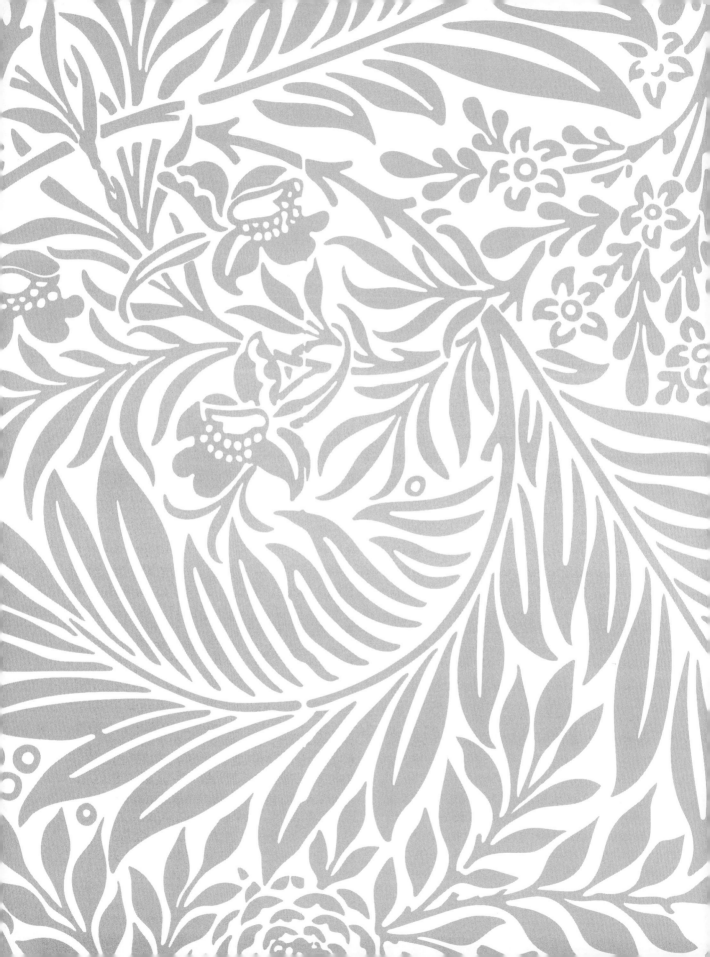

Notes

1. *Neijing* Nature-based Medicine is a clinical research methodology within Chinese medicine developed by Dr. Edward Neal at the Xinglin Institute and based on the application of the text of the *Huangdi neijing*.

2. What happened on this day has been widely reported and an explanation can be found in S. Odenwald, "The Day the Sun Brought Darkness", *NASA* (March 13, 2009). Accessed: www.nasa.gov/topics/earth/features/sun_darkness.html

3. Harvard professor Avi Loeb was reported as actually saying this: "Fast radio bursts are exceedingly bright given their short duration and origin at great distances, and we haven't identified a possible natural source with any confidence. An artificial origin is worth contemplating and checking." Harvard-Smithsonian Center for Astrophysics, "Could Fast Radio Bursts Be Powering Alien Probes?" *Science Daily.* (March 9, 2017). Retrieved September 5, 2021 from www.sciencedaily.com/releases/2017/03/170309120419.htm

4. K.M. Rajwade, "Possible Periodic Activity in the Repeating FRB 121102." *Monthly Notices of the Royal Astronomical Society.* 495, 3551-3558. (May 19, 2020).

5. This is concisely explained by E. Neal, "Introduction to Neijing Classical Acupuncture Part I: History and Basic Principles", *Journal of Chinese Medicine*, No. 100 (October 2012). It is one of the core concepts in *Neijing* Nature-based Medicine.

6. This is another core concept from *Neijing* Nature-based Medicine and is explained in abridged form by E. Neal, "Introduction to Neijing Classical Acupuncture Part I: History and Basic Principles", *Journal of Chinese Medicine*, No. 100 (October, 2012).

7. "Out of this basic dichotomy of generic developmental growth patterns arises a comprehensive and theoretically coherent construction and understanding of human anatomy." E. Neal, "Introduction to Neijing Classical Acupuncture Part II: Clinical Theory". *Journal of Chinese Medicine*, No. 102 (June 2013).

8. K. Creath et al, "What Biophoton Images of Plants Can Tell Us about Biofields and Healing", *Journal of Scientific Exploration* 19 (2005).

9. RP Bajpai, "Quantum Coherence of Biophotons and Living Systems", *Indian J Exp Biol.* (May 2003); 41(5):514-27. PMID: 15244274.

10. B. Bordoni, "Emission of Biophotons and Adjustable Sounds by the Fascial System: Review and Reflections for Manual Therapy", *Journal of Evidence-Based Integrative Medicine* Vol. 23 (2018): 1–6.

11. RV Wijk & EP Wijk, "An Introduction to Human Biophoton Emission", *Forsch Komplementarmed Klass Naturheilkd* 12(2) (April 2005): 77–83.

12. D Balasigamani et al, "Biophotons: Ultraweak Light Emission from Living Systems", *Current Opinion in Solid State and Materials Science* Vol. 2, Issue 2 (April 1997): 188–193.

13. This idea of *shenming* is heavily influenced by the work of Dr. Edward Neal. Neal explains it briefly in "Introduction to Neijing Classical Acupuncture Part II: Clinical Theory", *Journal of Chinese Medicine* No. 102 (June 2013).

14. *Shenming* is "believed to have the capacity to restructure the body back to a state of health along the lines of its original inception." Edward Neal, "Introduction to Neijing Classical Acupuncture Part III: Clinical Therapeutics", *Journal of Chinese Medicine* No. 104 (February 2014).

15. This is based on unpublished translations and interpretations of the *Huangdi neijing* by Dr. Edward Neal.

16. "In the Neijing, it is likely that the modern anatomical spleen was understood to be a 'left-sided liver'." Edward Neal, "Introduction to Neijing Classical Acupuncture Part III: Clinical Therapeutics", *Journal of Chinese Medicine* No. 104 (February 2014).

17. This is based on unpublished translations and interpretations of the *Huangdi neijing* by Edward Neal.

18. More details about Soulié de Morant's translations and interpretations can be found in D. Kendall, *Dao of Chinese Medicine: Understanding an Ancient Healing Art* (Oxford University Press, 2002).

19. Peter Unschuld, respected translator and expert on the *Huangdi neijing*, makes his opinion on this very clear: "It should be noted that the interpretation of qi 氣 as 'energy', so widespread in TCM literature today, lacks any historical basis." P. Unschuld & H. Tessenow, *Huang Di Nei Jing Su Wen: An Annotated Translation* (University of California Press, 2003).

20. "In Chinese, the character 'mai' (脈) is a basic anatomical term that simply means 'blood vessel'. E. Neal, "Introduction to Neijing Classical Acupuncture Part II: Clinical Theory", *Journal of Chinese Medicine* No. 102 (June 2013).

21. This is taken from an autopsy description in the *Huangdi neijing ling shu*, translated by P. Unschuld, *Huang Di Nei Jing Ling Shu: The Ancient Classic on Needle Therapy* (University of California Press, 2016): 12-311-7b.

22. These are the rivers, seas, and oceans that were used to describe each of the river systems in the *Huangdi neijing ling shu*:
Lung: Yellow river; large intestine: Yangtze river; stomach: Ocean and Seas; pancreas: Lakes and Marshes; heart: Ji river; small intestine: Huai river; bladder: Qing river; kidney: Ru river; heart ruler: Zhang river; sanjiao: Ta river; gallbladder: Wei river; and liver: Mian river. These are neatly listed in E.Neal, "Introduction to Neijing Classical Acupuncture Part II: Clinical Theory", *Journal of Chinese Medicine* No. 102 (June 2013).

23. ". . . the organ described by the character 脾 (pi – now translated as 'Spleen') originally described the modern anatomical pancreas." E. Neal, "Introduction to Neijing Classical Acupuncture Part III: Clinical Therapeutics", *Journal of Chinese Medicine* No. 104 (February 2014).

24. The term "xinbao" (心包) is ascribed to the coronary arteries from the perspective of *neijing* terminology. The pericardium is "a type of mo (膜) or 'membrane' and as such belongs to the tissue plane divisions of the East." E. Neal, "Introduction to Neijing Classical Acupuncture Part III: Clinical Therapeutics", *Journal of Chinese Medicine* No. 104 (February 2014).

25. This is detailed in chapter 77 of the *Huangdi neijing ling shu,* and here is a summary of the text: South Wind (Extremely weak wind) settles in the heart and vessels (rivers) and causes heat; Southwest Wind (Planning wind) settles in the pancreas and muscles and causes weakness; West Wind (Hard Wind) settles in the lung and the skin and causes dryness; Northwest Wind (Breaking wind) settles in the small intestine river and causes obstruction; North Wind (Extremely Hard Wind) settles in the kidney and bones, back, and shoulders and causes cold; Northeast Wind (Inauspicious Wind) settles in the large intestine and sides of ribs, armpit, and limb joints; East Wind (Infantile Wind) settles in the

liver and sinews and causes damp; Southeast Wind (Weak Wind) settle in the stomach and flesh and causes body weight.

Original text translated by P. Unschuld, *Huang Di Nei Jing Ling Shu: The Ancient Classic on Needle Therapy* (University of California Press, 2016): 12-311-7b.

26. The character for wind is 風 and the character for a common cold is 風邪 (literally "harmful wind"). Both are pronounced *kase*.

27. J. Fowler, "Dynamic Spread of Happiness in a Large Social Network: Longitudinal Analysis over 20 years in the Framingham Heart Study", *British Medical Journal* (December 2008): 337:a2338.

28. This is based on unpublished translations and interpretations of the *Huangdi neijing* by Dr. Edward Neal.

29. J. Li et al, "Improvement in Chewing Activity Reduces Energy Intake in One Meal and Modulates Plasma Gut Hormone Concentrations in Obese and Lean Young Chinese Men", *American Journal of Clinical Nutrition* (July 2, 2011).

30. K. Maruyama et al, "The Joint Impact on Being Overweight of Self-Reported Behaviours of Eating Quickly and Eating until Full: Cross-Sectional Survey", *British Medical Journal* 337 (October 21, 2008): a2002.

31. A. Trichopoulou, "Anatomy of Health Effects of Mediterranean Diet: Greek EPIC Prospective Cohort Study", *British Medical Journal* 338 (June 23, 2009): b2337.

32. This is taken from Chapter 22 of the *Huangdi neijing su wen*. Translated text taken from P. Unschuld & H. Tessenow, *Huang Di Nei Jing Su Wen: An Annotated Translation* (University of California Press, 2003): 22 22-149-1.

33. This is taken from Chapter 2 of the *Huangdi neijing su wen*. The translated text was taken from P. Unschuld, *Huang Di Nei Jing Su Wen: Nature, Knowledge, Imagery in an Ancient Chinese Medical Text* (University of California Press, 2003).

34. P. Unschuld & H. Tessenow, *Huang Di Nei Jing Ling Shu: The Ancient Classic on Needle Therapy* (University of California Press, 2016).

35. P. Unschuld & H. Tessenow, *Huang Di Nei Jing Ling Shu: The Ancient Classic on Needle Therapy* (University of California Press, 2016).

36. R. Van Dam, "Combined Impact of Lifestyle Factors on Mortality: Prospective Cohort Study on US Women", *British Medical Journal* 337 (September 16, 2008): a1440.

37. These stages in life are in chapter 1 of the *Huangdi neijing su wen* and the translated text taken from P. Unschuld, P & H. Tessenow, *Huang Di Nei Jing Su Wen: An Annotated Translation* (University of California Press, 2003): 22 22-149-1.

38. This research was in the Netherlands but applicable to many species and any countries. It can be found in K. Whittington, "Seasonal Mismatch: The Fight to Adapt to Advancing Spring", *Eyes on Environment. Scitable* (May 16, 2013).

39. Again this is one of many reports on this topic: E. Chang, "Observed and Projected Decrease in Northern Hemisphere Extratropical Cyclone Activity in Summer and Its Impacts on Maximum Temperature", *Geophys. Res. Lett.* 43 (2016): 2200–2208.

40. This is based on the *ko,* or controlling cycle of breath motion, and that the qualities have the capacity to both support and deplete each other. This cycle is that wood diminishes earth, earth diminishes water, water diminishes fire, fire diminishes metal, and metal diminishes wood.

41. R. Rivlin, "Keeping the Young-Elderly Healthy: Is It Too Late to Improve Our Health through Nutrition?" *American Journal of Clinical Nutrition* 86(5) (November 2007):1572S-6S.

42. This is based on unpublished translations and interpretations of the *Huangdi neijing* by Dr. Edward Neal.

43. This is explored in more detail in Clive Witham, *Holographic Gua sha: A Practical Microsystem Handbook* (Mangrove Press, 2019).

44. This is mentioned in Chapter 49 of the *Huangdi neijing ling shu* and is a very detailed projection of the body onto the face via the imagery of the structures of a city.

45. In the late 14th century to be exact, according to D. Tiran & P. Mackereth, *Clinical Reflexology: A Guide for Integrated Practice* (Churchill Livingstone, 2010).

46. This is mentioned in Chapter 63 of the *Huangdi neijing su wen*. You can find it in P. Unschuld, *Huang Di Nei Jing Su Wen: An Annotated Translation* (University of California Press, 2011): 63-146.

47. L. Huang, *Auricular Point Therapy* (Science and Technology Literature Publishing House, 2005).

48. An alternative sequence is in Clive Witham, *Holographic Gua sha: A Practical Microsystem Handbook* (Mangrove Press, 2019).

49. F. Cappuccio, "Sleep Duration and All-Cause Mortality: A Systematic Review and Meta-Analysis of Prospective Studies", *Sleep* 33(5) (May 1, 2010): 585–92.

50. G. Healy, "Sedentary Time and Cardio-Metabolic Biomarkers in US Adults: NHANES 2003–06", *European Heart Journal* 32(5) (March 2011): 590–7.

51. U. Siqueira, "Effectiveness of Aquatic Exercises in Women with Rheumatoid Arthritis: A Randomized, Controlled, 16-Week Intervention – The HydRA Trial", *Am J Phys Med Rehabil* 96(3) (March 2017): 167-175.

52. "Although generally structured on Chinese medical theory and influenced primarily by later imperial styles of medicine, in most cases the medicine the world now knows as TCM bears little resemblance to the style of medicine practised by classically trained physicians of earlier generations." E. Neal, "Introduction to Neijing Classical Acupuncture Part II: Clinical Theory", *Journal of Chinese Medicine* No. 102 (June 2013).

53. J. Thompson Coon, "Does Participating in Physical Activity in Outdoor Natural Environments Have a Greater Effect on Physical and Mental Wellbeing than Physical Activity Indoors? A Systematic Review", *Environmental Science and Technology* 45(5) (March 1, 2011): 1761–72.

54. H.Y. Chiu et al, "A Feasibility Randomized Controlled Crossover Trial of Home-Based Warm Footbath to Improve Sleep in the Chronic Phase of Traumatic Brain Injury", *J Neurosci Nurs.* 49(6) (2017): 380–385 (foot soak insomnia).

55. T.Akbaraly, "Dietary Pattern and Depressive Symptoms in Middle Age", *British Journal of Psychiatry* 195(5) (November 2009): 408–13.

56. M. Virtanen et al, "Overtime Work as a Predictor of Major Depressive Episode: A 5-Year Follow-Up of the Whitehall II Study", *PLoS One* 7(1) (2012): e30719.

57. D. Passali et al, "The International Study of the Allergic Rhinitis Survey: Outcomes from 4 Geographical Regions", *Asia Pacific Allergy* 8(1) (2018), e7.

58. D. Wallace, "The Diagnosis and Management of Rhinitis: An Updated Practice Parameters – Joint Task Force on Practice Parameters", *Journal of Allergy Clinical Immunology* 122 (2008): S1–S84.

59. T.A.E. Platts-Mills & L.J. Rosenwasser, "Chronic Sinusitis Consensus and the Way Forward", *Journal of Allergy Clinical Immunology* 114 (2004): 1359–1361.

60. S. Patel, "Effect of Visual Display Unit Use on Blink Rate and Tear Stability", *Optom Vis Sci.* 68(11) (November 1991): 888–92.

61. D. Nieman, "Upper Respiratory Tract Infection Is Reduced in Physically Fit and Active Adults", *British Journal of Sports Medicine* (November 1, 2010).

62. I. Paul, "Effect of Honey, Dextromethorphan, and No Treatment on Nocturnal Cough and Sleep Quality for Coughing Children and Their Parents", *Archives of Pediatrics and Adolescent Medicine* 161(12) (December 2007): 1140–6.

63. O. Enilari & S. Sinha, "The Global Impact of Asthma in Adult Populations", *Annals of Global Health* 85(1) (2019): 2.

64. A. Sherriff, "Association of Duration of Television Viewing in Early Childhood with the Subsequent Development of Asthma", *Thorax* 64(4) (April 2009): 321–5.

65. F. Borrelli et al, "Effectiveness and Safety of Ginger in the Treatment of Pregnancy-Induced Nausea and Vomiting", *Obstetrics & Gynecology* 105(4) (2005): 849-856.

66. H. Choi, "Soft Drinks, Fructose Consumption, and the Risk of Gout in Men: Prospective Cohort Study", *British Medical Journal* 336(7639) (February 9, 2008): 309–12.

67. Filho Rocha et al, "Essential Fatty Acids for Premenstrual Syndrome and Their Effect on Prolactin and Total Cholesterol Levels: A Randomized, Double Blind, Placebo-Controlled Study", *Reproductive Health* 8:2 (2011).

68. B. Blödt, "Effectiveness of App-Based Self-Acupressure for Women with Menstrual Pain Compared to Usual Care: A Randomized Pragmatic Trial", *American Journal of Obstetrics and Gynecology* Vol. 218, Issue 2, (2018): 227. e1-227 e9.

69. F. Saraç et al, "Early Menopause Association with Employment, Smoking, Divorced Marital Status and Low Leptin Levels", *Gynecological Endocrinology* (2010). [Epub ahead of print]

70. CASH, "Salt Awareness Week Survey Reveals High Levels of Salt in Takeaway Pizzas" (March 26, 2012). This is one of many common food items surveyed between 2008 and 2022 with high salt content that I could have included here, and you can read about them yourself at www.actiononsalt.org.uk /salt-surveys.

71. Putri Fithriyani et al, "Effect of Hydrotherapy Warm Red Ginger to Reduce Blood Pressure on Elderly at Panti Werdha Budi Luhur, Jambi", Indian *Journal of Public Health Research & Development* Vol. 11, Issue 3, (March 2020): 1968–1972.

72. J.A. Blumenthal et al, "Effects of the DASH Diet Alone and in Combination with Exercise and Weight Loss on Blood Pressure and Cardiovascular Biomarkers in Men and Women with High Blood Pressure: The ENCORE Study", *Archives of Internal Medicine 170* (2) (January 2010): 126–35.

73. National Diabetes Statistics Report 2020. US Department of Health and Human Services. CDC. www.cdc.gov/diabetes/pdfs/data/statistics /national-diabetes-statistics-report.pdf

74. J. Guan et al, "Clinical Application and Thinking of a Medicated Diet for Elderly Diabetic Patients", *Chin J Integr Med Cardio/Cerebrovasc Dis* 16 (2018): 376–7.

75. Y. Zhou, "Application of TCM Dietary Therapy in Elderly Type 2 Diabetes Mellitus Patients with Qi and Yin Deficiency", *Chin J Integr Nursing* Vol 3, Issue 10 (2017); 75–77.

76. S.R. Vakilinia et al, "Evaluation of the Efficacy of Warm Salt Water Foot-Bath on Patients with Painful Diabetic Peripheral Neuropathy: A Randomized Clinical Trial", *Complement Ther Med.* 49 (March 2020): 102325.

77. W.C. Knowler et al, Diabetes Prevention Program Research Group, "Reduction in the Incidence of Type 2 Diabetes with Lifestyle Intervention or Metformin," *N Engl J Med.* 346(6) (February 7 2002): 393–403.

78. Prospective Studies Collaboration, "Body-Mass Index and Cause-Specific Mortality in 900,000 Adults: Collaborative Analyses of 57 Prospective Studies", *The Lancet* 373(9669) (March 28, 2009): 1083–96.

Index

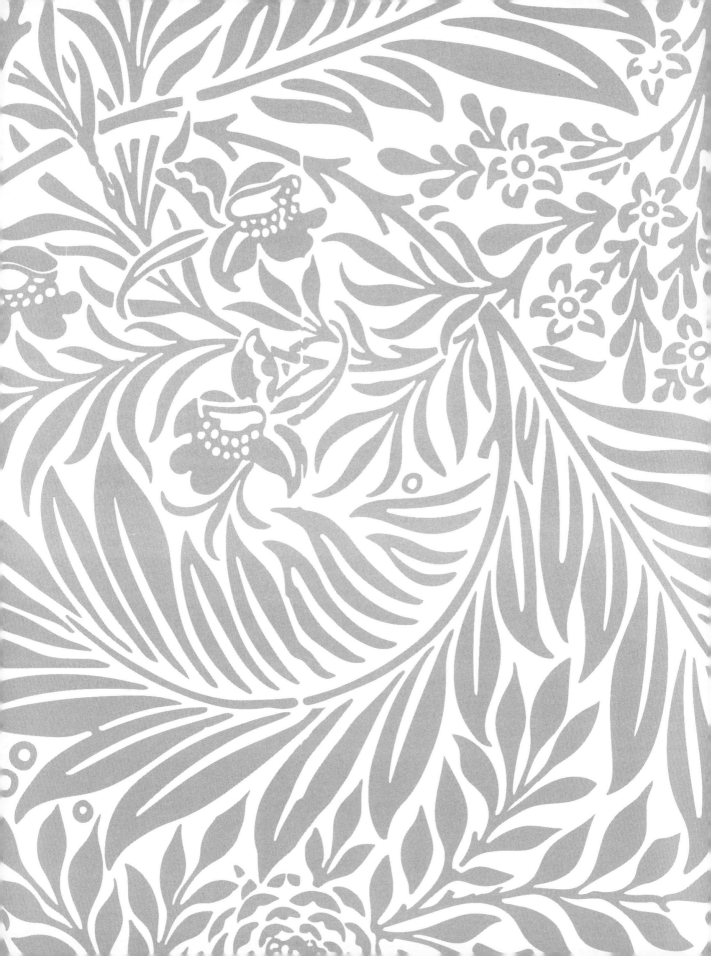

About the Author

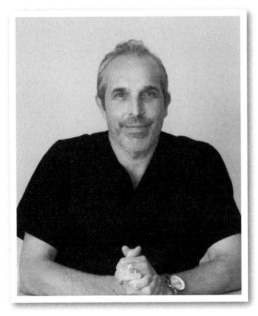

Photo by Keigo Witham

CLIVE WITHAM, L.Ac., M.Sc., is a licensed acupuncturist and qualified health promotion specialist. He has been practising Chinese medicine for more than 20 years, and for more than a decade, he ran a chronic illness clinic in North Africa. As director of the Komorebi Institute, he specializes in Ecology in Motion, a nature-based approach to Gua sha and Chinese medicine and promoting the knowledge of ancient Chinese healing as a viable, practical world medicine. The author of several popular books, including *Facial Gua Sha* and *Holographic Gua Sha*, he runs a health and research centre in Barcelona, Spain.

For more information see: www.clivewitham.com

Also of Interest from Findhorn Press

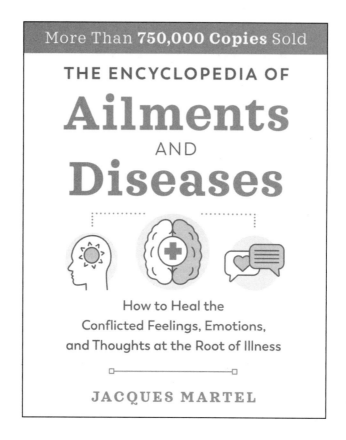

The Encyclopedia of Ailments and Diseases

by Jacques Martel

IN THIS REFERENCE AND HEALING TOOL, Jacques Martel explains how to uncover the conflicted conscious or unconscious feelings, thoughts, and emotions at the root of many illnesses and conditions. He offers healing prompts and affirmations to effect change for nearly 900 different ailments and diseases.

978-1-64411-189-5

Also of Interest from Findhorn Press

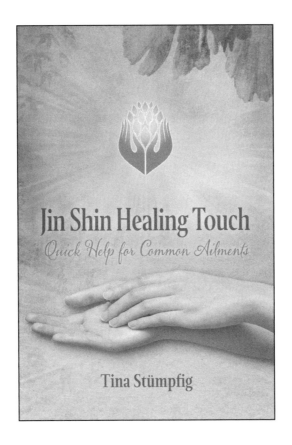

Jin Shin Healing Touch
by Tina Stümpfig

JIN SHIN JYUTSU is an ancient Japanese healing art akin to an easier form of acupressure. This full-colour guide details the 52 energy points of Jin Shin Jyutsu and explains the sequence of points to hold to address specific ailments, conditions, and injuries and stimulate the body's self-healing response.

Whether you are facing allergies, exhaustion, pain, or inflammation, the healing touch of Jin Shin Jyutsu offers a simple self-help tool that can quickly alleviate and soothe symptoms, kickstart the healing process, and improve overall health.

978-1-64411-076-8

FINDHORN PRESS

Life-Changing Books

Learn more about us and our books at
www.findhornpress.com

For information on the Findhorn Foundation:
www.findhorn.org

Rivers (Channels)

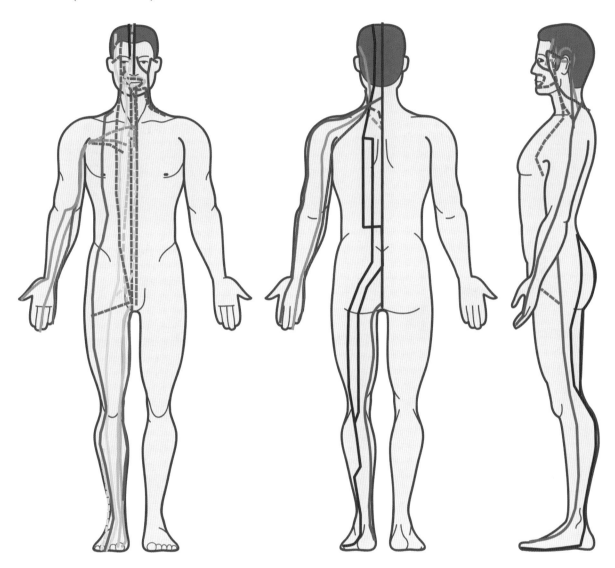

- ■ **light grey** – lung river system (ends at tip of thumb)
- ■ **dark grey** – large intestine river system (begins at tip of index finger)
- ■ **yellow** – stomach river system (ends at either side of middle toe)
- ■ **orange** – pancreas river system (begins at tip of big toe)
- ■ **red** – heart river system (finishes at tip of little finger)
- ■ **violet** – small intestine river system (begins at tip of little finger)
- ■ **pink** – heart ruler river system (ends at tip of middle finger)
- ■ **rose** – triple burner river system (begins at tip of ring finger)

- ■ **light blue** – kidney river system (begins below little toe)
- ■ **dark blue** – bladder river system (finishes at outside of foot at little toe)
- ■ **light green** – liver river system (begins at big toe)
- ■ **dark green** – gallbladder river system (finishes between fourth and fifth toes)
- ■ **brown** – ren reservoir (straight up front from between legs)
- ■ **black** – du reservoir (straight up back from between legs)

For more information see pages **38–44**.

The Areas on Your Head

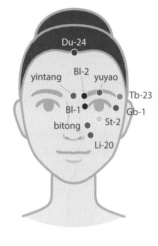

Du-24
yintang · Bl-2 · yuyao
Bl-1 · Tb-23
bitong · St-2 · Gb-1
Li-20

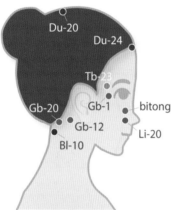

Du-20
Du-24
Tb-23
Gb-20 · Gb-1 · bitong
Gb-12 · Li-20
Bl-10

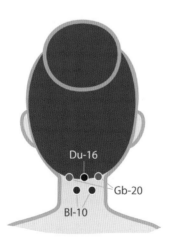

Du-16
Gb-20
Bl-10

For more information see page **117**.

The Areas on Your Neck and Shoulders

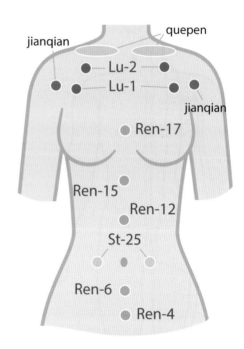

jianqian · quepen
Lu-2
Lu-1 · jianqian
Ren-17
Ren-15
Ren-12
St-25
Ren-6
Ren-4

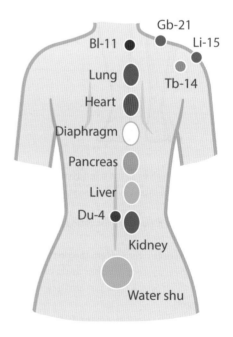

Gb-21
Bl-11 · Li-15
Lung · Tb-14
Heart
Diaphragm
Pancreas
Liver
Du-4
Kidney
Water shu

For more information see page **118**.

The Areas on Your Arms

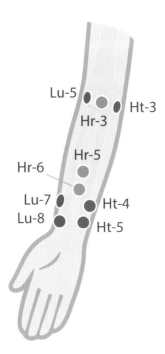

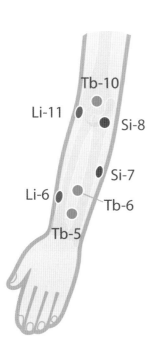

For more information see page **120**.

The Areas on Your Hands

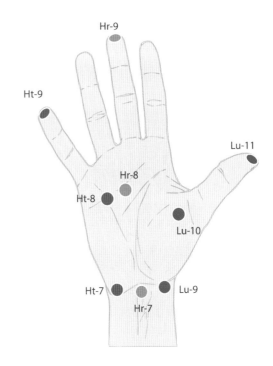

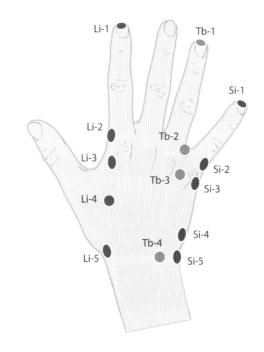

For more information see page **121**.

The Areas on Your Legs

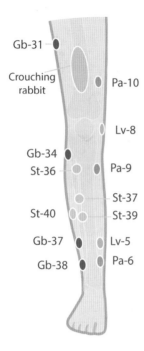

Gb-31

Crouching
rabbit

Pa-10

Lv-8

Gb-34
St-36

Pa-9

St-37
St-40
St-39

Gb-37
Lv-5

Gb-38
Pa-6

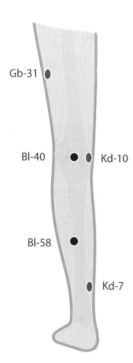

Gb-31

Bl-40
Kd-10

Bl-58

Kd-7

For more information see page **123**.

The Areas on Your Feet

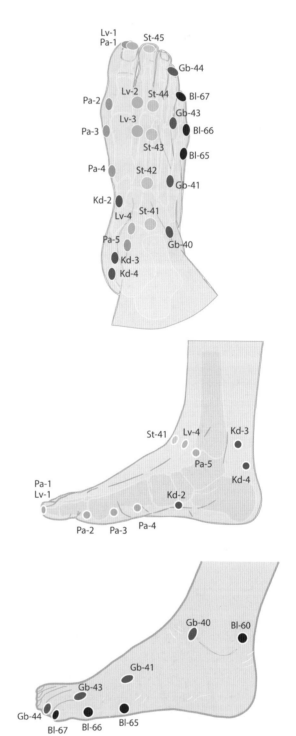

Lv-1
Pa-1
St-45

Gb-44

Lv-2
St-44
Bl-67
Pa-2

Lv-3
Gb-43

Pa-3
Bl-66

St-43
Bl-65

Pa-4
St-42

Gb-41

Kd-2

Lv-4
St-41

Pa-5
Gb-40

Kd-3

Kd-4

St-41
Lv-4
Kd-3

Pa-5

Kd-4

Pa-1
Lv-1

Kd-2

Pa-2
Pa-3
Pa-4

Gb-40
Bl-60

Gb-41

Gb-43

Gb-44

Bl-67
Bl-66
Bl-65

For more information see page **125**.